蒙医温针火针疗法

阿古拉 著

人民卫生出版社

·北京·

图书在版编目（CIP）数据

蒙医温针火针疗法 / 阿古拉著. —北京：人民卫
生出版社，2024.5

ISBN 978-7-117-36351-8

Ⅰ. ①蒙… Ⅱ. ①阿… Ⅲ. ①蒙医－温针疗法 Ⅳ.
①R291.2

中国国家版本馆 CIP 数据核字（2024）第 101346 号

人卫智网	www.ipmph.com	医学教育、学术、考试、健康，
		购书智慧智能综合服务平台
人卫官网	www.pmph.com	人卫官方资讯发布平台

蒙医温针火针疗法

Mengyi Wenzhen Huozhen Liaofa

著　　者：阿古拉
出版发行：人民卫生出版社（中继线 010-59780011）
地　　址：北京市朝阳区潘家园南里 19 号
邮　　编：100021
E - mail：pmph @ pmph.com
购书热线：010-59787592　010-59787584　010-65264830
印　　刷：北京瑞禾彩色印刷有限公司
经　　销：新华书店
开　　本：710×1000　1/16　　印张：15　　插页：2
字　　数：269 千字
版　　次：2024 年 5 月第 1 版
印　　次：2024 年 6 月第 1 次印刷
标准书号：ISBN 978-7-117-36351-8
定　　价：98.00 元

打击盗版举报电话：010-59787491　E-mail：WQ @ pmph.com
质量问题联系电话：010-59787234　E-mail：zhiliang @ pmph.com
数字融合服务电话：4001118166　E-mail：zengzhi @ pmph.com

著者简介

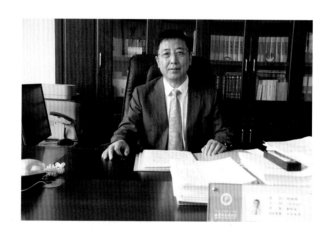

　　阿古拉（博·阿古拉），男，蒙古族，医学博士，1965年5月生，内蒙古扎赉特旗人，国家级非物质文化遗产——赞巴拉道尔吉温针、火针疗法代表性传承人，包头医学院党委书记、教授、硕士研究生导师，北京中医药大学、内蒙古医科大学博士研究生导师，第八届教育部科学技术委员会学部委员，中国民族医药学会教育分会会长、内蒙古自治区蒙医药学会副会长，《中国民族医药杂志》副主编、《中国蒙医药》杂志副主编。

　　长期从事蒙医传统疗法学基础与临床研究，完善了蒙医传统疗法学理论体系，提出"寒热平调""引病外除""整体调节"等蒙医传统疗法学的独特理论。传承蒙医药文化的同时，将蒙医药基础理论与现代科学技术相结合，对蒙医传统外治疗法进行深度挖掘与开发，开展大量的相关机制及临床疗效评价研究，为推动蒙医药关键技术现代化做出了重大贡献。为切实提高蒙医传统外治疗法的安全性和有效性，大力推进了蒙医传统外治疗法操作技术及器械、穴位定位、配方选方等的标准化建设，实现了科技成果转化，取得了显著的社会效益和经济效益。

　　先后主持国家自然科学基金、国家科技支撑计划重点项目、国家中医药管理局项目等重点科研课题，取得丰硕成果：以第一完成人身份获华夏医学科技奖二等奖，内蒙古自治区自然科学一等奖和三等奖、科技进步二等奖、教学成果一等奖和二等奖、中国图书奖、全国优秀教材三等奖、中国民族医药学会科学技术进步奖一等奖各 1 项等；以第一或通讯作者身份发表学术论文 203 篇（汉文100 篇、蒙文 77 篇、英文 23 篇、斯拉夫蒙文 3 篇）；主编出版专著、教材 20 部；以第一完成人身份获授权专利 12 项（3 项已成果转化）、计算机软件著作权 1 部。

　　先后被评为内蒙古自治区"草原英才"、杰出人才、劳动模范等；2011 年获批享受国务院政府特殊津贴，2015 年入选国家百千万人才工程，被授予"有突出贡献中青年专家"荣誉称号；培养博士研究生 33 名、硕士研究生 50 名；擅长采用蒙医特色疗法治疗风湿类疾病等疑难病，深受广大患者信赖。

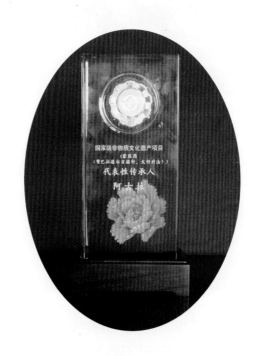

蒙医温针火针疗法是蒙医传统外治疗法的重要组成部分，临床应用较为广泛。蒙医温针疗法是用特制的针具在人体相应的穴位进行针刺，并在针柄上加热，使温热刺激通过针体传入体内，达到治疗疾病目的；蒙医火针疗法是先将特制的针具尖部在火上烧红后迅速针刺人体相应穴位，达到治疗疾病目的。针具主要用结实而富有弹性的金属制作，构造分针尖、针身、针根、针柄、针顶五个部分。蒙医温针火针疗法经过历代蒙医师家的不断实践、充实和发展，承载了宝贵、丰富的临床经验，具有简、便、验、廉、安全性高、实践性强、疗效独特等优点，治疗赫依性疾病、巴达干、风湿类疾病、寒性病等疗效稳定、可靠，受到医务工作者的重视和关注，具有良好的推广价值和广阔的发展前景。

蒙医温针火针疗法以蒙医"辨证施治"学说为指导，主要根据不同疾病的病因病机，并结合白脉分布、疼痛点、病变部位等具体情况辨证取穴。蒙医温针火针疗法辨证取穴方法多来源于临床经验，用穴少而精，疗效确切，临床上经常可以达到一针即验的疗效。蒙医温针火针疗法常用穴位有 259 个，治疗某种疾病时，一般选取相应主治功效的一个或几个穴位。

蒙医温针火针疗法是针刺与温灸相结合的一种外治疗法，具有温通经脉、调和气血、调理体素、增强抵抗力以防治疾病的作用。它通过针刺刺激、温热刺激及穴位功效的相互作用，对机体产生生物学效应，以调节机体的生理和病理状态，从而达到治疗疾病的目的。

蒙医温针火针疗法 2008 年被列入国家级非物质文化遗产代表性传统医药类项目名录，本人被评为该项目代表性传承人。我认真履行传承义务和责任，培养人才，提高学生的蒙医温针火针疗法基本技能和临床操作能力，使他们在工作中一展专门技能，普遍受到了当地患者的赞扬和信任。本书是关于蒙医温针火针疗法的一部专著，试图在总结本人及团队过去研究工作的基础上阐述蒙医温针火针疗法的基础理论、技术方法及应用实践，为蒙医传统疗法的开发应用及现代研究提供科学依据。本书分为上、中、下篇及附录，上篇主要介绍了蒙医温针火针疗法的作用、操作、适应证及注意事项、常用穴位、选穴原则等内容；中篇介绍了蒙医温针火针疗法在蒙医疗术科、蒙医内科及其他科室的临床应用；下篇介绍了蒙医温针火针疗法机制相关研究的内容；附录主要收载了蒙医温针疗法相关 SCI 数据库录入论文。

　　本书的编写工作得到了国家自然科学基金、国家非物质文化遗产保护专项、内蒙古自治区"草原英才"工程人才基金的资助，以及其他横向研究课题的支撑，特此向支持和关心本人及团队研究工作的所有单位和个人表示衷心的感谢。在编写过程中主要参考了明根巴雅尔编写的《五疗》《蒙医刺灸学》，策·苏荣扎布编写的《蒙医临床学》及巴·吉格木德编写的《蒙古医学简史》等著作，部分内容参考了有关单位和个人的研究成果，在此一并致谢。

　　本书内容在继承传统的基础上力求体现创新，编撰工作难度较大，再加上本人水平有限，虽几经改稿，仍恐存在错误和缺点，敬请广大读者批评指正。

阿古拉

2023 年 8 月于包头

目 录

下篇　机制研究

上篇

基础知识

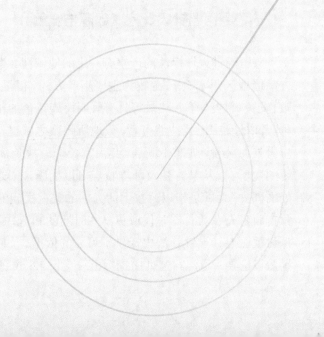

第一章

概　论

　　蒙医温针火针疗法是蒙医传统外治疗法的重要组成部分，在临床应用较为广泛。温针疗法先用特制的针具刺入人体相应的穴位，在其针柄上加热，使温热刺激通过针体传入人体内，达到治疗疾病的目的；火针疗法亦采用特制的针具，先将针尖部烧红，再刺入人体相应的穴位，达到治疗疾病的目的。目前，在临床应用中，蒙医温针疗法和火针疗法的作用与适应证基本一致，临床较多使用温针疗法，较少使用火针疗法。

　　历代蒙医的不断实践、充实和发展蒙医温针火针疗法，积累了丰富的临床经验。蒙医文献记载与现代临床实践证明，蒙医温针火针疗法治疗赫依性疾病、巴达干、风湿类疾病、寒性病等疗效稳定、可靠。蒙医温针火针疗法有简、便、验、廉、安全性高、实践性强、疗效独特等优点，具有悠久的历史、丰富的临床经验积累和宝贵的文献资源。蒙医温针火针疗法受到了医务工作者的重视和关注，具有良好的推广价值和广阔的发展前景。

一、蒙医温针火针疗法起源与发展

　　蒙医温针火针疗法的产生有一定的地域性。蒙古民族长期居住在寒冷的北方高原地区，以狩猎、游牧为主要生产方式，很早就掌握并运用温针、火针、热敷、艾灸、沙疗、羊砖热敷等具有鲜明民族特色的传统外治疗法。中医经典著作《黄帝内经》中记载："北方者，天地所闭藏之域也，其地高陵居，风寒冰冽，其民乐野处而乳食，脏寒生满病，其治宜灸焫。故灸焫者，亦从北方来。[1]"这里所说的"北方"，从其方位及环境特点可以推断，主要指蒙古高原一带，"其民乐野处而乳食"无疑是指以游牧生活为主的蒙古民族的祖先。近年来的考古学证明蒙古族祖先在新石器时代或更早些时期就制造并运用传统疗法专用针具，这对探讨蒙医温针火针疗法史提供了可靠的依据。如 1963 年内蒙古自治区锡林郭勒盟多伦县头道洼村遗址中挖掘出一支长 4.5cm 的石针[2]，其形状一端扁平，有半圆形刀，另一端呈锥形，中间手持处为四棱形，便于操作。又如 1978 年从内蒙古自治区伊克昭盟达拉特旗树林召发掘一支长 4.6cm，形状类似上述石针的青铜针 [3]。

古代蒙古族人在分猎物、解剖脏器等日常劳动中获得了丰富的动物机体结构方面的知识。如蒙古地区广为流传的民间故事《牛腰子》《骆驼的尾巴》《旱獭为何没有拇指》等，无不表明当时人们对动物机体结构的认识达到了很高的水平，同时以动物解剖知识来推测和比较人体的解剖结构。这对蒙医温针、火针等疗法的选穴及进针方法与技巧的形成起到了积极的促进作用。

蒙古民族在长期的劳动生产及实践中创造出适应地区自然环境特点的蒙医温针、火针等独特的外治疗法，并有意识地将这些技术运用于临床中，不断地继承、整理、研究和提高其理论及操作方法。自公元 16 世纪以来，蒙医学家进一步发展了温针火针疗法的理论及操作，如《四部甘露》一书中写道，"针刺疗法有寒针和热针两种"，并说明寒针只是针刺，热针则是针刺和烤灸相结合的火针疗法。蒙医针刺疗法经常与烤灸相结合，这是因蒙古寒冷地区多发寒证的具体需要而形成的。蒙医常用的针具大多数是银针（也有金针），故蒙医的针刺疗法称为"银针疗法"。[4]

随着现代蒙医学的进一步发展，蒙医温针火针疗法的理论体系和疗术渐趋完整，形成了独具特色的一种蒙医外治疗法。

二、蒙医温针火针疗法的适应证和禁忌证

1. 适应证　蒙医温针火针疗法的适应证主要包括赫依性疾病、巴达干性寒证、消化不良、痞块、瘀积病、水肿、肌肉麻木或肿胀、黄水病。如支气管哮喘、慢性胃炎、慢性结肠炎、失眠、偏头痛、慢性疲劳综合征、脑血管意外、面神经炎、面肌痉挛、三叉神经痛、坐骨神经痛、风湿、类风湿、肩周炎、脊柱炎、落枕、颈椎病、腰椎间盘突出症、腰肌扭伤、慢性腰肌劳损、退行性膝关节炎、耳鸣耳聋、鼻炎等。

2. 禁忌证　肝痞、脾痞渗漏引起的热性水肿，热痞扩张，心等脏腑热性病余邪未除及外伤等疾病，如由血和希拉引起的一切热性疾病，特别是肌肉、骨骼、脉络、脂肪等要害部位，老年人、婴幼儿以及病危者等，都禁忌使用温针火针疗法治疗。

三、蒙医温针火针疗法应用注意事项

要使蒙医温针火针疗法取得满意的效果，不仅要全面熟练地掌握温针火针疗法的内容，还要通晓其他相关的医疗知识。应用蒙医温针火针疗法时必须注意以下几个方面。

1. 治疗前应对患者做好解释工作，避免患者紧张；患者以坐位或卧位为宜，减少晕针事件的发生。

2. 注意用火安全，避免烧伤患者皮肤、头发、汗毛等部位或衣物，加热用具不用时立即切断电源或灭火处理。

3. 注意检查与维护针具，发现有缺损或折弯，不宜使用，以防意外。

4. 治疗前要严格消毒施术局部皮肤，以防感染。

5. 刺激量不宜过度，尤其对身体虚弱或寒热敏感者。

6. 温针火针治疗后针眼一般不需要特殊处理，只需要用干棉球按压针眼即可。

7. 温针火针治疗后针眼当天不要浸水，以防感染。

8. 温针火针治疗后1周少食辛发之物，如辛辣、海鲜等食物，宜食清淡，并注意休息，勿过劳。

参 考 文 献

[1] 黄帝内经素问 [M]. 北京：人民卫生出版社，1963：81.

[2] 甄志亚. 中国医学史 [M]. 上海：上海科学技术出版社，1984：5.

[3] 张厚墉. 关于内蒙古地区医学史中几个问题的考察 [J]. 陕西中医学院学报，1979，3（3）：45.

[4] 巴·吉格木德. 蒙古医学简史 [M]. 呼和浩特：内蒙古教育出版社，1997：90-91.

第二章

蒙医温针火针疗法的作用及机制

一、蒙医温针火针疗法的作用

蒙医温针火针疗法能抑制赫依、增强胃火、破痞块、助消化、散积消聚、排出脓血及黄水,治肌肉麻木或肿胀、水肿等。蒙医温针火针疗法在临床应用广泛,涉及临床各科、各系统疾病,包括慢性病、急性病,甚至有些恶性疾病。蒙医温针火针疗法的主要治疗作用,可概括为以下几个方面。

1. 消炎作用　大量临床实践及实验研究证明,蒙医温针火针疗法具有消炎作用。皮肤、黏膜、肌肉、关节,乃至内脏器官,由各种病因引起的急慢性炎症,均可用蒙医温针火针疗法治疗。

2. 镇痛作用　疼痛是一个极为复杂的问题,既是一种物质现象,又是一种精神现象。引起疼痛的原因有很多,损伤、炎症、缺血、痉挛、肌力不平衡、反射性,乃至精神因素,均可引起疼痛。应用蒙医温针火针疗法镇痛,要弄清病因,有针对性地进行治疗。如炎症性疼痛,以消炎治疗为主;缺血性和痉挛性疼痛,以改善缺血,消除痉挛为主;神经痛、神经炎,以阻断痛觉冲动传入,或以关闭疼痛闸门,激发镇痛物质的释放为主。

3. 镇静、促进睡眠　蒙医温针火针疗法能控制大脑皮层扩散性抑制,解除全身紧张状态,因而产生明显的镇静和促进睡眠的效果。

4. 兴奋神经肌肉　蒙医温针火针疗法能引起运动神经及肌肉兴奋,用于治疗周围性神经麻痹及肌肉萎缩,具有明显的兴奋神经和肌肉的效果。也能促使毛细血管扩张,增强局部皮肤和肌肉的营养供应,使肌肉萎缩得以改善,并促进损害组织的修复。

5. 缓解痉挛　蒙医温针火针疗法具有缓解痉挛作用,使牵张反射减弱和肌张力下降。

6. 软化瘢痕,松解粘连　蒙医温针火针疗法有软化瘢痕和松解粘连的作用,使肌腱、韧带、关节囊等组织延展性增加。

7. 影响机体免疫 蒙医温针火针疗法有增强和调节机体免疫的作用。

二、蒙医温针火针疗法的作用机制

蒙医温针火针疗法就是针刺与温灸相结合的一种外治疗法。它具有针刺与温灸的双重作用，能温通经脉、调和气血、调理体素、增强抵抗力，以防治疾病。它通过针刺刺激、温热刺激及穴位功效的相互作用，对机体产生一些生物学效应，以调节机体的生理和病理状态，从而达到治疗疾病的目的。

1. 改善血液循环 温针火针疗法使局部平均温度升高，改善局部血液循环，加强局部组织代谢，有利于炎症等病理反应的消失，并改善肌肉皮肤等正常组织的营养。温针火针疗法将针具加热到较高温度后，在皮肤上形成红、热、痛及轻微的水肿现象，对局部皮肤肌肉产生针刺与温灸的双重刺激，激活机体的应激性反应，释放出组胺样物质；同时变性坏死的组织溶解成蛋白而被吸收，可引起自身免疫反应，从而促使全身炎症因子释放及局部趋附，进一步导致局部血管的收缩与舒张，从而达到改善局部循环的目的。温针火针疗法通过刺激穴位，并通过神经上传至大脑，调节大脑皮层，解除脑血管痉挛，使脑血管扩张而降低脑血管阻力，改善脑循环。

2. 调节神经 - 内分泌 - 免疫网络 现代神经内分泌免疫学研究表明，外界任何物理或化学的刺激均可引起神经系统的应激，激活垂体体系，从而影响中枢神经系统对免疫系统的调控；而免疫细胞则可以释放神经肽和细胞因子，从而对中枢神经系统起到活性作用，最终引起人体内分泌的变化。从临床试验结果来看，白细胞减少症通过温针火针治疗后，白细胞数量上升，中性粒细胞的吞噬率、吞菌率和杀菌率都有所提高。说明温针火针疗法通过免疫激活反应调节神经 - 内分泌 - 免疫网络，对机体产生镇痛、提高抗病能力等治疗效应。

3. 调节神经递质与细胞因子含量 温针火针疗法有改善睡眠、安神、镇静的作用。通过蒙医温针火针刺激氯苯丙氨酸（PCPA）失眠大鼠的相应穴位后，观测大鼠的相关细胞因子、神经递质含量及 5- 羟色胺、多巴胺神经递质与其受体特异性结合率，发现蒙医温针火针疗法能够调节对睡眠起到重要作用的 5- 羟色胺、去甲肾上腺素、多巴胺、γ- 氨基丁酸（GABA）、谷氨酸、乙酰胆碱等神经递质的含量和细胞因子（白介素 -1β、白介素 -2、白介素 -6、肿瘤坏死因子 -α）含量，推测 5- 羟色胺能神经系统、GABA 能神经系统、细胞因子（白介素 -1、白介素 -2、白介素 -6、肿瘤坏死因子 -α）介导了蒙医温针火针疗法改善睡眠作用，从神经递质、细胞因子层面揭示了蒙医温针火针改善睡眠作用机制。

4. 影响自由基活性 温针火针疗法通过提高体内超氧化物歧化酶（SOD）活性，增强清除丙二醛（MDA）等氧化代谢产物的作用，升高一氧化氮（NO）含量和生物学活性，从而延缓组织器官衰老和老年病的发生。由于提高了自由基的清除能力，减少了自由基诱导的免疫器官细胞凋亡，从而延缓免疫器官萎缩和功能退化，提高机体免疫力。还有实验观察到，蒙医温针火针疗法能提高疲劳大鼠肝脏的抗氧化酶活性，以增加对自由基损伤的抵抗力和对自由基的清除，阻断脂质过氧化反应，保护细胞免受损伤，从而促进疲劳的恢复。

第三章

白脉与穴位

一、白脉

蒙医学将脑、脊髓及白脉统称为白脉。由胚胎时期从脐部生出的阴脉所形成，归五元中属水，故又称水脉。脑位于颅腔内，由无数支白脉形成。因此，脑有白脉之海或白脉之根之说。脑为司命赫依和能足巴达干所寓之处，又在二者支配下发挥掌管人体各系统器官的功能，是生命之根本。脑之滋养血液借普行赫依的作用，由心脉通过依存脉供给。脊髓导源于脑，系主白脉，从脑部脉的海洋里，像树根一样向下延伸传导的水脉有 19 条。由脊髓分支的白脉分内白脉（隐匿脉）和外白脉（明显脉）。

（一）内白脉（隐匿脉）

连接五脏六腑的 13 条白脉称为内白脉，又称隐匿脉。其中有与心脏和小肠相连的 4 条赫依脉，与肺、大肠、肝、胆相通的 4 条希拉脉，与脾、胃、肾、膀胱相通的 4 条巴达干脉，与精府相通的 1 条三根（赫依、希拉、巴达干）混合脉。

十三内白脉离于脑，随脊髓由枕骨大孔下行至各自的脊椎位时，向外循行与相关脏腑相连接。其分布见表 3-1。

表 3-1 内白脉（隐匿脉）分布

内白脉	连接脏腑	分出位置	脉数
赫依	心	至第 7 椎分左右两路运行与心脏相连	2
	小肠	至第 17 椎分左右两路运行与小肠相连	2
希拉	肺	至第 5 椎与肺相连	1
	大肠	至第 16 椎与大肠相连	1
	肝	至第 9 椎与肝相连	1
	胆	至第 10 椎与胆相连	1

续表

内白脉	连接脏腑	分出位置	脉数
巴达干	脾	至第11椎与脾相连	1
	胃	至第12椎与胃相连	1
	肾	至第14椎与肾相连	1
	膀胱	至第18椎与膀胱相连	1
三根混合脉	精府	至第13椎与精府相连	1

(二)外白脉(明显脉)

分布于四肢的6条白脉称为外白脉,又称明显脉。包括曲脉和珍宝脉、管脉。

1. 曲脉 分布于上肢的白脉,分左右两支。自枕骨大孔开始下行至第1椎,两支脉相交于此,隐入于里,在肱骨、肩胛骨之间,至此分为两支,一条自关节外出,经三角肌至肘部,一条自腋窝外侧出来,至肘部与另一条衔接,绕肘关节循拇指,汇集于掌心。

2. 珍宝脉 分布于上肢的白脉,分左右两支。始于脑下,经小尖脉尖端,于耳垂下外出,而隐入于锁骨处,向下运行,至腋窝内外出,经肘窝之内侧向下循行,通于无名指,至掌心与曲脉汇合。

3. 管脉 分布于下肢的白脉,分左右两支。管脉自脑分出,第1椎左右各约1寸处直接向下运行,至第5椎复入里与脊柱内之脉道相连接,至第12椎又向脊柱外循行,与精府和肾脏相通,称管脉精肾分支。再往下至第14椎分为4支(左右各2支),称管脉后支及前支,后支由第14椎外出,经尾骨、髋骨之间,然后越髋眼外出,经大腿外侧,到外踝、中趾,止于足心。前支由第14椎外出,自髋骨上显露,向下运行于大腿前内侧,沿膝关节、胫骨,与大趾之外侧相连,与后支汇集于足心。

二、穴位测定法

(一)手指测定法

手指测定法是以患者手指为标准,中指两关节中间的横纹的距离为1寸,或以患者拇指宽度为1寸(图3-1)等测定穴位的准确位置。这种测定法,对男女老少、高矮胖瘦人群均适用。在临床上测定施疗穴位时,根据人体各部骨骼的长度，以手指作测量单位，可量出许多同等长度的单位。如测定胫下穴位时，从膝关节到踝关节的距离以 16 寸计算，折半则成 8 寸，再把从踝关节以上 8 寸折半成 4 寸，由此确定外踝以上 3 寸（腓骨前缘）处为准确的针刺部位（图 3-2）。手指测定法常用周身距离测量见表 3-2。

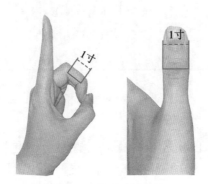

图 3-1　手指取寸示意图

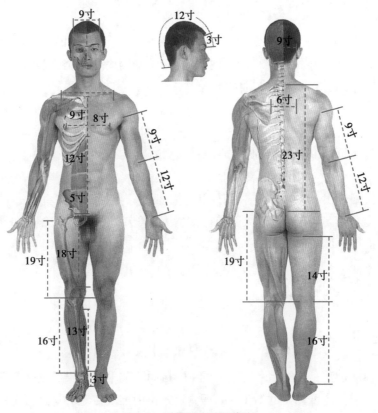

图 3-2　手指测定法示意图

表3-2　手指测定法常用周身距离测量表

区分部位	起止点	长度/寸	量法
头部	前发际正中至后发际正中	12	纵量
	眉间至前发际正中	3	纵量
	耳后两乳突之间	9	横量
胸腹部	胸骨上窝至剑胸结合中点	9	纵量
	剑胸结合中点至脐中	12	纵量
	脐中至耻骨联合上缘	5	纵量
	两乳头间的距离	8	横量
脊柱部	第一脊椎（第七颈椎）关节至尾骨	23	纵量
	两肩胛骨间	6	横量
上肢	腋窝横纹至肘横纹	9	纵量
	肘窝横纹至腕横纹	12	纵量
下肢	耻骨联合上缘至髌骨上缘	18	纵量
	胫骨结节至踝骨	13	纵量
	股骨大转子至腘横纹	19	纵量
	臀沟至腘横纹	14	纵量
	膝关节至外踝	16	纵量
	外踝至足底	3	纵量

（二）解剖学固定点测定法

解剖学固定点测定法是根据现代解剖学，按人体各部位解剖学位置，把看得见、摸得着的固定点作为测定施疗穴位的新方法。其特点是固定的部位明显而不移动，便于测定，易于掌握。以脊柱部的穴位为例，脊柱椎体关节组成包括7个颈椎关节、12个胸椎关节、5个腰椎关节、5个骶椎关节、4或5个尾椎。灸疗、针刺的穴位，从颈椎第7节（蒙医脊椎第1节）开始，每一脊椎下凹正中和从此点再向左、右各量1寸处，三穴并列。如：赫依穴位于第1脊椎下凹正中和从此点再向左、右各量1寸处，三穴并列，解剖学上的准确位置在第7颈椎棘突与第1胸椎棘突间隙正中和左、右两侧各量1寸；精府穴位于第13脊椎下凹正中，解剖学上准确位置在第12胸椎与第1腰椎棘突间隙正中和左、右两侧各量1寸处，三穴并列。心尖穴位于两侧乳头下1寸处，解剖学上准确位置在第5肋间隙,乳头直下。从上述几个穴位的测定法可以看出,蒙医传统疗法的穴位准确测定与解剖学有着密切的关系。

(三)简便测定法

穴位的简便测定法是根据人体表面最明显的标记或点、躯体的不同体位、器官特征等,迅速找到施治的部位或穴位的方法。如测定大腿穴,令患者站立,两手自然伸直放下后其中指尖处就是大腿穴(图 3-3);测定膝眼穴,令患者屈膝而坐,膝关节前下方两侧出现明显的凹陷正中就是膝眼穴(图 3-4);测定髋穴,令患者侧卧,将上侧腿屈曲,在臀肌部出现明显的陷凹,此凹就是髋穴,并在此凹上、下、左、右各量 1 寸处各有 1 穴(图 3-5);嗓窝穴位于嗓窝正中;黑白际穴位于两乳头连线与正中线交叉点上;等等。

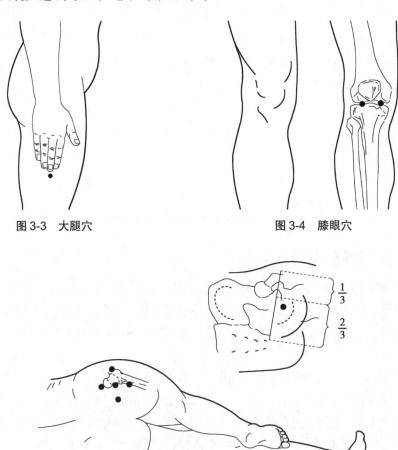

图 3-3 大腿穴　　　　　　　　　　　图 3-4 膝眼穴

图 3-5 髋穴

三、蒙医温针火针疗法常用穴位

（一）头颈部穴位（42穴）

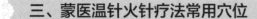

顶会穴

【出处】《蓝琉璃》。

【别名】顶中穴、吉朱格。

【穴位释义】顶，头顶；会，交会。

【定位】在头部，在前、后发际正中连线与两耳尖向上连线交叉处（图3-6）。本穴与中医针灸之"百会"穴是同一处。

【局部解剖】皮肤，皮下组织，帽状腱膜，筋膜下疏松组织。布有枕大神经，额神经的分支，左、右颞浅动脉、静脉及枕动、静脉吻合网。

【主治】赫依热、喑哑症、神志不清、失眠、记忆力减退、视力减弱、脱发、鼻出血、头痛、头晕、癫痫、抑郁症、癫狂症及妇女赫依瘀症、慢性疲劳等。

【操作】选用Ⅰ号或Ⅱ号蒙医银针，平刺0.5～1寸，温针给予针柄加热，温度38～42℃，留针15～20min。

火针或单针刺不加热，留针15～20min。

单灸，直接灸3～7炷或间接灸5～20min。

小儿慎刺。

【文献摘要】《蓝琉璃》：顶会穴是心穴，就是肉脉、骨脉、脑脉三脉会穴。

《四部医典·秘诀本》：赫依性头晕昏迷病灸顶会穴、后颈发穴、额穴。

【常用配穴】①配赫依穴，治赫依偏盛。②配心穴、黑白际穴、命脉穴，治心、命脉病。

【现代研究】（1）蒙医温针刺激顶会穴、赫依穴、心穴治疗失眠症的实验研究：①蒙医温针刺激顶会穴、赫依穴、心穴可以明显使失眠大鼠大脑兴奋性降低，蒙医温针促睡眠机制与其可以调节失眠大鼠大脑、下丘脑、海马组织中白介素-1（IL-1）、白介素-2（IL-2）、白介素-6（IL-6）、肿瘤坏死因子-α（TNF-α）、去甲肾上腺素（NE）、多巴胺（DA）、谷氨酸（Glu）、5-羟色胺（5-HT）、γ-氨基丁酸（GABA）、乙酰胆碱（ACh）含量密切相关。[1]②蒙医温针刺激顶会穴、赫依穴、心穴可使失眠大鼠下丘脑和部分前额皮质中升高的多巴胺含量降低，从而使大脑兴奋性降低，由此认为其促睡眠机制与其可以调节大鼠下丘脑及部分前额皮质多巴胺的含量密切相关。[2] ③蒙医温针刺激顶会穴、赫依穴、心穴可以明显降低失眠大鼠海马中谷氨酸含量和升高海马中 γ- 氨基丁酸、乙酰胆碱含量，从而使大脑兴奋性降低，由此认为，其促睡眠机制与其可以调节失眠大鼠海马中谷氨酸、γ- 氨基丁酸、乙酰胆碱含量密切相关。[3] ④蒙医温针刺激顶会穴、赫依穴、心穴对大鼠有镇静和改善睡眠作用。[4]

（2）蒙医温针刺激顶会穴、顶前穴、顶后穴治疗失眠症的实验研究：选顶会穴、顶前穴和顶后穴，用蒙医银针（针长为 9cm，针径为 0.85mm）斜刺顶会穴 1～2cm，再以蒙医疗术温针仪给针柄加热（温度为 40℃左右），留针加热时间为 20min。隔 4 天同样方法刺激顶前穴，再隔 3 天刺激顶后穴，14 天为 1 个疗程。治疗期间每晚睡前给患者煎服苏格木勒 -3 汤。有效率 97.5%。[5]

（3）蒙医温针刺激顶会穴治疗失眠症的实验研究：取顶会穴常规消毒后，2% 利多卡因 1ml 浅麻，自制银针斜刺透前顶穴，艾灸 3～5 壮不等，隔日 1 次，7 天为 1 个疗程。重者配合口服补心安神的自制蒙药。有效率 97.0%。[6]

（4）蒙医温针刺激顶会穴、心穴治疗慢性疲劳症的实验研究：①蒙医温针刺激顶会穴、心穴可以提高疲劳大鼠运动能力，与抑制亢进的下丘脑 - 垂体 - 肾上腺轴有关。[7] ②蒙医温针刺激顶会穴、心穴，通过降低运动性疲劳大鼠脑组织中单胺类神经递质含量而起到治疗作用，这可能是蒙医温针抗疲劳的作用机制之一。[8] ③蒙医温针刺激顶会穴、心穴，可降低运动性疲劳大鼠血清 TNF。[9]

（5）蒙医温针刺激顶会穴、命脉穴、心穴治疗慢性疲劳综合征的实验研究：选顶会穴、命脉穴和心穴，用蒙医银针（针长为 5cm，针径为 0.8mm）向后斜刺顶会穴 1.5～2cm，得气后以蒙医疗术温针仪离体表 1cm 处给针柄加热（温度在

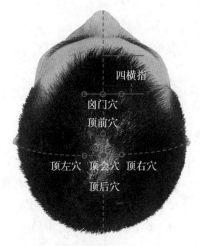

图 3-6

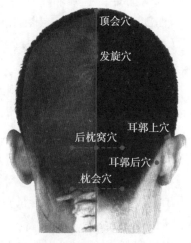

图 3-7

40～43℃），留针加热时间为 20～25min。隔 3 天同样方法刺激命脉穴，再隔 3 天刺激心穴，9 天为 1 个疗程。有效率 89.7%。[10]

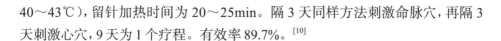

【出处】《蒙医疗术》《五疗》）。

【别名】前顶穴。

【穴位释义】穴在颅顶之前方，与顶后穴相对应。

【定位】在头部，在前、后发际正中连线顶会穴前方 1 寸处（图 3-6）。

【局部解剖】皮肤，皮下组织，帽状腱膜，筋膜下疏松组织。布有额神经的分支，左、右颞浅动、静脉和额动、静脉的吻合网。

【主治】胸闷、顶心痛、神志不清、失眠、记忆力减退、视力减弱、脱发、鼻出血、头痛、头晕、癫痫、抑郁症、癫狂症、浮肿、高血压等。

【操作】选用Ⅰ号或Ⅱ号蒙医银针，平刺 0.5～1 寸，温针给予针柄加热，温度 38～42℃，15～20min。

火针或单针刺不加热，留针 15～20min。

单灸，直接灸 3～7 炷或间接灸 5～20min。

小儿慎刺。

【文献摘要】《蒙医疗术》《五疗》）：顶前穴是肝脉结；针灸顶前穴主治"萨"病、半身麻木、头痛、头晕、目眩、癫痫、精神病、脑血管意外后肢体瘫痪。

【出处】《蒙医疗术》《五疗》）。

【别名】后顶穴。

【穴位释义】穴在颅顶之后方，与顶前穴相对应。

【定位】在头部，在前、后发际正中连线顶会穴后方 1 寸处（图 3-6）。

【局部解剖】皮肤，皮下组织，帽状腱膜，筋膜下疏松组织。布有枕大神经以及枕动、静脉和颞前动、静脉的吻合网。

【主治】失眠、心烦、头痛、头晕、癫痫、抑郁症、癫狂症、浮肿、高血压等。

【操作】选用Ⅰ号或Ⅱ号蒙医银针，平刺 0.5～1 寸，温针给予针柄加热，温度 38～42℃，15～20min。

火针或单针刺不加热，留针 15～20min。

单灸，直接灸 3～7 炷或间接灸 5～20min。

小儿慎刺。

【文献摘要】《蒙医疗术》(《五疗》):顶后穴是肾脉结。

顶右穴

【出处】《蒙医疗术》(《五疗》)。

【别名】顶会右穴。

【穴位释义】穴在颅顶之右方,与顶左穴相对应。

【定位】在头部,在两耳尖向上连线顶会穴右方 1 寸处(图 3-6)。

【局部解剖】皮肤,皮下组织,帽状腱膜,筋膜下疏松组织。布有枕动、静脉,颞前动、静脉顶支和眶上动、静脉的吻合网,有枕大神经、耳颞神经及眶上神经的分支。

【主治】由肺刺痛产生热邪、面部眼睑浮肿、癫狂、昏厥等。

【操作】选用 I 号或 II 号蒙医银针,平刺 0.5～1 寸,温针给予针柄加热,温度 38～42℃,15～20min。

火针或单针刺不加热,留针 15～20min。

单灸,直接灸 3～7 炷或间接灸 5～20min。

小儿慎刺。

【文献摘要】《蒙医疗术》(《五疗》):顶右穴是肺脉结。

顶左穴

【出处】《蒙医疗术》(《五疗》)。

【别名】顶会左穴。

【穴位释义】穴在颅顶之左方,与顶右穴相对应。

【定位】在头部,在两耳尖向上连线顶会穴左方 1 寸处(图 3-6)。

【局部解剖】皮肤,皮下组织,帽状腱膜,筋膜下疏松组织。布有枕动、静脉,颞前动、静脉顶支和眶上动、静脉的吻合网,有枕大神经、耳颞神经及眶上神经的分支。

【主治】心烦躁扰不安、恶寒等。

【操作】选用 I 号或 II 号蒙医银针,平刺 0.5～1 寸,温针给予针柄加热,温度 38～42℃,15～20min。

火针或单针刺不加热,留针 15～20min。

单灸,直接灸 3～7 炷或间接灸 5～20min。

小儿慎刺。

【文献摘要】《蒙医疗术》(《五疗》):顶左穴是心脉结。

囟门穴

【出处】《蓝琉璃》。

【别名】朝克桑。

【穴位释义】囟，指囟门。在颅骨冠状缝和矢状缝交叉处，婴儿时脑髓不充，头骨不合，俗称囟门，年长囟门渐合。

【定位】在头部，前发际正中直上四横指处有 1 穴，从此点再向左右量 1 寸各有 1 穴，三穴并列（图 3-6）。中间穴与中医针灸之"囟会"穴是同一处。

【局部解剖】皮肤，皮下组织，帽状腱膜，筋膜下疏松组织。布有额神经及左、右颞浅动、静脉和额动脉、静脉的吻合网。

【主治】赫依而致的头晕、癫痫病、晕厥等。

【操作】选用Ⅰ号或Ⅱ号蒙医银针，平刺 0.5～1 寸，温针给予针柄加热，温度 38～42℃，15～20min。

火针或单针刺不加热，留针 15～20min。

单灸，直接灸 3～5 炷或间接灸 5～20min。

小儿慎刺。

【文献摘要】《蒙药正典》：囟门穴在额头发际上四指处施灸可医脑疾所致健忘，头晕等。

《蒙医疗术》（《五疗》）：囟门穴是颅骨缝"三会"。

发旋穴

【出处】《蒙医临床学》。

【穴位释义】穴在头顶发旋处。

【定位】在头部，位于头顶发旋正中（图 3-7）。

【局部解剖】皮肤，皮下组织，帽状腱膜。布有耳颞神经的分支及颞浅动、静脉。

【主治】瘟疫、热证、胸闷昏沉、全身麻木不适与巩膜黄染等。

【操作】选用Ⅰ号或Ⅱ号蒙医银针，直刺 0.3～0.5 寸或平刺 0.5～1 寸，温针给予针柄加热，温度 38～42℃，15～20min。

火针或单针刺不加热，留针 15～20min。

单灸，直接灸 3～7 炷或间接灸 5～20min。

小儿慎刺。

后枕窝穴

【出处】《蒙医临床学》。

【别名】枕三组穴。

【穴位释义】主穴在后枕窝。

【定位】在头部,枕外隆凸的上缘凹陷处1穴,在其左右两侧1寸处各有1穴,三穴并列(图3-7)。中间穴与中医针灸之"脑户"穴是同一处。

【局部解剖】皮肤,皮下组织,左、右枕额肌枕腹之间,筋膜下疏松组织。布有枕大神经的分支和枕动、静脉的分支或属支。

【主治】颈项发僵、头痛、舌头肿胀等。

【操作】选用Ⅰ号或Ⅱ号蒙医银针,平刺0.5~1寸,温针给予针柄加热,温度38~42℃,15~20min。

火针或单针刺不加热,留针15~20min。

单灸,直接灸3~5炷或间接灸10~15min。

小儿慎刺。

枕会穴

【出处】《蒙医临床学》。

【穴位释义】主穴在后颈窝上。

【定位】在颈部,枕外隆凸直下,两侧斜方肌之间凹陷中有1穴,其左右两侧1寸处各有1穴,三穴并列(图3-7)。中间穴与中医针灸之"风府"穴是同一处。

【局部解剖】皮肤,皮下组织,左、右斜方肌腱之间,项韧带(左、右头半棘肌之间),左右头后大、小直肌之间。浅层分布有枕大神经和第三枕神经的分支及枕动、静脉的分支或属支;深层分布有枕下神经的分支。

【主治】赫依性头痛与头晕、昏迷昏厥、颈项发僵、低头受限、腰部僵痛等。

【操作】中间穴:伏案正坐,使头微前倾,项肌放松,选用Ⅰ号或Ⅱ号蒙医银针,向下颌方向缓慢刺入0.5~1寸,针尖不可向上,以免刺入枕骨大孔,误伤延髓;两侧穴:选用Ⅰ号或Ⅱ号蒙医银针,向下颌方向斜刺入0.5~1寸。温针给予针柄加热,温度38~42℃,10~15min。

火针或单针刺不加热,留针15~20min。

单灸,直接灸3~5炷或间接灸10~15min。

小儿慎刺。

前额穴 ᠮᠠᠩᠨᠠᠢ

【出处】《蒙医临床学》。

【穴位释义】穴在前额正中。

【定位】在头部,位于前额正中线发际处(图3-8)。

【局部解剖】皮肤,皮下组织,帽状腱膜,筋膜下疏松组织。布有额神经的分支和额动、静脉的分支或属支。

【主治】眼昏蒙症,疫病致发狂等。

【操作】选用Ⅰ号或Ⅱ号蒙医银针,平刺0.5～1寸,温针给予针柄加热,温度38～42℃左右,10～15min。

火针或单针刺不加热,留针15～20min。

单灸,直接灸1～3炷或间接灸5～10min。

小儿慎刺。

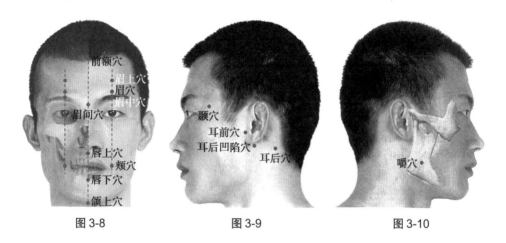

图3-8   图3-9   图3-10

眉间穴 ᠬᠥᠮᠥᠰᠭᠡ

【出处】《蒙医临床学》。

【穴位释义】穴在两眉中间。

【定位】在面部,位于两眉毛内侧端中间的凹陷中(图3-8)。本穴与中医针灸之"印堂"穴是同一处。

【局部解剖】皮肤,皮下组织,降眉间肌。布有额神经的分支,滑车上神经,眼动脉的分支,额动脉及伴行的静脉。

【主治】巩膜及皮肤黄染、头痛、鼻出血等。

【操作】选用Ⅰ号或Ⅱ号蒙医银针,向下平刺 0.3～0.5 寸,温针给予针柄加热,温度 38℃左右,3～5min。

火针或单针刺不加热,留针 15～20min。

单灸,直接灸 3～5 炷或间接灸 10～15min。

小儿慎刺。

眉上穴

【出处】《蒙医临床学》。

【穴位释义】穴在眉毛以上。

【定位】在头部,位于眼眉上 1 寸,瞳孔直上,左右各有 1 穴(图 3-8)。本穴与中医针灸之"阳白"穴是同一处。

【局部解剖】皮肤,皮下组织,额肌。浅层分布有眶上神经颞浅动脉;深层分布有面神经颞支,眶上动脉。

【主治】头痛、赤眼病等。

【操作】选用Ⅰ号或Ⅱ号蒙医银针,平刺 0.3～0.5 寸,温针给予针柄加热,温度 38℃左右,3～5min。

火针或单针刺不加热,留针 15～20min。

单灸,间接灸 5～10min。

小儿慎刺。

眉穴

【出处】《蒙医临床学》。

【穴位释义】穴在眼眉上缘。

【定位】在面部,位于眉上缘正中,左右各有 1 穴(图 3-8)。

【局部解剖】皮肤,皮下组织,眼轮匝肌,枕额肌额腹。布有眶上神经外侧支,面神经的分支和眶上动、静脉的外侧支。

【主治】视力模糊、心迷、头痛、眼眶痛等。

【操作】选用Ⅰ号或Ⅱ号蒙医银针,向上或左右平刺 0.3～0.5 寸,或直刺 0.1～0.3 寸,温针给予针柄加热,温度为 38℃左右,3～5min。

火针或单针刺不加热,留针 15～20min。

单灸,间接灸 3～5min。

小儿慎刺。

眉中穴 ᠮᡝᠯ᠌ᠵᡝᡳ

【出处】《蒙医临床学》。

【穴位释义】穴在眼眉中。

【定位】在头部,位于瞳孔直上,眉毛中,左右各有 1 穴(图 3-8)。本穴与中医针灸之"鱼腰"穴是同一处。

【局部解剖】皮肤,皮下组织,眼轮匝肌,枕额肌额腹。布有眶神经外侧支,面神经的分支和眶上动、静脉的外侧支。

【主治】巩膜、皮肤染黄及鼻出血等。

【操作】选用 I 号或 II 号蒙医银针,平刺 0.3～0.5 寸或直刺 0.1～0.2 寸,温针给予针柄加热,温度为 38℃左右,3～5min。

火针或单针刺不加热,留针 15～20min。

小儿慎刺。

颞穴 ᠲᠣᠯᠣᡤᠠᡳ

【出处】《蒙医临床学》。

【穴位释义】穴在颞部。

【定位】在头部,位于眉梢与目外眦之间,向后约一横指的凹陷处,左右各有 1 穴(图 3-9)。本穴与中医针灸之"太阳"穴是同一处。

【局部解剖】皮肤,皮下组织,眼轮匝肌,颞筋膜,颞肌。布有颞神经的分支颧面神经,面神经的颧支和颞支,下颌神经的颞神经和颞浅动、静脉的分支或属支。

【主治】头痛、头晕、胸闷昏沉等赫依血引起的病症。

【操作】选用 I 号或 II 号蒙医银针,直刺或斜刺 0.3～0.5 寸,温针给予针柄加热,温度为 38℃左右,3～5min。

火针或单针刺不加热,留针 15～20min。

单灸,间接灸 3～5min。

小儿慎刺。

耳前穴 ᠴᡳᡥᡳᠨ

【出处】《蒙医临床学》。

【穴位释义】穴在耳朵前。

【定位】在面部,耳屏前,位于耳屏间切迹与下颌骨髁状突的后缘间之凹陷处，左右各有 1 穴（图 3-9）。本穴与中医针灸之"听会"穴是同一处。

【局部解剖】皮肤，皮下组织，布有颞前动、静脉的耳前支，面神经及三叉神经第三支的耳颞神经。

【主治】口眼㖞斜、昏厥、淋巴结肿胀、牙痛、耳鸣等。

【操作】选用 I 号或 II 号蒙医银针，微张口，直刺 0.5～0.8 寸，温针给予针柄加热，温度为 38℃左右，3～5min。

火针或单针刺不加热，留针 15～20min。

单灸，间接灸 5～10min。

小儿慎刺。

耳后穴

【出处】《蒙医临床学》。

【穴位释义】穴在耳朵后。

【定位】在头部，位于耳后乳突的后方凹陷中，左右各有 1 穴（图 3-9）。本穴与中医针灸之"完骨"穴是同一处。

【局部解剖】皮肤，皮下组织，胸锁乳突肌。浅层分布有枕小神经，耳大神经，耳后动、静脉的分支；深层有副神经，颈神经丛肌支，枕动脉，颈深动、静脉。

【主治】耳鸣、牙痛、偏头痛等。

【操作】选用 I 号或 II 号蒙医银针，斜刺 0.5～0.8 寸，温针给予针柄加热，温度为 38℃左右，3～5min。

火针或单针刺不加热，留针 15～20min。

可不针刺，单灸，间接灸 5～10min。

小儿慎刺。

嚼穴

【出处】《蒙医临床学》。

【穴位释义】穴在腮部。

【定位】在面部，位于下颌角前方一横指凹陷处（张嘴时出现凹陷），左右各有 1 穴（图 3-10）。本穴与中医针灸之"颊车"穴是同一处。

【局部解剖】皮肤，皮下组织，笑肌，咬肌。浅层分布有耳大神经分支，耳颞神经（下颌神经分支）；深层分布有面神经下颌支，下颌神经咬肌支，面神经。

【主治】口眼㖞斜、耳鸣、张口困难等。

【操作】选用 I 号或 II 号蒙医银针，直刺 0.3～0.5 寸或向口角方向斜刺 0.5～

1寸,温针给予针柄加热,温度为38℃左右,3~5min。

火针或单针刺不加热,留针15~20min。

单灸,间接灸5~10min。

小儿慎刺。

颊穴

【出处】《蒙医临床学》。

【穴位释义】穴在颊部。

【定位】在面部,位于口角外侧,上直对瞳孔,左右各有1穴(图3-8)。本穴与中医针灸之"地仓"穴是同一处。

【局部解剖】皮肤,皮下组织,口轮匝肌,颊肌。浅层分布有眶下神经,下颌神经的分支,颊神经;深层分布有面神经颊支,面动、静脉分支或属支。

【主治】口颊㖞斜、流涎等。

【操作】选用Ⅰ号或Ⅱ号蒙医银针,向外上方平刺0.5~1寸,温针给予针柄加热,温度为38℃左右,3~5min。

火针或单针刺不加热,留针15~20min。

单灸,间接灸5~10min。

小儿慎刺。

唇上穴

【出处】《蒙医临床学》。

【别名】人中穴。

【穴位释义】穴在鼻柱正下,嘴唇正上。

【定位】在面部,位于人中沟的上1/3与中1/3的交点处(图3-8)。本穴与中医针灸之"水沟"穴是同一处。

【局部解剖】皮肤,皮下组织,口轮匝肌。布有眶下神经的分支和上唇动、静脉。

【主治】舌肿而不能言语、昏迷、昏厥等。

【操作】选用Ⅰ号或Ⅱ号蒙医银针,向上斜刺0.3~0.5寸,温针给予针柄加热,温度为38℃左右,3~5min。

火针或单针刺不加热,留针15~20min。

单灸,间接灸5~10min。

小儿慎刺。

唇下穴 ᠊ᠠ᠊᠊ᠠ

【出处】《蒙医临床学》。

【别名】嘴唇窝穴。

【穴位释义】穴在下嘴唇正下。

【定位】在面部,位于颏唇沟的正中凹陷处(图3-8)。本穴与中医针灸之"承浆"穴是同一处。

【局部解剖】皮肤,皮下组织,口轮匝肌,降下唇肌。布有下牙槽神经的终支颏神经和颏动、静脉。

【主治】赫依性口吃、神志模糊等。

【操作】选用Ⅰ号或Ⅱ号蒙医银针,直刺0.3~0.5寸或斜刺0.5~1寸,温针给予针柄加热,温度38℃左右,3~5min。

火针或单针刺不加热,留针15~20min。

单灸,间接灸5~10min。

小儿慎刺。

颌上穴 ᠊ᠠ᠊᠊ᠠ

【出处】《蒙医临床学》。

【穴位释义】穴在下颌。

【定位】在面部,位于下颌骨下缘正中处,即颏下点(图3-8)。

【局部解剖】皮肤,皮下组织,口轮匝肌,降下唇肌。布有下牙槽神经的终支颏神经和颏动、静脉。

【主治】舌肿、失语、牙痛等。

【操作】选用Ⅰ号或Ⅱ号蒙医银针,直刺0.3~0.5寸或平刺0.5~1寸,温针给予针柄加热,温度为38℃左右,3~5min。

火针或单针刺不加热,留针15~20min。

单灸,间接灸5~10min。

小儿慎刺。

耳郭上穴 ᠊ᠠ᠊

【出处】《蒙医临床学》。

【别名】达日格乐穴。

【穴位释义】穴在耳郭上缘,左右各有1穴。

【定位】在头部,位于耳郭直上入发际处(图3-7)。

【局部解剖】皮肤,皮下组织,耳上肌,颞肌。浅层分布有耳颞神经皮支;深层分布有耳颞神经肌支,颞浅动、静脉耳前支。

【主治】头痛、头晕、耳朵疼痛等。

【操作】选用Ⅰ号或Ⅱ号蒙医银针,平刺0.3～0.5寸,温针给予针柄加热,温度为38℃左右,3～5min。

火针或单针刺不加热,留针15～20min。

可单灸,间接灸5～10min。

小儿慎刺。

耳郭后穴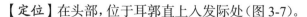

【出处】《蒙医临床学》。

【穴位释义】穴在耳朵后。

【定位】在头部,位于耳郭直后一横指处,左右各有1穴(图3-7)。

【局部解剖】皮肤,皮下组织,耳后肌。浅层分布有耳大神经,枕小神经;深层分布有面神经耳后支,耳后动、静脉分支。

【主治】颈项发僵、头痛、颈部两侧僵痛等。

【操作】选用Ⅰ号或Ⅱ号蒙医银针,平刺0.3～0.5寸,温针给予针柄加热,温度为38℃左右,3～5min。

火针或单针刺不加热,留针15～20min。

可单灸,间接灸5～10min。

小儿慎刺。

耳后凹陷穴

【出处】《蒙医临床学》。

【穴位释义】穴在耳垂后方。

【定位】在颈部,位于耳垂后方,乳突下端前方凹陷中,左右各有1穴(图3-9)。本穴与中医针灸之"翳风"穴是同一处。

【局部解剖】皮肤,皮下组织,腮腺。浅层分布有耳大神经,面神经耳支,耳后静脉;深层分布有面神经干,颈外动脉的分支,耳后动脉,翼静脉丛。

【主治】头痛、胸闷昏沉、口吃等。

【操作】选用Ⅰ号或Ⅱ号蒙医银针,直刺0.5～1寸,温针给予针柄加热,温度为38℃左右,3～5min。

火针或单针刺不加热,留针 15～20min。

可单灸,间接灸 5～10min。

小儿慎刺。

(二)胸腹部穴位(64穴)

心主脉穴 ꯁꯢꯀꯢꯃꯖ

【出处】《四部医典·秘诀本》。

【别名】命脉心穴、命脉与心脏之合穴、颈窝穴、嗓窝穴、苏如格尼格。

【穴位释义】穴在胸骨上窝正中,颈喉结下 2 寸处,内当肺系。

【定位】在颈前区,胸骨上窝中央,前正中线上(图3-11)。本穴与中医针灸之"天突"穴是同一处。

【局部解剖】皮肤,皮下组织,左、右胸锁乳突肌腱(两胸骨头)之间,胸骨柄颈静脉切迹上方,左、右胸骨甲状肌,气管前间隙。浅层布有锁骨上内侧神经,皮下组织内有颈阔肌和颈静脉弓;深层有头臂干、左颈总动脉、主动脉弓和头臂静脉等重要结构。

【主治】心绞痛、呃逆、咽喉阻塞巴达干、巴达干性病、赫依性心颤、呕吐、浮肿等。

【操作】选用Ⅱ号或Ⅲ号蒙医银针,先直刺,当针尖超过胸骨柄内缘后,即向下沿胸骨柄后缘、气管前缘缓慢向下刺入 0.5～1 寸,温针给予针柄加热,温度 38～40℃,10～15min。

火针或单针刺不加热,留针 15～20min。

可单灸,直接灸 1～3 炷或间接灸 5～15min。

小儿慎刺。

【文献摘要】《四部医典·秘诀本》:嗓窝是命脉和心的交会穴,施灸可治心绞痛、呃逆、咽喉阻塞。

《蒙古学百科全书·医学》:热邪隐伏于心等脏腑者,禁灸此穴。

【常用配穴】①配顶会穴或赫依穴,治赫依偏盛病。②配胃穴,治胃病。③配赫依穴或心穴,治赫依性颤悸症。④配黑白际穴,治咽喉阻塞巴达干、呕吐。

黑白际穴 ꯀꯢꯃꯖꯖ

【出处】《四部医典·论述本》。

【别名】嘎日那格扎木。

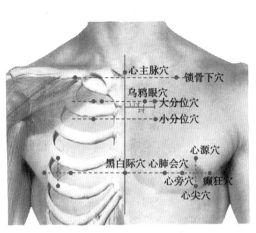

图 3-11

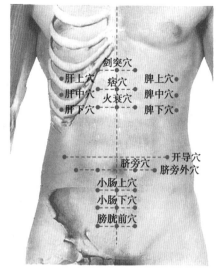

图 3-12

【穴位释义】胸中两乳间,穴在两乳间凹陷中。

【定位】在胸部,横平第四肋间,前正中线上(图 3-11)。本穴与中医针灸之"膻中"穴是同一处。

【局部解剖】皮肤,皮下组织,胸骨体。主要分布有第四肋间神经前皮支和胸廓内动、静脉的穿支。

【主治】心悸、心颤、心前区不适、心烦不安等。

【操作】选用Ⅱ号或Ⅲ号蒙医银针,直刺 0.3～0.5 寸或平刺 0.5～1 寸,温针给予针柄加热,温度 38～40℃,10～15min。

火针或单针刺不加热,留针 15～20min。

可单灸,直接灸 1～3 炷或间接灸 5～15min。

小儿慎刺。

【文献摘要】《四部医典•论述本》:心脏黄水病可服用阿嘎如 -8 味,再灸黑白际穴、顶会穴、心穴。

《蒙古学百科全书•医学》:热邪隐伏于心及肾脏以及其他脏腑有热象者,禁灸此穴。

【常用配穴】①配赫依穴,治赫依偏盛病。②配心穴及命脉穴,治心脏病。

剑突穴

【出处】《四部医典•论述本》。

【别名】兰桑。

【穴位释义】穴在剑突下，上临心界。

【定位】在腹部前正中线上，剑突尖下 1 寸有 1 穴，其左右两侧 1 寸处各有 1 穴，三穴并列（图 3-12）。中间穴与中医针灸之"巨阙"穴是同一处。

【局部解剖】皮肤，皮下组织，腹白线，腹横筋膜，腹膜外脂肪，壁腹膜。浅层主要有第七胸神经前支的前皮支和腹壁浅静脉；深层主要有第七胸神经前支的分支。

【主治】胃痛、胸痛、巴达干黏液增多而积于剑突下成痞证等。

【操作】选用Ⅱ号或Ⅲ号蒙医银针，直刺 0.3～0.5 寸或向下斜刺 0.5～1 寸，温针给予针柄加热，温度 38～40℃，10～15min。

火针或单针刺不加热，留针 15～20min。

可单灸，直接灸 1～3 炷或间接灸 5～15min。

小儿慎刺。

【文献摘要】《四部医典·论述本》："阿尤鲁海"尖就是"阿尤鲁海"窝上角，即嗓窝下角下 7 寸处。

《珍集》：巴达干病、"阿尤鲁海"巴达干引起的胃萎缩时，灸剑突穴为主，"阿尤鲁海"巴达干病还可吸烧盐剂和催吐剂，再灸剑突穴。

【常用配穴】①配痞穴，治剑突痞证。②配火衰穴，治胃火衰败证。

【现代研究】蒙医温针刺激火衰穴、胃穴、剑突穴、痞穴等穴位治疗单纯性肥胖症：用蒙医银针（直径为 0.8mm，针身为 60mm）刺入火衰穴、胃穴、剑突穴、痞穴等穴位后接蒙医 RZ-I 型电热针治疗仪，温度为 45℃左右（电流为 150～180mA），为防止灼伤针刺部位，在被灸穴位皮肤和电热针治疗仪灸头之间放置隔热纸层。总有效率 90.10%。[11]

痞穴 ᠬᠡᠷᠡᠭᠦᠷ

【出处】《四部医典·论述本》。

【别名】痞瘤穴、再桑。

【穴位释义】痞，指痞证；穴在剑突穴下。

【定位】在腹部前正中线上，剑突尖下 2 寸有 1 穴，其左右两侧 1 寸处各有 1 穴，三穴并列（图 3-12）。中间穴与中医针灸之"中脘"穴是同一处。

【局部解剖】皮肤，皮下组织，腹白线，腹横筋膜，腹膜外脂肪，壁腹膜。浅层主要有第七胸神经前支的前皮支和腹壁浅静脉的属支；深层主要有第七胸神经前支的分支。

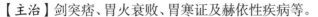

【主治】剑突痞、胃火衰败、胃寒证及赫依性疾病等。

【操作】选用Ⅱ号或Ⅲ号蒙医银针，直刺 0.5～1 寸，温针给予针柄加热，温度 38～40℃，10～15min。

火针或单针刺不加热，留针 15～20min。

可单灸，直接灸 1～3 炷或间接灸 5～15min。

小儿慎刺。

【文献摘要】《蒙古学百科全书·医学》：在胃热时，对本穴禁灸或放热针。肝大时，行针刺要注意，并不要将针刺入腹腔中。

【常用配穴】①配火衰穴，治胃火衰败。②配胃穴，治胃痞。

火衰穴

【出处】《四部医典·论述本》。

【别名】米力雅玛桑。

【穴位释义】火衰，指胃火衰减；本穴主要治疗胃火衰减。

【定位】在腹部前正中线上，剑突尖下 3 寸有 1 穴，其左右两侧 1 寸处各有 1 穴，三穴并列（图 3-12）。中间穴与中医针灸之"下脘"穴是同一处。

【局部解剖】皮肤，皮下组织，腹白线，腹横筋膜，腹膜外脂肪，壁腹膜。浅层主要有第八胸神经前支的前皮支和腹壁浅静脉的属支；深层主要有第八胸神经前支的分支。

【主治】主治胃火衰败和剑突痞、胃寒证及赫依性疾病等。

【操作】选用Ⅱ号或Ⅲ号蒙医银针，直刺 0.5～1 寸，温针给予针柄加热，温度 38～40℃，10～15min。

火针或单针刺不加热，留针 15～20min。

可单灸，直接灸 1～3 炷或间接灸 5～15min。

小儿慎刺。

【文献摘要】《蒙古学百科全书·医学》：胃或肝胆热，对本穴禁止施灸和放热针。

【常用配穴】①配剑突穴，治胃巴达干病。②配剑突穴、痞穴、胃穴，治食管癌和胃癌。

脐旁穴

【出处】《四部医典·秘诀本》。

【别名】回肠穴、龙德日。

【穴位释义】穴在脐旁。

【定位】在腹部，脐窝正中左右两侧1寸处各有1穴，二穴对称（图3-12）。

【局部解剖】皮肤，皮下组织，腹直肌鞘前壁，腹直肌，腹直肌鞘后壁。浅层分布有肋间神经前皮支，腹壁浅动、静脉；深层分布有肋间神经，肋间动脉，腹壁上下动、静脉吻合支。

【主治】大肠痞、大肠赫依病引起的腹胀或肠鸣、泄泻、消化不良等。

【操作】选用Ⅱ号或Ⅲ号蒙医银针，直刺0.5～1寸，温针给予针柄加热，温度38～40℃，10～15min。

火针或单针刺不加热，留针15～20min。

可单灸，直接灸1～3炷或间接灸5～15min。

小儿慎刺。

【文献摘要】《四部医典·秘诀本》：脐窝左右各一寸处是脐旁穴，灸治结肠痞、腹鸣、常腹泻。

【常用配穴】①配盲肠穴，治大肠痞证。②配大肠穴，治大肠赫依病。

脐旁外穴

【出处】《珍集》。

【别名】盲肠穴、龙普格桑。

【穴位释义】穴在脐旁外。

【定位】在腹部，脐窝正中左右两侧2寸处各有1穴，二穴对称（图3-12）。本穴与中医针灸之"天枢"穴是同一处。

【局部解剖】皮肤，皮下组织，腹直肌鞘前壁，腹直肌，腹直肌鞘后壁。浅层分布有肋间神经前皮支，腹壁浅动、静脉；深层分布有肋间神经，肋间动脉，腹壁上下动、静脉吻合支。

【主治】大肠痞、腹胀肠鸣、泄泻、消化不良等。

【操作】选用Ⅱ号或Ⅲ号蒙医银针，直刺0.5～1寸，温针给予针柄加热，温度38～40℃，10～15min。

火针或单针刺不加热，留针15～20min。

可单灸，直接灸1～3炷或间接灸5～15min。

小儿慎刺。

【文献摘要】《珍集》：结肠赫依病服石榴方剂，再灸脐旁外穴。

《蒙古学百科全书·医学》：患者过饱或饥饿时禁灸此穴。

【常用配穴】配回肠穴、大肠穴，治大肠病。

小肠上穴 ᠪᠠᠭᠠ ᠭᠡᠳᠡᠰᠤ

【出处】《四部医典·论述本》。

【别名】珠独德桑。

【穴位释义】主治小肠病，在小肠下穴之上。

【定位】在腹部，脐窝正中下 1 寸有 1 穴，其左右两侧 1 寸处各有 1 穴，三穴并列（图 3-12）。中间穴与中医针灸之"阴交"穴是同一处。

【局部解剖】皮肤，皮下组织，腹白线，腹横筋膜，腹膜外脂肪，壁腹膜。浅层主要有第十一胸神经前支的前皮支，脐周静脉网；深层主要有第十一胸神经前支的分支。

【主治】小肠寒性赫依病和泄泻等。

【操作】选用Ⅱ号或Ⅲ号蒙医银针，直刺 0.5～1 寸，温针给予针柄加热，温度 38～40℃，10～15min。

火针或单针刺不加热，留针 15～20min。

可单灸，直接灸 1～3 炷或间接灸 5～15min。

小儿慎刺。

【文献摘要】《四部医典·论述本》：小肠绞痛时，用汤酒送服阿魏剂，再用热盐外敷。温和导泻法治疗，再灸小肠上穴和小肠穴。

《蒙古学百科全书·医学》：患者过饱或饥饿时禁灸此穴。

小肠下穴 ᠶᠡᡐᡝ ᠭᠡᠳᠡᠰᠤ

【出处】《四部医典·论述本》。

【别名】珠玛德桑。

【穴位释义】主治小肠病，在小肠上穴之下。

【定位】在腹部，脐窝正中下 2 寸有 1 穴，其左右两侧 1 寸处各有 1 穴，三穴并列（图 3-12）。中间穴与中医针灸之"石门"穴是同一处。

【局部解剖】皮肤，皮下组织，腹白线，腹横筋膜，腹膜外脂肪，壁腹膜。浅层主要有第十胸神经前支的前皮支和腹壁浅静脉的属支；深层主要有第十一胸神经前支的分支。

【主治】小肠寒性赫依病和泄泻等。

【操作】选用Ⅱ号或Ⅲ号蒙医银针，直刺 0.5～1 寸，温针给予针柄加热，温度 38～40℃，10～15min。

火针或单针刺不加热，留针 15～20min。

可单灸,直接灸1～3炷或间接灸5～15min。

小儿慎刺。

【文献摘要】《蒙古学百科全书·医学》:患者过饱或饥饿时禁灸此穴。

【常用配穴】配小肠上穴,治小肠寒性疾病。

膀胱前穴

【出处】《蒙医疗术》(《五疗》)。

【别名】膀胱穴Ⅱ。

【穴位释义】穴在腹部,主治膀胱病。

【定位】在腹部,脐窝正中下3寸有1穴,其左右两侧1寸处各有1穴,三穴并列(图3-12)。中间穴与中医针灸之"关元"穴是同一处。

【局部解剖】皮肤,皮下组织,腹白线,腹横筋膜,腹膜外脂肪,壁腹膜。浅层主要有第十二胸神经前支的前皮支和腹壁浅动、静脉的分支或属支;深层主要有第十二胸神经前支的分支。

【主治】寒性赫依引起的小便不利或尿频等。

【操作】选用Ⅱ号或Ⅲ号蒙医银针,直刺0.5～1寸,温针给予针柄加热,温度38～40℃,10～15min。

火针或单针刺不加热,留针15～20min。

可单灸,直接灸1～3炷或间接灸5～15min。

小儿慎刺。

【文献摘要】《蒙古学百科全书·医学》:患者月经期、怀孕期禁灸此穴。

【常用配穴】配膀胱穴,治寒性尿频和小便不利。

开导穴

【出处】《四部医典·秘诀本》。

【穴位释义】开导,指开通道路。

【定位】在腹部,距离前正中线五横指处,与髂前上棘平行,左右各有1穴,二穴对称(图3-12)。

【局部解剖】皮肤,皮下组织,腹直肌鞘前壁,腹直肌,腹直肌鞘后壁。浅层分布有肋间神经前皮支,腹壁前动、静脉;深层分布有肋间神经,肋间动脉,腹壁上下动、静脉分支或属支。

【主治】睾丸肿胀,寒性尿频、尿闭等。

【操作】选用Ⅱ号或Ⅲ号蒙医银针,直刺0.5～1寸,温针给予针柄加热,温度 38～40℃，10～15min。

火针或单针刺不加热，留针 15～20min。

可单灸，直接灸 1～3 炷或间接灸 5～15min。

小儿慎刺。

【文献摘要】《蒙古学百科全书·医学》：注意针刺时切不可进针过深。

心源穴

【出处】《蒙医疗术》（《五疗》）。

【定位】在胸部，两侧乳头向上各 1 寸（横平第三肋间，前正中线旁开 4 寸）处各有 1 穴，二穴对称（图 3-11）。本穴与中医针灸之"膺窗"穴是同一处。

【局部解剖】皮肤，皮下组织，胸大肌，胸小肌，肋间外肌，肋间内肌。浅层分布有锁骨上神经中间支，肋间神经前皮支；深层分布有胸前神经，胸肩峰动、静脉分支与属支，肋间神经，肋间动脉；再深层分布有壁层胸膜与肺。

【主治】赫依性心病等。

【操作】选用Ⅱ号或Ⅲ号蒙医银针，直刺 0.5～0.8 寸，温针给予针柄加热，温度 38～40℃，10～15min。

火针或单针刺不加热，留针 15～20min。

可单灸，直接灸 1～3 炷或间接灸 5～10min。

小儿慎刺。

锁骨下穴

【出处】《蒙医疗术》（《五疗》）。

【别名】锁下窝穴。

【穴位释义】穴在锁骨下。

【定位】在胸部，两侧锁骨下缘凹陷正中（约前正中线旁开 4 寸）各有 1 穴，二穴对称（图 3-11）。本穴与中医针灸之"气户穴"穴是同一处。

【局部解剖】皮肤，皮下组织，胸大肌，第一肋间外肌。浅层分布有锁骨上神经中间支；深层分布有胸前神经，腋动脉及其分支，胸肩峰动脉。

【主治】胸闷、手臂酸麻等。

【操作】选用Ⅱ号或Ⅲ号蒙医银针，沿肋间隙向外斜刺 0.5～0.8 寸，温针给予针柄加热，温度 38～40℃，10～15min。

火针或单针刺不加热，留针 15～20min。

可单灸，直接灸 1～3 炷或间接灸 5～10min。

小儿慎刺。

癫狂穴

【出处】《蒙医疗术》（《五疗》）。

【别名】乳外穴。

【穴位释义】主治癫狂之穴。

【定位】在胸部，两侧乳头向外 1 寸（横平第四肋间隙，前正中线旁开 5 寸）处各有 1 穴，二穴对称（图 3-11）。本穴与中医针灸之"天池"穴是同一处。

【局部解剖】皮肤，皮下组织，胸大肌，胸小肌，肋间外肌，肋间内肌。浅层分布有第四肋间神经外侧皮支，胸腹壁静脉，女性皮下组织还有乳房等组织；深层分布有胸前神经肌支，第四肋间神经及胸外侧动、静脉分支和属支。

【主治】赫依性失语、气短、赫依或黄水浸入命脉所引起的各种病。

【操作】选用Ⅱ号或Ⅲ号蒙医银针，直刺 0.5～0.8 寸，温针给予针柄加热，温度 38～40℃，10～15min。

火针或单针刺不加热，留针 15～20min。

可不针刺单灸，直接灸 1～3 炷或间接灸 5～10min。

小儿慎刺。

乌鸦眼穴

【出处】《蒙医临床学》。

【定位】在胸部，胸骨上窝中央直下 2.5 寸，再向左右 1.1 寸处各有 1 穴，二穴对称（图 3-11）。

【局部解剖】皮肤，皮下组织，胸大肌。浅层分布有第二肋间神经的前皮支，胸廓内动、静脉的穿支；深层分布有胸内、外神经的分支。

【主治】心脏赫依引起的癫狂病等。

【操作】选用Ⅱ号或Ⅲ号蒙医银针，沿肋间隙向外斜刺 0.5～0.8 寸，温针给予针柄加热，温度 38～40℃，10～15min。

火针或单针刺不加热，留针 15～20min。

可单灸，直接灸 1～3 炷或间接灸 5～10min。

小儿慎刺。

心尖穴

【出处】《蒙医疗术》（《五疗》）。

【定位】在胸部，两侧乳头向下 1 寸（横平第五肋间隙，前正中线旁开 4 寸）处各有 1 穴，二穴对称（图 3-11）。本穴与中医针灸之"乳根"穴是同一处。

【局部解剖】皮肤，皮下组织，胸大肌，肋间外肌，肋间内肌。浅层分布有肋间神经皮支，胸腹壁静脉；深层分布有胸前神经，肋间神经，肋间后动、静脉，胸外侧动、静脉分支与属支。

【主治】胸痛、咳嗽等。

【操作】选用Ⅱ号或Ⅲ号蒙医银针，沿肋间隙向外斜刺 0.5～0.8 寸，温针给予针柄加热，温度 38～40℃，10～15min。

火针或单针刺不加热，留针 15～20min。

可单灸，直接灸 1～3 炷或间接灸 5～10min。

小儿慎刺。

【文献摘要】《蒙医疗术》《五疗》：心尖穴是排出瘀积于心包之黄水的穴位。

心旁穴 ᠵᠢᠷᠦᠬᠡᠨ

【出处】《蒙医疗术》《五疗》。

【定位】在胸部，两侧乳头向内 1 寸（横平第四肋间隙，前正中线旁开 3 寸）处各有 1 穴，二穴对称（图 3-11）。

【局部解剖】皮肤，皮下组织，胸大肌。浅层分布有第四肋间神经皮支，胸廓内动、静脉的穿支；深层分布有胸内、外侧神经的分支。

【主治】胸痛、黄水积于心脏、赫依气瘀积于心等。

【操作】选用Ⅱ号或Ⅲ号蒙医银针，斜刺或平刺 0.5～0.8 寸，温针给予针柄加热，温度 38～40℃，10～15min。

火针或单针刺不加热，留针 15～20min。

可单灸，直接灸 1～3 炷或间接灸 5～10min。

小儿慎刺。

心肺会穴 ᠵᠢᠷᠦᠬᠡᠨ

【出处】《蒙医疗术》《五疗》。

【别名】心肺穴。

【定位】在胸部，两侧乳头向内 2 寸（横平第四肋间隙，前正中线旁开 2 寸）处各有 1 穴，二穴对称（图 3-11）。本穴与中医针灸之"神封"穴是同一处。

【局部解剖】皮肤，皮下组织，胸大肌。浅层分布有第四肋间神经皮支，胸廓内动、静脉的穿支；深层分布有胸内、外侧神经的分支。

【主治】胸痛，咳嗽，心肺巴达干性、寒性病和赫依病等。

【操作】选用Ⅱ号或Ⅲ号蒙医银针，斜刺或平刺 0.5～0.8 寸，温针给予针柄加热，温度 38～40℃，10～15min。

火针或单针刺不加热，留针 15～20min。

可单灸，直接灸 1～3 炷或间接灸 5～10min。

小儿慎刺。

大分位穴

【出处】《蒙医疗术》（《五疗》）。

【定位】在胸部，胸骨上窝正中（心主脉穴）直下 2.5 寸，再向两侧各 2 寸（横平第二肋间隙，前正中线旁开 2 寸）处有 1 穴，二穴对称（图 3-11）。本穴与中医针灸之"神藏"穴是同一处。

【局部解剖】皮肤，皮下组织，胸大肌。浅层分布有第二肋间神经的前皮支，胸廓内动、静脉的穿支；深层分布有胸内、外侧神经的分支。

【主治】胸部郁气、心绞痛、胸部胀满、呼吸短促等。

【操作】选用Ⅱ号或Ⅲ号蒙医银针，斜刺或平刺 0.5～0.8 寸，温针给予针柄加热，温度 38～40℃，10～15min。

火针或单针刺不加热，留针 15～20min。

可单灸，直接灸 1～3 炷或间接灸 5～10min。

小儿慎刺。

小分位穴

【出处】《蒙医疗术》（《五疗》）。

【定位】在胸部，胸骨上窝正中（心主脉穴）直下 3.5 寸，再向两侧 2 寸（横平第三肋间隙，前正中线旁开 2 寸）处各有 1 穴，二穴对称（图 3-11）。本穴与中医针灸之"灵墟"穴是同一处。

【局部解剖】皮肤，皮下组织，胸大肌。浅层分布有第三肋间神经的前皮支，胸廓内动、静脉的穿支；深层分布有胸内、外侧神经的分支。

【主治】胸部郁气、心绞痛、胸部胀满、呼吸短促等。

【操作】选用Ⅱ号或Ⅲ号蒙医银针，斜刺或平刺 0.5～0.8 寸，温针给予针柄加热，温度 38～40℃，10～15min。

火针或单针刺不加热，留针 15～20min。

可单灸，直接灸 1～3 炷或间接灸 5～10min。

小儿慎刺。

肺旁穴

【出处】《蒙医疗术》《五疗》。

【定位】在胸部,两腋窝横纹前端直下 1 寸为上穴,再直下 1 寸为中穴,更直下 1 寸为下穴。两侧对称,共 6 穴(图 3-13)。

【局部解剖】皮肤,皮下组织,前锯肌,肋间外肌。浅层分布有第五、六、七肋间神经外侧皮支和胸腹壁静脉;深层分布有胸长神经的分支,第五、六、七肋间神经和第五、六、七肋间动、静脉。

【主治】胸肋胀痛、肺旁痞证等。

【操作】选用Ⅱ号或Ⅲ号蒙医银针,斜刺 0.5～0.8 寸,温针给予针柄加热,温度 38～40℃,10～15min。

火针或单针刺不加热,留针 15～20min。

可单灸,直接灸 1～3 炷或间接灸 5～10min。

小儿慎刺。

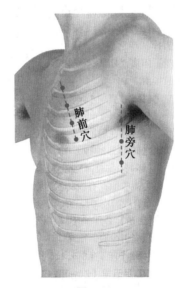

图 3-13

肺前穴

【出处】《蒙医疗术》《五疗》。

【定位】在胸部,两侧乳头向外一横指,再向上一横指处(肋间)为第一穴;

第一穴向内 1 寸,再向上 1 寸处(肋间)为第二穴;第二穴向内一横指半,向上 1 寸处(肋间)为第三穴;第三穴向内一横指半,向上 1 寸处(肋间)为第四穴。两侧对称,共 8 穴(图 3-13)。

【局部解剖】皮肤,皮下组织,胸大肌。浅层分布有第三、四肋间神经外侧皮支;深层分布有胸内、外侧神经分支,胸外侧动、静脉的分支或属支。

【主治】胸肋胀痛、子肺痞证等。

【操作】选用Ⅱ号或Ⅲ号蒙医银针,斜刺 0.5～0.8 寸,温针给予针柄加热,温度 38～40℃,10～15min。

火针或单针刺不加热,留针 15～20min。

可单灸,直接灸 1～3 炷或间接灸 5～10min。

小儿慎刺。

肝上穴

【出处】《蒙医疗术》(《五疗》)。

【定位】在胸部,位于右侧乳头向下 3 寸(横平第七肋间隙,前正中线旁开 4 寸)处。女性在右锁骨中线与第七肋间隙交点处(图 3-12)。

【局部解剖】皮肤,皮下组织,腹外斜肌,肋间胸外肌,肋间内肌。浅层分布有第七肋间神经前皮支;深层分布有第七肋间神经和动脉。

【主治】胃炎、胆囊炎、胃肝痞证等。

【操作】选用Ⅱ号或Ⅲ号蒙医银针,斜刺或平刺 0.5～0.8 寸,不可深刺,以免伤及内部脏器。温针给予针柄加热,温度 38～40℃,10～15min。

火针或单针刺不加热,留针 15～20min。

可单灸,直接灸 1～3 炷或间接灸 5～10min。

小儿慎刺。

肝中穴

【出处】《蒙医疗术》(《五疗》)。

【定位】在胸部,位于右侧乳头向下 4 寸(横平第八肋间隙,前正中线旁开 4 寸)处。女性在右锁骨中线与第八肋间隙交点处(图 3-12)。

【局部解剖】皮肤,皮下组织,腹外斜肌,肋间胸外肌,肋间内肌。浅层分布有第八肋间神经前皮支;深层分布有第八肋间神经和动脉。

【主治】胃炎、胆囊炎、肝中部痞证等。

【操作】选用Ⅱ号或Ⅲ号蒙医银针,斜刺或平刺 0.5～0.8 寸,不可深刺,以免伤及内部脏器。温针给予针柄加热，温度 38～40℃，10～15min。

火针或单针刺不加热，留针 15～20min。

可单灸，直接灸 1～3 炷或间接灸 5～10min。

小儿慎刺。

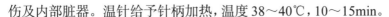

肝下穴

【出处】《蒙医疗术》《五疗》。

【定位】在胸部，位于右侧乳头向下 5 寸（横平第九肋间隙，前正中线旁开 4 寸）处。女性在右锁骨中线与第九肋间隙交点处（图 3-12）。

【局部解剖】皮肤，皮下组织，腹外斜肌，肋间胸外肌，肋间内肌。浅层分布有第九肋间神经前皮支；深层分布有第九肋间神经和动脉。

【主治】胃炎、胆囊炎、肝下部痞证等。

【操作】选用Ⅱ号或Ⅲ号蒙医银针，斜刺或平刺 0.5～0.8 寸，不可深刺，以免伤及内部脏器。温针给予针柄加热，温度 38～40℃，10～15min。

火针或单针刺不加热，留针 15～20min。

可单灸，直接灸 1～3 炷或间接灸 5～10min。

小儿慎刺。

脾上穴

【出处】《蒙医疗术》《五疗》。

【定位】在胸部，位于左侧乳头向下 3 寸（横平第七肋间隙，前正中线旁开 4 寸）处。女性在左锁骨中线与第七肋间隙交点处（图 3-12）。

【局部解剖】皮肤，皮下组织，腹外斜肌，肋间胸外肌，肋间内肌。浅层分布有第七肋间神经前皮支；深层分布有第七肋间神经和动脉。

【主治】胃炎、脾胃间痞证等。

【操作】选用Ⅱ号或Ⅲ号蒙医银针，斜刺或平刺 0.5～0.8 寸，不可深刺，以免伤及内部脏器。温针给予针柄加热，温度 38～40℃，10～15min。

火针或单针刺不加热，留针 15～20min。

可单灸，直接灸 1～3 炷或间接灸 5～10min。

小儿慎刺。

脾中穴

【出处】《蒙医疗术》《五疗》。

【定位】在胸部,位于左侧乳头向下 4 寸(横平第八肋间隙,前正中线旁开 4 寸)处。女性在左锁骨中线与第八肋间隙交点处(图 3-12)。

【局部解剖】皮肤,皮下组织,腹外斜肌,肋间胸外肌,肋间内肌。浅层分布有第八肋间神经前皮支;深层分布有第八肋间神经和动脉。

【主治】胃炎、脾中部痞证等。

【操作】选用Ⅱ号或Ⅲ号蒙医银针,斜刺或平刺 0.5～0.8 寸,不可深刺,以免伤及内部脏器。温针给予针柄加热,温度 38～40℃,10～15min。

火针或单针刺不加热,留针 15～20min。

可单灸,直接灸 1～3 炷或间接灸 5～10min。

小儿慎刺。

脾下穴

【出处】《蒙医疗术》(《五疗》)。

【定位】在胸部,位于左侧乳头向下 5 寸(横平第九肋间隙,前正中线旁开 4 寸)处。女性在左锁骨中线与第九肋间隙交点处(图 3-12)。

【局部解剖】皮肤,皮下组织,腹外斜肌,肋间胸外肌,肋间内肌。浅层分布有第九肋间神经前皮支;深层分布有第九肋间神经和动脉。

【主治】胃炎、脾下部痞证等。

【操作】选用Ⅱ号或Ⅲ号蒙医银针,斜刺或平刺 0.5～0.8 寸,不可深刺,以免伤及内部脏器。温针给予针柄加热,温度 38～40℃,10～15min。

火针或单针刺不加热,留针 15～20min。

可单灸,直接灸 1～3 炷或间接灸 5～10min。

小儿慎刺。

(三)背部穴位(83穴)

肩上穴

【出处】《蒙医疗术》(《五疗》)。

【穴位释义】穴在肩上部。

【定位】在三角肌区,位于第七颈椎棘突与肩峰连线中点,肩部最高处,两侧对称(图 3-14)。

【局部解剖】皮肤,皮下组织,斜方肌,肩胛提肌,冈下肌。浅层分布有颈横动、静脉分支;深层分布有腋神经和桡神经。

【主治】胁痛、咳嗽等症。

【操作】选用Ⅲ号或Ⅳ号蒙医银针，直刺0.5～0.8寸，温针给予针柄加热，温度38～42℃，10～15min。

火针或单针刺不加热，留针15～20min。

可单灸，直接灸1～5炷或间接灸5～20min。

小儿慎刺。

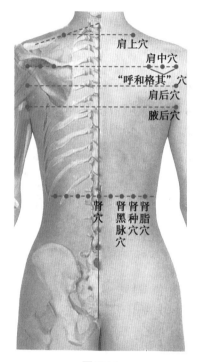

图 3-14

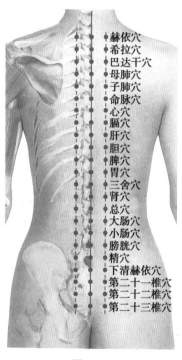

图 3-15

肩中穴

【出处】《蒙医传统疗法大成》。

【穴位释义】穴在肩胛正中。

【定位】在肩胛部，位于两肩胛骨正中（冈下窝中央凹陷处，与第四胸椎相平），左右各有1穴，两穴对称（图3-14）。与中医针灸之"天宗"穴是同一处。

【局部解剖】皮肤，皮下组织，冈下肌。浅层有第四、第五胸神经后支的皮支重叠分布和伴行的动、静脉；深层分布有肩胛上神经的分支，肩胛动脉网。

【主治】白脉病、肩关节疼痛、半身麻木等。

【操作】选用Ⅰ号或Ⅱ号蒙医银针,直刺或斜刺 0.5～1 寸,温针给予针柄加热,温度 38～42℃,15～20min。

火针或单针刺不加热,留针 15～20min。

可单灸,直接灸 1～5 炷或间接灸 5～20min。

小儿慎刺。

"呼和格其"穴 ᠬᠥᠬᠡᠭᠡᠴᠢ

【出处】《蒙医疗术》(《五疗》)。

【别名】青穴。

【定位】在肩部,于肩中穴左右两侧各 1 寸处分别有 1 穴,两肩共 4 穴(图 3-14)。

【局部解剖】皮肤、皮下组织、冈下肌。浅层有第四、第五胸神经后支的皮支重叠分布和伴行的动、静脉;深层分布有肩胛上神经的分支,肩胛动脉网。

【主治】肋间痛、嗳气频作、呃逆、胸骨疼痛、胸胀、肺部诸症等。

【操作】选用Ⅰ号或Ⅱ号蒙医银针,斜刺 0.5～1 寸,温针给予针柄加热,温度 38～42℃,15～20min。

火针或单针刺不加热,留针 15～20min。

可单灸,直接灸 1～5 炷或间接灸 5～20min。

小儿慎刺。

赫依穴 ᠬᠡᠢ

【出处】《四部医典·秘诀本》。

【别名】第一椎穴、隆桑、安洞当布。

【穴位释义】主治赫依病的穴位。

【定位】位于后正中线上,第七颈椎棘突下凹陷中及左右 1 寸处各有 1 穴,三穴并列(图 3-15)。中间穴与中医针灸之"大椎"穴是同一处。

【局部解剖】中间穴位:皮肤,皮下组织,棘上韧带,棘间韧带。浅层主要有第七颈神经后支的内侧支和棘突间皮下静脉丛;深层有棘突间的椎外(后)静脉丛和第七颈神经后支的分支。两侧穴位:皮肤,皮下组织,斜方肌,菱形肌,头夹肌。浅层有第七颈神经后支的皮支及伴行的动、静脉;深层有副神经,肩胛背神经的分支,颈动、静脉分支。

【主治】癫狂、心悸、激荡、哑结、夜不安寐、舌苔灰白、颈项强直等赫依性疾病。

【操作】选用Ⅰ号或Ⅱ号蒙医银针,中间穴位直刺 0.5 寸,两侧穴位斜刺

0.5～1寸,温针给予针柄加热,温度38～42℃,15～20min。

火针或单针刺不加热,留针15～20min。

可单灸,直接灸1～5炷或间接灸5～20min。

小儿慎刺。

【文献摘要】《蒙古学百科全书·医学》:如三穴并灸,则对老年患者最有效。而且对渗于骨骼的陈旧热、呼吸急促、大汗淋漓、腰背僵硬疼痛、心烦不宁、食欲不振以及对平息赫依病,疗效显著。

希拉穴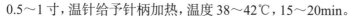

【出处】《四部医典·秘诀本》。

【别名】第二椎穴、热依桑。

【穴位释义】主治希拉病的穴位。

【定位】在脊柱区,位于后正中线上,第一胸椎棘突下凹陷中及左右1寸处各有1穴,三穴并列(图3-15)。中间穴与中医针灸之"陶道"穴是同一处。

【局部解剖】中间穴:皮肤,皮下组织,棘上韧带,棘间韧带。浅层主要有第一胸神经后支的内侧支和伴行的动、静脉;深层有棘突间的椎外(后)静脉丛,第一胸神经后支的分支和第一肋间后动、静脉背侧支的分支或属支。两侧穴位:皮肤,皮下组织,斜方肌,菱形肌,上后锯肌,竖脊肌。浅层有第一、二胸神经后支的内侧皮支及伴行的第一肋间动、静脉后支;深层有副神经,肩胛背神经及肩胛背动、静脉分支。

【主治】寒希拉诸病,心慌、胸闷等。

【操作】选用Ⅰ号或Ⅱ号蒙医银针,中间穴位直刺0.5寸,两侧穴位斜刺0.5～1寸,温针给予针柄加热,温度38～42℃,15～20min。

火针或单针刺不加热,留针15～20min。

可单灸,直接灸1～5炷或间接灸5～20min。

小儿慎刺。

【文献摘要】《蒙古学百科全书·医学》:如三穴并灸,可治热邪渗于内、瘿疾、上身沉重及寒性希拉诸症等。肝胆热和热邪隐伏于脏腑时,禁灸此穴。

巴达干穴

【出处】《四部医典·秘诀本》。

【别名】第三椎穴、巴达干桑。

【穴位释义】主治巴达干病的穴位。

【定位】在脊柱区,位于后正中线上,第二胸椎棘突下凹陷中及左右 1 寸处各有 1 穴,三穴并列(图 3-15)。

【局部解剖】中间穴:皮肤,皮下组织,棘上韧带,棘间韧带。浅层主要有第二胸神经后支的内侧支和伴行的动、静脉;深层有棘突间的椎外(后)静脉丛,第二胸神经后支的分支和第二肋间后动、静脉背侧支的分支或属支。两侧穴位:皮肤,皮下组织,斜方肌,菱形肌,上后锯肌,竖脊肌。浅层有第二、三胸神经后支的内侧皮支及伴行的肋间动、静脉背侧的内侧支;深层有副神经,肩胛背神经,第二、三胸神经后支及肩胛背动、静脉分支。

【主治】赫依寒症及巴达干、希拉亢盛扩散于肺、心、头及胸部等。

【操作】选用 Ⅰ 号或 Ⅱ 号蒙医银针,中间穴位直刺 0.5 寸,两侧穴位斜刺 0.5～1 寸,温针给予针柄加热,温度 38～42℃,15～20min。

火针或单针刺不加热,留针 15～20min。

可单灸,直接灸 1～5 炷或间接灸 5～20min。

小儿慎刺。

【文献摘要】《蒙古学百科全书·医学》:如三穴并灸,对巴达干增盛、鼻塞不通、赫依热导致的口舌干燥有疗效。

【现代研究】蒙医温针刺激巴达干穴等结合芒针治疗腰椎间盘脱出症的研究:蒙医温针刺激脊柱三穴、水痞穴、闭孔穴、髋臼穴、配穴、巴达干穴、脊柱肾穴、股外侧穴、腘窝穴、肌腹穴等穴位,结合芒针治疗腰椎间盘脱出症,总有效率为 96%。[12]

母肺穴

【出处】《四部医典·秘诀本》。

【别名】第四椎穴、鲁玛桑。

【穴位释义】主治母肺病的穴位。

【定位】在脊柱区,位于后正中线上,第三胸椎棘突下凹陷中及左右 1 寸处各有 1 穴,三穴并列(图 3-15)。中间穴与中医针灸之"身柱"穴是同一处。

【局部解剖】中间穴:皮肤,皮下组织,棘上韧带,棘间韧带。浅层主要有第三胸神经后支的内侧支和伴行的动、静脉;深层有棘突间的椎外(后)静脉丛,第三胸神经后支的分支和第三肋间后动、静脉背侧支的分支或属支。两侧穴位:皮肤,皮下组织,斜方肌,菱形肌,上后锯肌,竖脊肌。浅层有第三、四胸神经后支的内侧皮支及伴行的肋间动、静脉背侧的内侧支;深层有副神经,肩胛背神经,第三、四胸神经后支及肩胛背动、静脉分支。

【主治】目中流泪及肺赫依病、巴达干病等。

【操作】选用Ⅰ号或Ⅱ号蒙医银针,中间穴位直刺 0.5 寸,两侧穴位斜刺 0.5～1 寸,温针给予针柄加热,温度 38～42℃,15～20min。

火针或单针刺不加热,留针 15～20min。

可单灸,直接灸 1～5 炷或间接灸 5～20min。

小儿慎刺。

【文献摘要】《蒙古学百科全书·医学》:如三穴并灸,则治味觉不灵、肺病、胸刺痛、肺陈热等病有效。

【常用配穴】①配赫依穴,治赫依偏盛病。②配子肺穴、治肺痼疾咳嗽。

子肺穴

【出处】《四部医典·秘诀本》。

【别名】第五椎穴、罗布桑。

【穴位释义】主治子肺病的穴位。

【定位】在脊柱区,位于后正中线上,第四胸椎棘突下凹陷中及左右 1 寸处各有 1 穴,三穴并列(图 3-15)。

【局部解剖】中间穴:皮肤,皮下组织,棘上韧带,棘间韧带。浅层主要有第四胸神经后支的内侧支和伴行的动、静脉;深层有棘突间的椎外(后)静脉丛,第四胸神经后支的分支和第四肋间后动、静脉背侧支的分支或属支。两侧穴位:皮肤,皮下组织,斜方肌,菱形肌,上后锯肌,竖脊肌。浅层有第四、五胸神经后支的内侧皮支及伴行的动、静脉背侧的内侧支;深层有副神经,肩胛背神经,第四、五胸神经后支及肩胛背动、静脉分支。

【主治】流泪等眼疾、子肺病、赫依病及巴达干病。

【操作】选用Ⅰ号或Ⅱ号蒙医银针,中间穴位直刺 0.5 寸,两侧穴位斜刺 0.5～1 寸,温针给予针柄加热,温度 38～42℃,15～20min。

火针或单针刺不加热,留针 15～20min。

可单灸,直接灸 1～5 炷或间接灸 5～20min。

小儿慎刺。

【文献摘要】《蒙古学百科全书·医学》:如三穴并灸,对肺赫依病引起的频咳、出血、瘟疫后期神志昏迷或癫狂、胸背刺痛、四肢颤抖、恶心呕吐等症,亦有较好的治疗效果。

【常用配穴】①配赫依穴,治赫依偏盛病。②配母肺穴,治肺痼疾咳嗽。

命脉穴 ᠵᠢᠷᠦᠬᠡ

【出处】《四部医典·秘诀本》。

【别名】第六椎穴、苏如格扎桑。

【穴位释义】主治命脉病的穴位。

【定位】在脊柱区,位于后正中线上,第五胸椎棘突下凹陷中及左右1寸处各有1穴,三穴并列(图3-15)。中间穴与中医针灸之"神道"穴是同一处。

【局部解剖】中间穴:皮肤,皮下组织,棘上韧带,棘间韧带。浅层主要有第五胸神经后支的内侧支和伴行的动、静脉;深层有棘突间的椎外(后)静脉丛,第五胸神经后支的分支和第五肋间后动、静脉背侧支的分支或属支。两侧穴位:皮肤,皮下组织,斜方肌,菱形肌下缘,竖脊肌。浅层有第五、六胸神经后支的内侧皮支及伴行的动、静脉背侧的内侧支;深层有副神经,第五、六胸神经后支。

【主治】身重、健忘、全身皮疹、心脏黄水症、头重疼痛等。

【操作】选用Ⅰ号或Ⅱ号蒙医银针,中间穴位直刺0.5寸,两侧穴位斜刺0.5～1寸,温针给予针柄加热,温度38～42℃,15～20min。

火针或单针刺不加热,留针15～20min。

可单灸,直接灸1～5炷或间接灸5～20min。

小儿慎刺。

【文献摘要】《珍集》云:心悸病、心赫依刺痛病灸命脉穴、心穴、心母穴、心旁穴。

《蒙古学百科全书·医学》:本穴为心、命脉病的常用穴位,并且对心血管疾病、脑神经疾病有良好的疗效,但脏器热或心热隐伏者,于本穴禁灸和热性针刺。

【常用配穴】①配心穴,治心脏巴达干寒性病和赫依性病。②配赫依穴、黑白际穴,治癫狂症或昏厥症。

心穴 ᠵᠢᠷᠦᠬᠡ

【出处】《四部医典·秘诀本》。

【别名】第七椎穴、宁桑。

【穴位释义】主治心脏病的穴位。

【定位】在脊柱区,位于后正中线上,第六胸椎棘突下凹陷中及左右1寸处各有1穴,三穴并列(图3-15)。中间穴与中医针灸之"灵台"穴是同一处。

【局部解剖】中间穴:皮肤,皮下组织,棘上韧带,棘间韧带。浅层主要有第六胸神经后支的内侧支和伴行的动、静脉；深层有棘突间的椎外（后）静脉丛，第六胸神经后支的分支和第六肋间后动、静脉背侧支的分支或属支。两侧穴位：皮肤，皮下组织，斜方肌，背阔肌，竖脊肌。浅层有第六、七胸神经后支的内侧皮支及伴行的动、静脉背侧的内侧支；深层有副神经，第六、七胸神经后支。

【主治】心悸、心慌、癫狂、昏厥、巴达干、赫依性病（赫依性心病）、失眠、谵妄、纳呆及味觉不灵、心烦神异、黄水或赫依窜于主脉、胸胁胀闷等。

【操作】选用Ⅰ号或Ⅱ号蒙医银针，中间穴位直刺0.5寸，两侧穴位斜刺0.5～1寸，温针给予针柄加热，温度38～42℃，15～20min。

火针或单针刺不加热，留针15～20min。

可不针刺单灸，直接灸1～5炷或间接灸5～20min。

小儿慎刺。

【文献摘要】《四部医典•秘诀本》云：心悸和心黄水病可灸或针刺心穴。

《蒙古学百科全书•医学》：治疗心、脑、神经疾病时也常灸此穴。

【常用配穴】①配赫依穴，治赫依性心刺痛。②配命脉穴、黑白际穴，治心赫依引起的晕厥。③配顶会穴、赫依穴，治赫依性癫狂症。

膈穴

【出处】《四部医典•秘诀本》。

【别名】第八椎穴、沁日依桑。

【穴位释义】主治膈肌的穴位。

【定位】在脊柱区，位于后正中线上，第七胸椎棘突下凹陷中及左右1寸处各有1穴，三穴并列（图3-15）。中间穴与中医针灸之"至阳"穴是同一处。

【局部解剖】中间穴：皮肤，皮下组织，棘上韧带，棘间韧带。浅层主要有第七胸神经后支的内侧支和伴行的动、静脉；深层有棘突间的椎外（后）静脉丛，第七胸神经后支的分支和第七肋间后动、静脉背侧支的分支或属支。两侧穴位：皮肤，皮下组织，斜方肌，背阔肌，竖脊肌。浅层有第七、八胸神经后支的内侧皮支及伴行的动、静脉背侧的内侧支；深层有副神经，第七、八胸神经后支。

【主治】胸胁刺痛、胸闷厌烦等。

【操作】选用Ⅰ号或Ⅱ号蒙医银针，中间穴位直刺0.5寸，两侧穴位斜刺0.5～1寸，温针给予针柄加热，温度38～42℃，15～20min。

火针或单针刺不加热，留针15～20min。

可不针刺单灸，直接灸1～5炷或间接灸5～20min。

小儿慎刺。

【文献摘要】《四部医典·论述本》云：由肝病引起的膈肌病可先放肝脉血，再灸膈穴。

《蒙古学百科全书·医学》：三穴并灸，对胁部刺痛、巴达干侵于肝膈和膈、膈部酸痛有疗效。

肝穴

【出处】《四部医典·秘诀本》。

【别名】第九椎穴、亲桑。

【穴位释义】主治肝脏病的穴位。

【定位】在脊柱区，位于后正中线上，第八胸椎棘突下凹陷中及左右 1 寸处各有 1 穴，三穴并列（图 3-15）。

【局部解剖】中间穴：皮肤，皮下组织，棘上韧带，棘间韧带。浅层主要有第八胸神经后支的内侧支和伴行的动、静脉；深层有棘突间的椎外（后）静脉丛，第八胸神经后支的分支和第八肋间后动、静脉背侧支的分支或属支。两侧穴位：皮肤，皮下组织，斜方肌，背阔肌，竖脊肌。浅层有第八、九胸神经后支的内侧皮支及伴行的动、静脉背侧的内侧支；深层有副神经，第八、九胸神经后支。

【主治】嗳气、呕吐、膈部酸痛、肝痞、肝巴达干或赫依病、肝血外溢、肝萎缩等。

【操作】选用Ⅰ号或Ⅱ号蒙医银针，中间穴位直刺 0.5 寸，两侧穴位斜刺 0.5～1 寸，温针给予针柄加热，温度 38～42℃，15～20min。

火针或单针刺不加热，留针 15～20min。

可不针刺单灸，直接灸 1～5 炷或间接灸 5～20min。

小儿慎刺。

【文献摘要】《蒙古学百科全书·医学》：如三穴并灸，对肝病引起的吐酸水、赫依性刺痛、肝肿胀或胀痛、淋浊带血等病有疗效。

胆穴

【出处】《四部医典·秘诀本》。

【别名】第十椎穴、如比桑。

【穴位释义】主治胆囊病的穴位。

【定位】在脊柱区，位于后正中线上，第九胸椎棘突下凹陷中及左右 1 寸处各有 1 穴，三穴并列（图 3-15）。中间穴与中医针灸之"筋缩"穴是同一处。

【局部解剖】皮肤，皮下组织，棘上韧带，棘间韧带。浅层主要有第九胸神经后支的内侧支和伴行的动、静脉；深层有棘突间的椎外（后）静脉丛，第九胸神经后支的分支和第九肋间后动、静脉背侧支的分支或属支。两侧穴位：皮肤，皮下组织，斜方肌，背阔肌，竖脊肌。浅层有第九、十胸神经后支的内侧皮支及伴行的肋间动、静脉背侧的内侧支；深层有副神经，第九、十胸神经后支。

【主治】不消化病、目黄、胆痞病、呕吐胆汁、胃火衰竭、食欲减退、经常性头痛等。

【操作】选用Ⅰ号或Ⅱ号蒙医银针，中间穴位直刺0.5寸，两侧穴位斜刺0.5～1寸，温针给予针柄加热，温度38～42℃，15～20min。

火针或单针刺不加热，留针15～20min。

可不针刺单灸，直接灸1～5炷或间接灸5～20min。

小儿慎刺。

【文献摘要】《蒙古学百科全书·医学》：在一般情况下，不能三穴并灸。只有在胆腑肿胀时方可三穴并灸。

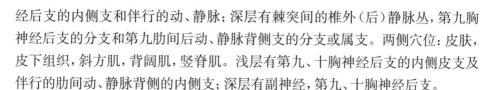

脾穴

【出处】《四部医典·秘诀本》。

【别名】第十一椎穴、撒日桑。

【穴位释义】主治脾脏病的穴位。

【定位】在脊柱区，位于后正中线上，第十胸椎棘突下凹陷中及左右1寸处各有1穴，三穴并列（图3-15）。中间穴与中医针灸之"中枢"穴是同一处。

【局部解剖】中间穴：皮肤，皮下组织，棘上韧带，棘间韧带。浅层主要有第十胸神经后支的内侧支和伴行的动、静脉；深层有棘突间的椎外（后）静脉丛，第十胸神经后支的分支和第十肋间后动、静脉背侧支的分支或属支。两侧穴位：皮肤，皮下组织，背阔肌，竖脊肌。浅层有第十、十一胸神经后支的内侧皮支及伴行的肋间动、静脉背侧的内侧支；深层有副神经，第十、十一胸神经后支。

【主治】脾胃发胀作鸣、身体沉重、多寐嗜睡等。

【操作】选用Ⅰ号或Ⅱ号蒙医银针，中间穴位直刺0.5寸，两侧穴位斜刺0.5～1寸，温针给予针柄加热，温度38～42℃，15～20min。

火针或单针刺不加热，留针15～20min。

可不针刺单灸，直接灸1～5炷或间接灸5～20min。

小儿慎刺。

【文献摘要】《蒙古学百科全书·医学》：如三穴并灸，则治腹胀作鸣、胃病、呕吐、消化不良，颜面发黑枯萎等症。

【常用配穴】配赫依胃穴、大肠穴，治长期腹胀、泡沫黏液样泄泻及大便失禁。

胃穴

【出处】《四部医典·秘诀本》。

【别名】第十二椎穴、普比桑。

【穴位释义】主治胃病的穴位。

【定位】在脊柱区，位于后正中线上，第十一胸椎棘突下凹陷中及左右 1 寸处各有 1 穴，三穴并列（图 3-15）。中间穴与中医针灸之"脊中"穴是同一处。

【局部解剖】中间穴：皮肤，皮下组织，棘上韧带，棘间韧带。浅层主要有第十一胸神经后支的内侧支和伴行的动、静脉；深层有棘突间的椎外（后）静脉丛，第十一胸神经后支的分支和第十一肋间后动、静脉背侧支的分支或属支。两侧穴位：皮肤，皮下组织，背阔肌，竖脊肌。浅层有第十一、十二胸神经后支的内侧皮支及伴行的动、静脉；深层有第十一、十二胸神经后支的肌支，相应的肋间后动、静脉分支。

【主治】胃火衰败、胸口巴达干、腰背强直与僵硬、眼眶疼痛、久泻等。

【操作】选用 I 号或 II 号蒙医银针，中间穴位直刺 0.5 寸，两侧穴位斜刺 0.5～1 寸，温针给予针柄加热，温度 38～42℃，15～20min。

火针或单针刺不加热，留针 15～20min。

可单灸，直接灸 1～5 炷或间接灸 5～20min。

小儿慎刺。

【文献摘要】《蒙古学百科全书·医学》：如三穴并灸，则对胃巴达干寒症、呕吐、陈旧性希拉病有治疗效果。

【常用配穴】①配火衰穴，治胃火衰病、慢性胃炎、胃下垂。②配痞穴、剑突穴，治胃痞。

三舍穴

【出处】《四部医典·秘诀本》。

【别名】第十三椎穴、精府穴、萨木色桑。

【穴位释义】三舍，指男女生殖器官，即贮藏精血，传宗接代之腑，与胃、小肠、大肠、胆囊、膀胱并称为六腑。本穴是主治三舍病的穴位。

【定位】在脊柱区，位于后正中线上，第十二胸椎棘突下凹陷中及左右 1 寸处各有 1 穴，三穴并列（图 3-15）。

【局部解剖】中间穴：皮肤，皮下组织，棘上韧带，棘间韧带。浅层主要有第十二胸神经后支的内侧支和伴行的动、静脉；深层有棘突间的椎外（后）静脉丛，第十二胸神经后支的分支和第十二肋间后动、静脉背侧支的分支或属支。两侧穴位：皮肤，皮下组织，背阔肌，竖脊肌。浅层有第十二胸神经和第一腰神经后支的皮支及伴行的动、静脉；深层有第十二胸神经和第一腰神经后支的肌支，相应的肋间后动、静脉分支。

【主治】遗精、月经过多、子宫肌瘤、心神不安、赫依增盛、腹胀、大便秘结、不能仰或俯卧、脐部左右腹鸣等。

【操作】选用Ⅰ号或Ⅱ号蒙医银针，中间穴位直刺0.5寸，两侧穴位斜刺0.5～1寸，温针给予针柄加热，温度38～42℃，15～20min。

火针或单针刺不加热，留针15～20min。

可单灸，直接灸1～5炷或间接灸5～20min。

小儿慎刺。

【文献摘要】《蒙古学百科全书·医学》：如三穴并灸，可治一切子宫病和男子阳痿等症。

【常用配穴】配肾穴，治肾病、子宫病。

肾穴

【出处】《四部医典·秘诀本》。

【别名】第十四椎穴、卡拉玛桑。

【穴位释义】主治肾病的穴位。

【定位】在脊柱区，位于后正中线上，第一腰椎棘突下凹陷中及左右1寸处各有1穴，三穴并列（图3-15）。中间穴与中医针灸之"悬枢"穴是同一处。

【局部解剖】中间穴：皮肤，皮下组织，棘上韧带，棘间韧带。浅层主要有第一腰神经后支的内侧支和伴行的动、静脉；深层有棘突间的椎外（后）静脉丛，第一腰神经后支的分支和第一腰动、静脉背侧支的分支或属支。两侧穴位：皮肤，皮下组织，背阔肌，竖脊肌。浅层有第一、二腰神经后支的皮支及伴行的动、静脉；深层有第一、二腰神经后支的肌支和肋下动、静脉分支。

【主治】肾寒证、下腹部疼痛、精液发凉和射精剧痛等。

【操作】选用Ⅰ号或Ⅱ号蒙医银针，中间穴位直刺0.5寸，两侧穴位斜刺0.5～1寸，温针给予针柄加热，温度38～42℃，15～20min。

火针或单针刺不加热，留针15～20min。

可单灸，直接灸1～5炷或间接灸5～20min。

小儿慎刺。

【文献摘要】《四部医典·论述本》：肾"达日干"病，灸突出椎上下，椎间施火针治疗。

《四部医典·秘诀本》：第十四椎是肾穴，灸此可治肾病。

《蒙古学百科全书·医学》：如三穴并灸，对肾脂寒凝和腰部疼痛、小便不利、男女外阴肿胀、阳痿、泄泻等症，均有治疗作用。

【现代研究】蒙医温针刺激肾穴、肾黑脉穴、肾精穴、髋穴、大腿穴、腓肠肌穴治疗腰椎间盘突出症：取肾穴、肾黑脉穴、肾精穴、髋穴、大腿穴、腓肠肌穴，使用蒙医温针仪加热，治疗时间30min。日1次，1周5次，10次为1疗程。治疗30例，下肢放射性酸痛消失，行走正常（痊愈）24例；下肢行走困难减轻，比较有力（有效）6例。[13]

总穴

【出处】《四部医典·秘诀本》。

【别名】第十五椎穴、脏腑总穴、"独那都"。

【穴位释义】对脏腑病有综合治疗作用的穴位。

【定位】在脊柱区，位于后正中线上，第二腰椎棘突下凹陷中及左右1寸处各有1穴，三穴并列（图3-15）。中间穴与中医针灸之"命门"穴是同一处。

【局部解剖】中间穴：皮肤，皮下组织，棘上韧带，棘间韧带。浅层主要有第二腰神经后支的内侧支和伴行的动、静脉；深层有棘突间的椎外（后）静脉丛，第二腰神经后支的分支和第二腰动、静脉背侧支的分支或属支。两侧穴位：皮肤，皮下组织，背阔肌筋膜和胸腰筋膜浅层。浅层有第二、三腰神经后支的皮支及伴行的动、静脉；深层有第二、三腰神经后支的肌支和相应的腰动、静脉分支。

【主治】肾寒性赫依症、体黑黄疸病、不孕症、疲倦、脐周疼痛等病。

【操作】选用Ⅰ号或Ⅱ号蒙医银针，中间穴位直刺0.5寸，两侧穴位斜刺0.5～1寸，温针给予针柄加热，温度38～42℃，15～20min。

火针或单针刺不加热，留针15～20min。

可单灸，直接灸1～5炷或间接灸5～20min。

小儿慎刺。

【文献摘要】《蒙古学百科全书·医学》：如肾、精府热时，禁灸本穴。

【常用配穴】①配肾穴，治肾寒或赫依。②配三舍穴，治子宫寒或赫依。

大肠穴

【出处】《四部医典·秘诀本》。

【别名】第十六椎穴、"龙桑"。

【穴位释义】主治大肠病的穴位。

【定位】在脊柱区，位于后正中线上，第三腰椎棘突下凹陷中及左右1寸处各有1穴，三穴并列（图3-15）。

【局部解剖】中间穴：皮肤，皮下组织，棘上韧带，棘间韧带。浅层主要有第三腰神经后支的内侧支和伴行的动、静脉；深层有棘突间的椎外（后）静脉丛，第三腰神经后支的分支和第三腰动、静脉背侧支的分支或属支。两侧穴位：皮肤，皮下组织，胸腰筋膜浅层，竖脊肌。浅层有第三、四腰神经后支的皮支和伴行的动、静脉；深层有第三、四腰神经后支的肌支及相应动、静脉的分支。

【主治】腹胀肠鸣、痞块、矢气频作、阴道灼痛、小便不利、痔疮等。

【操作】选用Ⅰ号或Ⅱ号蒙医银针，中间穴位直刺0.5寸，两侧穴位斜刺0.5～1寸，温针给予针柄加热，温度38～42℃，15～20min。

火针或单针刺不加热，留针15～20min。

可单灸，直接灸1～5炷或间接灸5～20min。

小儿慎刺。

【文献摘要】《蒙古学百科全书·医学》：如三穴并灸，对大便秘结、腹胀、肛门松弛、泄泻、站立时腰痛、消化不良、大肠作鸣等症亦有治疗效果。

小肠穴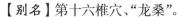

【出处】《四部医典·秘诀本》。

【别名】第十七椎穴、"珠玛依桑"。

【穴位释义】主治小肠病的穴位。

【定位】在脊柱区，位于后正中线上，第四腰椎棘突下凹陷中及左右1寸处各有1穴，三穴并列（图3-15）。中间穴与中医针灸之"腰阳关"穴是同一处。

【局部解剖】中间穴：皮肤，皮下组织，棘上韧带，棘间韧带。浅层主要有第四腰神经后支的内侧支和伴行的动、静脉；深层有棘突间的椎外（后）静脉丛，第四腰神经后支的分支和第四腰动、静脉背侧支的分支或属支。两侧穴位：皮肤，皮下组织，胸腰筋膜浅层，竖脊肌。浅层有第四、五腰神经后支的皮支和伴行的动、静脉；深层有第四、五腰神经后支的肌支及相应动、静脉的分支。

【主治】小肠痞块、寒性赫依引起的腹泻、大便带泡沫及黏液等。

【操作】选用Ⅰ号或Ⅱ号蒙医银针，中间穴位直刺0.5寸，两侧穴位斜刺0.5～1寸，温针给予针柄加热，温度38～42℃，15～20min。

火针或单针刺不加热，留针15～20min。

可单灸,直接灸 1~5 炷或间接灸 5~20min。

小儿慎刺。

【文献摘要】《四部医典·秘诀本》:肠绞痛时服用对症药剂,结合使用敷疗、温和导泻疗法,再灸小肠穴。

《蒙古学百科全书·医学》:如三穴并灸,对陈旧热、泄泻黏液性便、内痞症、气短、小便不利等症有疗效。

膀胱穴

【出处】《四部医典·秘诀本》。

【别名】第十八椎穴、膀胱后穴、"岗桑"。

【穴位释义】主治膀胱病的穴位。

【定位】在脊柱区,位于后正中线上,第五腰椎棘突下凹陷中及左右 1 寸处各有 1 穴,三穴并列(图 3-15)。

【局部解剖】中间穴:皮肤,皮下组织,棘上韧带,棘间韧带。浅层主要有第五腰神经后支的内侧支和伴行的动、静脉;深层有棘突间的椎外(后)静脉丛,第五腰神经后支的分支和第五腰动、静脉背侧支的分支或属支。两侧穴位:皮肤,皮下组织,胸腰筋膜浅层,竖脊肌。浅层有第五腰神经和第一骶神经后支的皮支和伴行的动、静脉;深层有第五腰神经和第一骶神经后支的肌支及相应动、静脉的分支。

【主治】膀胱石症(结石)、因寒性赫依而引起的小便不利或尿频、膝关节发冷疼痛等。

【操作】选用Ⅰ号或Ⅱ号蒙医银针,中间穴位直刺 0.5 寸,两侧穴位斜刺 0.5~1 寸,温针给予针柄加热,温度 38~42℃,15~20min。

火针或单针刺不加热,留针 15~20min。

可单灸,直接灸 1~5 炷或间接灸 5~20min。

小儿慎刺。

【文献摘要】《蒙古学百科全书·医学》:如三穴并灸,对尿频、尿道灼热、阴茎勃起肿胀、闭经、脐周疼痛、产后赫依等病有疗效。

精穴

【出处】《四部医典·秘诀本》。

【别名】第十九椎穴、"库比桑"。

【穴位释义】主治遗精等病的穴位。

【定位】在骶区，位于后正中线上，第一骶椎棘突下凹陷中及左右1寸处各有1穴，三穴并列（图3-15）。

【局部解剖】中间穴：皮肤，皮下组织，棘上韧带，棘间韧带。浅层主要有第一骶神经后支的内侧支和伴行的动、静脉；深层有棘突间的椎外（后）静脉丛，第一骶神经后支的分支和第一骶动、静脉背侧支的分支或属支。两侧穴位：皮肤，皮下组织，胸腰浅筋膜层，腰大肌，竖脊肌。浅层有臀中皮神经；深层有臀下神经分支和第一骶神经后支的肌支及臀上动、静脉的分支。

【主治】遗精、腰痛、前俯后仰皆困难、腰臀部肌肉僵硬、下身沉重、起身困难等。

【操作】选用Ⅰ号或Ⅱ号蒙医银针，中间穴位直刺0.3寸，两侧穴位斜刺0.5～0.8寸，温针给予针柄加热，温度38～42℃，15～20min。

火针或单针刺不加热，留针15～20min。

可单灸，直接灸1～5炷或间接灸5～20min。

小儿慎刺。

【文献摘要】《蒙古学百科全书·医学》：如三穴并灸，对尿道和腰部疼痛、便秘、四肢强直、行走困难、气短而促、口唇下垂、身乏无力、血便等，均有治疗效果。

下清赫依穴

【出处】《四部医典·秘诀本》。

【别名】第二十椎穴、"独日色拉龙桑"。

【穴位释义】主治下清赫依病的穴位。

【定位】在骶区，位于后正中线上，第二骶椎棘突下凹陷中及左右1寸处各有1穴，三穴并列（图3-15）。

【局部解剖】中间穴：皮肤，皮下组织，棘上韧带，棘间韧带。浅层主要有第二骶神经后支的内侧支和伴行的动、静脉；深层有棘突间的椎外（后）静脉丛，第二骶神经后支的分支和第二骶动、静脉背侧支的分支或属支。两侧穴位：皮肤，皮下组织，腰大肌，竖脊肌。浅层有臀中皮神经；深层有臀下神经分支和第二骶神经后支的肌支及臀上动、静脉的分支。

【主治】矢气不通、大便秘结或下泻泡沫黏液样便等。

【操作】选用Ⅰ号或Ⅱ号蒙医银针，中间穴位直刺0.3寸，两侧穴位斜刺0.5～0.8寸，温针给予针柄加热，温度38～42℃，15～20min。

火针或单针刺不加热，留针15～20min。

可单灸,直接灸 1～5 炷或间接灸 5～20min。

小儿慎刺。

【文献摘要】《蒙古学百科全书·医学》:三穴并灸,对腰骶部疼痛、髋关节痛、泄泻、气喘、由赫依引起的喑哑等症均有很好的疗效。

第二十一椎穴

【出处】《蒙医刺灸学》。

【定位】在骶区,位于后正中线上,第三骶椎棘突下凹陷中及左右 1 寸处各有 1 穴,三穴并列(图 3-15)。

【局部解剖】皮肤,皮下组织,骶尾背侧韧带,骶管。浅层主要分布有第三骶神经的后支;深层有尾丛。

【主治】肾腰僵硬疼痛、髋眼部刺痛、腹泻、肛周疾病、气短等。

【操作】选用 I 号或 II 号蒙医银针,中间穴位直刺 0.3 寸,两侧穴位斜刺 0.5～0.8 寸,温针给予针柄加热,温度 38～42℃,15～20min。

可单针刺不加热,留针 15～20min。

可单灸,直接灸 1～5 炷或间接灸 5～20min。

小儿慎刺。

第二十二椎穴

【出处】《蒙医刺灸学》。

【定位】在骶区,位于后正中线上,第四骶椎棘突下凹陷中及左右 1 寸处各有 1 穴,三穴并列(图 3-15)。

【局部解剖】皮肤,皮下组织,骶尾背侧韧带,骶管。浅层主要分布有第四骶神经的后支;深层有尾丛。

【主治】尿闭、尿不尽、闭经、空虚热证、赫依病等。

【操作】选用 I 号或 II 号蒙医银针,中间穴位直刺 0.3 寸,两侧穴位斜刺 0.5～0.8 寸,温针给予针柄加热,温度 38～42℃,15～20min。

火针或单针刺不加热,留针 15～20min。

可单灸,直接灸 1～5 炷或间接灸 5～20min。

小儿慎刺。

第二十三椎穴

【出处】《蒙医刺灸学》。

【定位】在骶区，位于后正中线上，第五骶椎棘突下凹陷中及左右1寸处各有1穴，三穴并列（图3-15）。

【局部解剖】皮肤，皮下组织，骶尾背侧韧带，骶管。浅层主要分布有第五骶神经的后支；深层有尾丛。

【主治】腰肾剧痛、胡言乱语、腹泻等。

【操作】选用Ⅰ号或Ⅱ号蒙医银针，中间穴位直刺0.3寸，两侧穴位斜刺0.5～0.8寸，温针给予针柄加热，温度38～42℃，15～20min。

火针或单针刺不加热，留针15～20min。

可单灸，直接灸1～5炷或间接灸5～20min。

小儿慎刺。

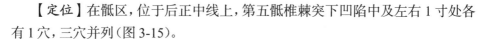

肾黑脉穴

【出处】《四部医典·秘诀本》。

【别名】"卡拉扎那格布桑"。

【定位】在背部腰区，第一腰椎棘突下凹陷旁开2寸左右各有1穴，两穴对称（图3-14）。

【局部解剖】皮肤，皮下组织，背阔肌，竖脊肌。浅层有第一、二腰神经后支的皮支及伴行的动、静脉；深层有第一、二腰神经后支的肌支和相应的肋下动、静脉分支。

【主治】肾寒性病及赫依性病等。

【操作】选用Ⅰ号或Ⅱ号蒙医银针，直刺0.5～0.8寸，温针给予针柄加热，温度38～42℃，15～20min。

火针或单针刺不加热，留针15～20min。

可单灸，直接灸1～5炷或间接灸5～20min。

小儿慎刺。

【文献摘要】《四部医典·秘诀本》：第十四椎左右各一寸处为肾黑脉穴，治疗肾寒赫依。

《蒙古学百科全书·医学》：肾热隐伏时，禁施热针。

肾和穴

【出处】《四部医典·秘诀本》。

【别名】"卡拉巴热依桑"。

【定位】在背部腰区，第一腰椎棘突下凹陷旁开3寸左右各有1穴，两穴对称（图 3-14）。本穴与中医针灸之"肓门"穴是同一处。

【局部解剖】皮肤，皮下组织，背阔肌，下后锯肌，竖脊肌。浅层有第一、二腰神经后支的皮支及伴行的动、静脉；深层有第一、二腰神经后支的肌支及腰背动、静脉的分支。

【主治】肾寒性病及赫依性病等。

【操作】选用Ⅰ号或Ⅱ号蒙医银针，直刺 0.5～0.8 寸，温针给予针柄加热，温度 38～42℃，15～20min。

火针或单针刺不加热，留针 15～20min。

可单灸，直接灸 1～5 炷或间接灸 5～20min。

小儿慎刺。

【文献摘要】《蒙古学百科全书·医学》：肾热隐伏时禁施热针。

肾脂穴

【出处】《四部医典·秘诀本》。

【别名】"卡拉扎拉桑"。

【定位】在背部腰区，第一腰椎棘突下凹陷旁开 4 寸左右各有 1 穴，两穴对称（图 3-14）。

【局部解剖】皮肤，皮下组织，背阔肌，下后锯肌，髂肋肌。浅层有第十二胸神经后支的外侧支及伴行的动、静脉；深层有第十二胸神经后支的肌支。

【主治】肾脂症块及肾寒性赫依病等。

【操作】选用Ⅰ号或Ⅱ号蒙医银针，直刺 0.5～0.8 寸，温针给予针柄加热，温度 38～42℃，15～20min。

火针或单针刺不加热，留针 15～20min。

可单灸，直接灸 1～5 炷或间接灸 5～20min。

小儿慎刺。

【文献摘要】《蒙古学百科全书·医学》：肾热隐伏时禁施热针。

（四）上肢部穴位（24 穴）

肩穴

【出处】《蒙医疗术》《五疗》。

【穴位释义】穴在肩峰上。

【定位】在三角肌区，肩峰外侧缘前端与肱骨大结节凹陷中（上臂平举或上举,位于肩关节前窝中),两侧对称(图3-16)。本穴与中医针灸之"肩髃"穴是同一处。

【局部解剖】皮肤,皮下组织,三角肌,三角肌下囊,冈上肌腱。浅层分布有锁骨上神经外侧支,腋神经皮支;深层分布有腋神经肌支,肩胛上神经,胸肩峰动脉,旋肱后动脉。

【主治】肩关节痛及关节肿胀、上肢白脉病等。

【操作】选用Ⅲ号或Ⅳ号蒙医银针,直刺或向下斜刺0.8~1.5寸,温针给予针柄加热,温度38~42℃,15~20min。

火针或单针刺不加热,留针15~20min。

可单灸,直接灸1~5炷或间接灸5~20min。

小儿慎刺。

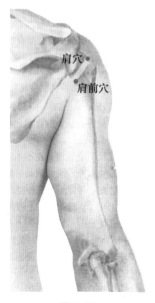

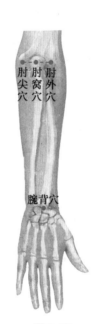

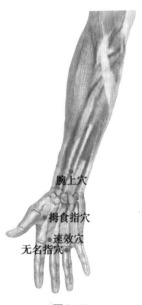

图3-16　　　　　　　　图3-17　　　　　　　　图3-18

肩前穴

【出处】《蒙医疗术》(《五疗》)。

【穴位释义】穴在肩前部。

【定位】位于肩前部,腋前皱襞与肩前角连线的正中,两侧对称(图3-16)。

【局部解剖】皮肤,皮下组织。分布有肩峰动、静脉,旋肱前后动、静脉,锁骨上神经后支，深部有腋神经。

【主治】肩关节酸痛或断裂样剧痛，肩关节以下麻木或手臂不能抬举等。

【操作】选用Ⅱ号或Ⅲ号蒙医银针，直刺 0.5～1 寸，温针给予针柄加热，温度 38～42℃，15～20min。

火针或单针刺不加热，留针 15～20min。

可单灸，直接灸 1～5 炷或间接灸 5～20min。

小儿慎刺。

肩后穴

【出处】《蒙医疗术》（《五疗》）。

【穴位释义】穴在肩后部。

【定位】在肩胛区，位于腋后纹头直上 1 寸处，两侧对称（图 3-14）。本穴与中医针灸之"臑俞"穴是同一处。

【局部解剖】皮肤，皮下组织，斜方肌，冈下肌。浅层分布有锁骨上外侧神经；深层分布有腋神经，肩胛上神经，肩胛上动、静脉的分支或属支，旋肱后动、静脉分支或属支。

【主治】降于肩关节之黄水病等。

【操作】选用Ⅲ号或Ⅳ号蒙医银针，直刺 0.8～1.2 寸，温针给予针柄加热，温度 38～42℃，15～20min。

火针或单针刺不加热，留针 15～20min。

可单灸，直接灸 1～5 炷或间接灸 5～20min。

小儿慎刺。

腋后穴

【出处】《蒙医疗术》（《五疗》）。

【穴位释义】穴在腋窝后方。

【定位】位于腋后纹头处，两侧对称（图 3-14）。

【局部解剖】皮肤，皮下组织，斜方肌，冈下肌。浅层分布有锁骨上外侧神经；深层分布有腋神经，肩胛上神经，肩胛上动、静脉的分支或属支，旋肱后动、静脉分支或属支。

【主治】胸闷，上肢酸痛不能上举及麻木等。

【操作】选用Ⅲ号或Ⅳ号蒙医银针，直刺 0.8～1.2 寸，温针给予针柄加热，温度 38～42℃，15～20min。

火针或单针刺不加热，留针 15～20min。

可单灸，直接灸 1～5 炷或间接灸 5～20min。

小儿慎刺。

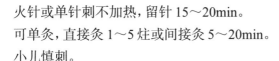

肘窝穴

【出处】《蒙医疗术》(《五疗》)。

【穴位释义】穴在肘窝。

【定位】在肘区，位于肘横纹正中，两侧对称(图 3-17)。

【局部解剖】皮肤，皮下组织，肱桡肌，肱肌。浅层分布有前臂后皮神经；深层分布有桡神经，桡侧副动、静脉，桡侧返动、静脉。

【主治】降于肘关节的黄水病等。

【操作】选用Ⅱ号或Ⅲ号蒙医银针，直刺 0.5～1 寸，温针给予针柄加热，温度 38～42℃，15～20min。

火针或单针刺不加热，留针 15～20min。

可单灸，直接灸 1～5 炷或间接灸 5～20min。

小儿慎刺。

肘尖穴

【出处】《蒙医疗术》(《五疗》)。

【穴位释义】穴在肘尖。

【定位】位于尺骨鹰嘴上方，两侧对称(图 3-17)。

【局部解剖】皮肤，皮下组织，肱三头肌。浅层分布有前臂后皮神经；深层分布有桡神经肌支，肱深动脉。

【主治】各种骨病等。

【操作】选用Ⅰ号或Ⅱ号蒙医银针，直刺 0.5～1 寸，温针给予针柄加热，温度 38～42℃，15～20min。

火针或单针刺不加热，留针 15～20min。

可单灸，直接灸 1～5 炷或间接灸 5～20min。

小儿慎刺。

肘外穴

【出处】《蒙医传统疗法》。

【穴位释义】穴在肘外侧。

【定位】在肘区,位于肘横纹外端,两侧对称(图3-17)。

【局部解剖】皮肤,皮下组织,肱桡肌,肱肌。浅层分布有前臂后皮神经;深层分布有桡神经,桡侧副动、静脉,桡侧返动、静脉。

【主治】降于肘关节的黄水病等。

【操作】选用Ⅱ号或Ⅲ号蒙医银针,直刺0.8～1.2寸,温针给予针柄加热,温度38～42℃,15～20min。

火针或单针刺不加热,留针15～20min。

可单灸,直接灸1～5炷或间接灸5～20min。

小儿慎刺。

腕上穴

【出处】《蒙医疗术》(《五疗》)。

【穴位释义】穴在腕以上。

【定位】在前臂前区,腕掌侧远端横纹上2寸,掌长肌腱与桡侧腕屈肌腱之间,两侧对称(图3-18)。本穴与中医针灸之"内关"穴是同一处。

【局部解剖】皮肤,皮下组织,掌长肌腱与桡侧腕屈肌腱之间,旋前方肌。浅层分布有前臂内、外侧皮神经和前臂正中静脉;深层分布有正中神经干及其伴行的正中动脉,骨间前动脉。

【主治】谵语、幻视、视力减退及骨骼疾病等。

【操作】选用Ⅰ号或Ⅱ号蒙医银针,直刺0.5～1寸,温针给予针柄加热,温度38～42℃,15～20min。

火针或单针刺不加热,留针15～20min。

可单灸,直接灸1～5炷或间接灸5～20min。

小儿慎刺。

腕背穴

【出处】《蒙医传统疗法》。

【穴位释义】穴在手腕背侧。

【定位】在腕后区,位于尺骨茎突与三角骨之间的凹陷处,两侧对称(图3-17)。本穴与中医针灸之"阳谷"穴是同一处。

【局部解剖】皮肤,皮下组织,尺侧腕伸肌腱与小指伸肌腱之间。浅层分布有前臂后皮神经,贵要静脉属支;深层分布有骨间后神经与动脉的分支。

【主治】降于腕关节的黄水引起的手麻或腕关节肿痛等。

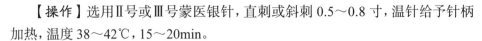

【操作】选用Ⅱ号或Ⅲ号蒙医银针，直刺或斜刺 0.5～0.8 寸，温针给予针柄加热，温度 38～42℃，15～20min。

火针或单针刺不加热，留针 15～20min。

可单灸，直接灸 1～5 炷或间接灸 5～20min。

小儿慎刺。

速效穴

【出处】《蒙医刺灸学》。

【穴位释义】本穴具有见效快之特点。

【定位】在掌区，位于手掌正中，握拳时，中指尖处（横平第三掌指关节近端，第二、三掌骨之间偏于第三掌骨），两侧对称（图 3-18）。本穴与中医针灸之"劳宫"穴是同一处。

【局部解剖】皮肤，皮下组织，掌腱膜，指浅、深屈肌腱。浅层分布有正中神经掌皮支；深层分布有正中神经的分支指掌侧固有神经，尺神经的掌深支，掌浅弓及其分支，指掌侧总动脉和掌深弓及其分支掌心动脉。

【主治】牙痛、手心发热等。

【操作】选用Ⅰ号或Ⅱ号蒙医银针，直刺 0.3～0.5 寸，温针给予针柄加热，温度 38～42℃，15～20min。

火针或单针刺不加热，留针 15～20min。

可单灸，直接灸 1～5 炷或间接灸 5～20min。

小儿慎刺。

无名指穴

【出处】《蒙医疗术》（《五疗》）。

【定位】在掌区，位于第四掌指关节正中，两侧对称（图 3-18）。

【局部解剖】皮肤，皮下组织，掌腱膜，第四蚓状肌，指深浅屈肌腱，骨间肌。浅层分布有尺神经掌支；深层分布有第四掌侧固有神经及指掌侧总动、静脉。

【主治】各种皮肤病等。

【操作】选用Ⅰ号蒙医银针，直刺 0.2～0.4 寸，温针给予针柄加热，温度 38～42℃，15～20min。

火针或单针刺不加热，留针 15～20min。

可单灸，直接灸 1～5 炷或间接灸 5～20min。

小儿慎刺。

拇食指穴 ᠬᠤᠷᠤᠭᠤ

【出处】《蒙医疗术》《五疗》。

【定位】位于手背，第一、二掌骨之间，约平第二掌骨中点处，两侧对称（图3-18）。本穴与中医针灸之"合谷"穴是同一处。

【局部解剖】有拇收肌横头；有手背静脉网，腧穴近侧正当桡动脉从手背穿向手掌之处；布有桡神经浅支的掌背侧神经，深部有正中神经的指掌侧固有神经。

【主治】疫热及肝血热所致的眼病等。

【操作】选用Ⅰ号或Ⅱ号蒙医银针，斜刺0.5～0.8寸，温针给予针柄加热，温度38～42℃，15～20min。

火针或单针刺不加热，留针15～20min。

可单灸，直接灸1～5炷或间接灸5～20min。

小儿慎刺。

（五）下肢部穴位（46穴）

髋穴 ᠨᠢᠳᠤ

【出处】《亲·却吉扎拉申三著》。

【别名】吉德贡。

【穴位释义】穴近髋关节。

【定位】在臀区，股骨大转子最凸点与骶骨裂孔的连线的外1/3与内2/3交点处及上、下、左、右量1寸处各有1穴，一侧5穴，两侧对称，共10穴（侧卧，伸下腿，上腿屈髋膝取穴）（图3-19）。中间穴与中医针灸之"环跳"穴是同一处。

【局部解剖】皮肤，皮下组织，臀大肌。浅层分布有臀上皮神经，臀下皮神经，髂骨下神经，股外侧皮神经；深层分布有坐骨神经，股后皮神经，臀下动、静脉。

【主治】半身麻木疼痛、白乎杨、腰腿痛、下肢强直或拘急等。

【操作】选用Ⅳ号或Ⅴ号蒙医银针，直刺1.5～3寸，温针给予针柄加热，温度38～42℃，15～20min。

火针或单针刺不加热，留针15～20min。

可单灸，直接灸3～7炷或间接灸5～20min。

小儿慎刺。

【文献摘要】《亲·却吉扎拉申三著》：尾骨向臀部量一虎口处是髋穴，或肾种穴上十六指处是髋穴，其上、下、左、右量一寸处各有一穴，共五穴。治大腿外侧及小腿黄水之穴位。

《蒙古学百科全书·医学》：据临床观察，在该穴施热针，对腰腿痛、降于腰椎间或髋关节的黄水病、白脉病疗效显著。隐伏热时禁施热针。

【常用配穴】①配肾穴，治腰痛、肾寒性赫依病。②配大腿穴或膝眼穴，治关节黄水病。

【现代研究】（1）温针刺激髋穴、大腿穴、腘穴等部位治疗慢性期腰椎间盘突出症：在腰部患处阿是穴及下肢白脉走行的髋穴（"色古金"穴）、大腿穴（"古雅"穴）、腘穴（"达黑莫"穴）、腓肠肌穴（"宝拉青高勒"穴）、腓肠肌下穴（"宝拉青道日"穴）、胫下穴（"嘎达日峡阿日"穴）等穴位中每次选出1～3个穴位，用蒙医特制银针（针体直径0.8～1.0mm，针柄用细银丝紧密的螺旋形缠绕，针端尖而不锐，针柄长度5～6cm，针身总长度为6cm、8cm、10cm、12cm等4种规格，适合于人体各不同部位）针刺，将大约1cm长灸炷悬于针柄上点燃，热温（以患者能忍受的温度为宜，直到灸炷燃完为止，类似点燃1～3次，使热度通过针身传入体内而达到治疗目的，留针20～30分钟），隔日1次治疗，14天为1个疗程。有效率90%，治愈率24%。[14]

（2）蒙医温针治疗坐骨神经痛的临床观察：选髋穴，蒙医温针治疗坐骨神经痛，每5天治疗1次，10天为1个疗程。治愈率与有效率为56.67%与96.67%。[15]

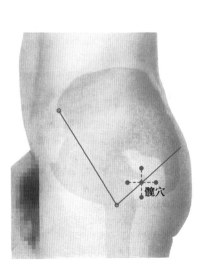

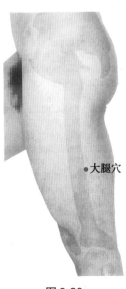

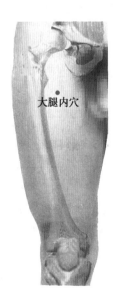

| 图 3-19 | 图 3-20 | 图 3-21 |

大腿穴 ᠵᠦᠷᠡ

【出处】《四部医典·秘诀本》。

【别名】拉叶齐苏乐。

【穴位释义】穴在大腿部。

【定位】在股部,直立垂手,掌心贴于大腿时,中指尖所指凹陷中,髂胫束后缘(稍屈膝,大腿稍内收提起,可显露髂胫束)。左右两侧对称,共2穴(图3-20)。本穴与中医针灸之"风市"穴是同一处。

【局部解剖】皮肤,皮下组织,髂胫束,股外侧肌,股中间肌。浅层分布有股外侧皮神经;深层分布有股神经的肌支,旋股外侧动脉降支的肌支。

【主治】腰胯酸痛,降于大腿外侧肌肉的黄水等。

【操作】选用Ⅲ号或Ⅳ号蒙医银针,直刺1～2寸,温针给予针柄加热,温度38～42℃,15～20min。

火针或单针刺不加热,留针15～20min。

可单灸,直接灸3～7炷或间接灸5～20min。

小儿慎刺。

【文献摘要】《四部医典·秘诀本》:髋五穴和小腿"苏扎嘎"、大腿"苏扎嘎"为黄水槽,针刺这些点位可以治寒赫依。

【常用配穴】①配肾穴和髋穴,治腰痛、肾寒性赫依病。②配髋穴和膝眼穴,治腰腿痛、关节黄水病。

大腿内穴 ᠵᠦᠷᠡ

【出处】《蒙医疗术》(《五疗》)。

【穴位释义】穴在大腿内侧。

【定位】在股前区,腹股沟斜纹正中直下三横指处。左右两侧对称,共2穴(图3-21)。

【局部解剖】皮肤,皮下组织,长收肌,短收肌,大收肌。浅层分布有股神经前皮支,大隐静脉;深层分布有闭孔神经的前支和后支,股深动、静脉的肌支,旋股内侧动、静脉的股支。

【主治】降于大腿内侧的黄水及寒性痞块,大便秘结等症。

【操作】选用Ⅲ或Ⅳ号蒙医银针,直刺0.8～1.2寸,温针给予针柄加热,温度38～42℃,15～20min。

火针或单针刺不加热,留针15～20分钟。

可单灸,直接灸 3～7 炷或间接灸 5～20 分钟。

小儿慎刺。

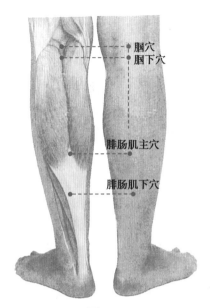

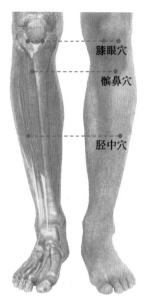

图 3-22   图 3-23

腘穴 ᠬᠣᠨ᠎ᠠ

【出处】《蒙医疗术》(《五疗》)。

【穴位释义】穴在腘窝。

【定位】在膝后区,腘窝横纹正中。左右两侧对称,共 2 穴(图 3-22)。本穴与中医针灸之"委中"穴是同一处。

【局部解剖】皮肤,皮下组织,腓肠肌内、外侧头之间。浅层分布有股后皮神经和小隐静脉;深层分布有胫神经,腓肠内侧皮神经起始端及腘动、静脉。

【主治】不消化、痢疾、泄泻泡沫黏液便及颈项筋拘挛等症。

【操作】选用Ⅲ号或Ⅳ号蒙医银针,直刺 1～1.5 寸,温针给予针柄加热,温度 38～42℃,15～20min。

火针或单针刺不加热,留针 15～20min。

可单灸,直接灸 3～7 炷或间接灸 5～20min。

小儿慎刺。

腘下穴 ᠪᠥᠭᠡᠷᠡ

【出处】《蒙医疗术》(《五疗》)。

【穴位释义】穴在腘窝下。

【定位】在小腿后区,腘窝横纹下一横指。左右两侧对称,共2穴(图3-22)。

【局部解剖】皮肤,皮下组织,腓肠肌,比目鱼肌。浅层分布有股后皮神经,腓肠内侧皮神经及小隐静脉;深层分布有胫神经及腘动、静脉。

【主治】关节痛等症。

【操作】选用Ⅱ号或Ⅲ号蒙医银针,直刺0.5~1.2寸,温针给予针柄加热,温度38~42℃,15~20min。

火针或单针刺不加热,留针15~20min。

可单灸,直接灸3~7炷或间接灸5~20min。

小儿慎刺。

腓肠肌主穴 ᠪᠥᠭᠡᠷᠡ

【出处】《蒙医疗术》(《五疗》)。

【穴位释义】穴在腓肠肌上部。

【定位】在小腿后区,腓肠肌两肌腹与肌腱交角处。左右两侧对称,共2穴(图3-22)。本穴与中医针灸之"承山"穴是同一处。

【局部解剖】皮肤,皮下组织,腓肠肌,比目鱼肌。浅层分布有腓肠内侧皮神经分支及小隐静脉;深层分布有胫神经,腓肠内侧神经干及胫后动、静脉。

【主治】颈项强直和活动受限、肛门病、出血、黄水疮等。

【操作】选用Ⅲ号或Ⅳ号蒙医银针,直刺1~1.5寸,温针给予针柄加热,温度38~42℃,15~20min。

火针或单针刺不加热,留针15~20min。

可单灸,直接灸3~7炷或间接灸5~20min。

小儿慎刺。

腓肠肌下穴 ᠪᠥᠭᠡᠷᠡ

【出处】《蒙医疗术》(《五疗》)。

【穴位释义】穴在腓肠肌上部。

【定位】在小腿后区,腓肠肌主穴直下2寸处,腓骨与跟腱之间。左右两侧对称,共2穴(图3-22)。

【局部解剖】皮肤,皮下组织,腓骨短肌,趾长屈肌。浅层分布有腓肠神经分支及小隐静脉;深层分布有腓浅神经,胫神经及腓后动脉分支。

【主治】腓肠肌萎缩及颈项强直、疼痛。

【操作】选用Ⅱ号或Ⅲ号蒙医银针,直刺0.5～1寸,温针给予针柄加热,温度38～42℃,15～20min。

火针或单针刺不加热,留针15～20min。

可单灸,直接灸3～7炷或间接灸5～20min。

小儿慎刺。

胫中穴

【出处】《蒙医疗术》(《五疗》)。

【穴位释义】穴在胫骨中段。

【定位】在小腿外侧,外踝尖上8寸,胫骨前肌的外缘。左右两侧对称,共2穴(图3-23)。本穴与中医针灸之"丰隆"穴是同一处。

【局部解剖】皮肤,皮下组织,趾长伸肌,踇长伸肌,小腿骨间膜,胫骨后肌。浅层分布有腓肠外侧皮神经;深层分布有腓深神经,胫前动、静脉;小腿骨间膜深面有胫神经,腓动脉。

【主治】膝关节酸痛或麻痛、足趾间糜烂等。

【操作】选用Ⅲ号或Ⅳ号蒙医银针,直刺1～1.5寸,温针给予针柄加热,温度38～42℃,15～20min。

火针或单针刺不加热,留针15～20min。

可单灸,直接灸3～7炷或间接灸5～20min。

小儿慎刺。

胫下穴

【出处】《蒙医疗术》(《五疗》)。

【穴位释义】穴在胫骨下段。

【定位】在小腿外侧,外踝尖上3寸,腓骨前缘。左右两侧对称,共2穴(图3-24)。本穴与中医针灸之"悬钟"穴是同一处。

【局部解剖】皮肤,皮下组织,趾长伸肌,小腿骨间膜。浅层分布有腓肠外侧皮神经,腓浅神经;深层分布有腓深神经,胫前动脉;再深层可分布有腓动、静脉干。

【主治】阳痿、遗精及踝关节疼痛等症。

【操作】选用Ⅱ号或Ⅲ号蒙医银针，直刺 0.8～1 寸，温针给予针柄加热，温度 38～42℃，15～20min。

火针或单针刺不加热，留针 15～20min。

可单灸，直接灸 3～7 炷或间接灸 5～20min。

小儿慎刺。

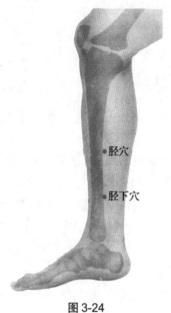

图 3-24

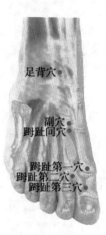

图 3-25

足背穴

【出处】《蒙医疗术》(《五疗》)。

【穴位释义】穴在足背。

【定位】在踝区，踝关节前面中央凹陷中，踇长伸肌腱与趾长伸肌腱之间。左右两侧对称，共 2 穴（图 3-25）。本穴与中医针灸之"解溪"穴是同一处。

【局部解剖】皮肤，皮下组织，踇长伸肌腱，趾长伸肌腱。浅层分布有足背内侧皮神经，足背皮下神经；深层分布有腓深神经，足背动、静脉。

【主治】阳痿、遗精及踝关节疼痛等症。

【操作】选用Ⅱ号或Ⅲ号蒙医银针，直刺 0.5～1 寸，温针给予针柄加热，温度 38～42℃，15～20min。

火针或单针刺不加热，留针 15～20min。

可单灸，直接灸 3～7 炷或间接灸 5～20min。

小儿慎刺。

胫穴 ᠱᠢᠶᠠ

【出处】《蒙医疗术》(《五疗》)。

【穴位释义】穴在胫骨部。

【定位】在小腿内侧,内踝尖上7寸,胫骨内侧面的中央。左右两侧对称,共2穴(图3-24)。本穴与中医针灸之"中都"穴是同一处。

【局部解剖】皮肤,皮下组织,胫骨骨面。分布有隐神经的小腿内侧皮支,大隐静脉。

【主治】月经淋漓不止及下身诸病。

【操作】选用Ⅱ号或Ⅲ号蒙医银针,直刺0.5～0.8寸,温针给予针柄加热,温度38～42℃,15～20min。

火针或单针刺不加热,留针15～20min。

可单灸,直接灸3～7炷或间接灸5～20min。

小儿慎刺。

髌鼻穴 ᠱᠢᠶᠠ

【出处】《蒙医疗术》(《五疗》)。

【穴位释义】穴在髌骨附近。

【定位】在髌骨下缘2寸处。左右两侧对称,共2穴(图3-23)。

【局部解剖】皮肤,皮下组织,胫骨前肌,趾长伸肌,小腿骨间膜,胫骨后肌。浅层分布有腓肠外侧皮神经;深层分布有腓深神经肌支,腓前动脉;小腿骨间膜深面有胫神经,胫后动、静脉分支或属支。

【主治】腓肠肌萎缩及腰腿痛、分娩后流血过多等症。

【操作】温针选用Ⅲ号或Ⅳ号蒙医银针,直刺1～1.5寸,给予针柄加热,温度为38～42℃,15～20min。

火针或单针刺不加热,留针15～20min。

可单灸,直接灸3～7炷或间接灸5～20min。

小儿慎刺。

膝眼穴 ᠱᠢᠶᠠ

【出处】《蒙医疗术》(《五疗》)。

【穴位释义】穴在膝眼处。

【定位】在膝部，髌韧带内侧凹陷和髌韧带外侧凹陷处各有 1 穴，左右两侧对称，共 4 穴（图 3-23）。内侧膝眼穴与中医针灸之"内膝眼"穴是同一处；外侧膝眼穴与中医针灸之"犊鼻"穴是同一处。

【局部解剖】内侧膝眼穴：皮肤，皮下组织，髌韧带与髌内侧支持带之间，膝关节囊，翼状皱襞。浅层分布有隐神经的髌下支和股神经的前皮支；深层分布有膝关节动、静脉网。外侧膝眼穴：皮肤，皮下组织，膝关节囊，翼状皱襞。浅层分布有腓肠外侧皮神经，股前皮神经；深层分布有胫神经，腓总神经的膝关节支，膝关节动、静脉网。

【主治】胃病、消化不良、肌肉酸痛麻木、膝痛等症。

【操作】内侧膝眼穴：选用Ⅱ号或Ⅲ号蒙医银针，从前向后外与额状面成 45°角斜刺 0.5～1 寸，给予针柄加热，温度 38～42℃，15～20min；外侧膝眼穴：选用Ⅲ号或Ⅳ号蒙医银针，向后内斜刺 0.8～1.5 寸，温针给予针柄加热，温度 38～42℃，15～20min。

火针或单针刺不加热，留针 15～20min。

可单灸，直接灸 3～7 炷或间接灸 5～20min。

小儿慎刺。

【现代研究】(1) 温针刺激膝眼穴结合康复训练治疗膝关节骨性关节炎：①取额博都格因尼都（内外膝眼）、宏戈尔（足三里）、希乐卡因博乐其尔（相当于阴陵泉）。操作：用 90 号细银针（直径 0.8mm、长度 40mm，含银量 85%）刺入穴位，待得气后，稍往外拉出 3～5mm，在针柄上加直径 10mm、长 5～8mm 艾柱，下端点燃或用酒精棉球闪火烧针，针柄微红或患者有灼热感后，继续留针 10～15 分钟。康复训练：仰卧位的双桥运动；仰卧位的直腿抬高运动；侧卧位的髋关节外展运动；仰卧膝关节内收运动；俯卧位的膝关节伸展运动；俯卧位的膝关节及腘窝收缩运动；扶物下蹲；仰卧位的空蹬自行车运动。双下肢交替，每日 2 遍，每次 20 个。每日针刺 1 次，10 次为 1 个疗程，连续治疗 2 个疗程，疗程间休息 3 天，康复训练不停止。疗效：优 83.07%，良 9.23%，可 6.15%，差 1.53%。[16] ②患者半卧位，屈膝关节 90°，用特定的银针，常规消毒后刺入膝眼穴，将约 1cm 直径艾绒穿入针柄捏好后点燃艾绒，艾绒燃尽，待针柄冷却后起针。康复训练：患者仰卧位直腿抬高，仰卧内收膝关节、伸展膝关节，侧卧外展髋关节，空蹬运动，扶物下蹲，等等。双下肢交替，每日 2 遍，每次 20 个，根据患肢情况，合理安排时间和训练次数。每 3 日治疗 1 次，3 次为 1 个疗程，治疗 2 个疗程。有效率 95.20%，治愈率 6.90%。[17]

(2) 温针刺激膝眼穴治疗膝关节骨质增生：取膝眼、阿是穴常规消毒，利多卡因局部麻醉后，刺入温针，得气后将针留在一定深度，于针柄上插小枣大的艾条，然后在下端点燃，直到艾条烧完为止，为了防止艾火脱落灼伤皮肤，可以在穴位区垫放硬纸片等隔离。每穴点 1～3 壮，3 天 1 次，辅以膝关节周围阳陵泉、足三里、阴陵泉等穴位。10 天为 1 个疗程，平均治疗 2 个疗程。治愈率：73.00%，显效：20.00%，好转：5.00%，无效：3.00%。[18]

（3）温针刺激膝眼穴等穴位治疗膝骨性关节炎：取膝眼穴（内外膝眼），强身穴（与中医足三里对应），胫内侧穴（与中医阴陵泉穴对应），先用银针先快后慢向膝关节腔后内斜刺，刺入内外膝眼穴，进针长度 1～1.5 寸，强身穴、胫内侧穴，可用银针也可用毫针，针尖垂直于穴位皮肤，先快后慢进针，进针深度 1～1.5 寸，待得气后向外拉出 2mm 左右用酒精棉球闪火烧针加热（或在针柄上加直径 10mm、长 5～8mm 艾柱，点燃下端），针柄微红或患者有灼热感后停止烧针，继续留针 20min，再重复烧针加热 1 次，待针柄冷却后出针，按住针眼 5～10s。如未出血用碘伏棉球再次消毒穴位即可，如有出血则止血后消毒。蒙医综合临床症状疗效评价：临床控制，总评分值下降率≥95%；显效：70%≤总评分值下降率＜95%；有效：30%≤总评分值下降率＜70%；无效：总评分值下降率＜30%。疼痛疗效评价治愈，疼痛缓解率≥75%；显效：50%≤疼痛缓解率＜75%；有效：25%≤疼痛缓解率＜50%；无效：疼痛缓解率＜25%。[19]

踇趾间穴

【出处】《蒙医疗术》（《五疗》）。

【定位】在足背，踇趾、次趾夹缝向脚背方向上 1 寸处（第 1、2 跖骨底结合部前方凹陷中），左右两侧对称，共 2 穴（图 3-25）。本穴与中医针灸之"太冲"穴是同一处。

【局部解剖】皮肤，皮下组织，踇长伸肌腱与趾长伸肌腱之间，踇短伸肌腱的外侧，第 1 骨间背侧肌。浅层分布有足背静脉网，足背内侧皮神经等；深层分布有腓深神经和第 1 趾背动、静脉。

【主治】降于足部的黄水、腿酸痛或强直痛、腹扩张、尿频等症。

【操作】选用Ⅰ号或Ⅱ号蒙医银针，直刺 0.5～0.8 寸，温针给予针柄加热，温度 38～42℃，15～20min。

火针或单针刺不加热，留针 15～20min。

可单灸，直接灸 1～5 炷或间接灸 5～20min。

小儿慎刺。

副穴 ᠳᠡᠳ

【出处】《蒙医疗术》《五疗》。

【定位】在足背,位于踇趾间穴直上 0.5 寸处,左右两侧对称,共 2 穴(图 3-25)。

【局部解剖】皮肤,皮下组织,踇长伸肌腱外缘。浅层分布有足背静脉网,第一跖背侧动脉,腓深神经的跖背侧神经;深层分布有胫神经、足底内侧神经。

【主治】痛风、痹病、睾丸肿胀等症。

【操作】选用 I 号蒙医银针,直刺 0.5~0.8 寸,温针给予针柄加热,温度 38~42℃,15~20min。

火针或单针刺不加热,留针 15~20min。

可单灸,直接灸 1~5 炷或间接灸 5~20min。

小儿慎刺。

踇趾第一穴 ᠭᠣᠣᠵᠢᠢᠨ ᠲᠡᠷᠢᠭᠦᠨ ᠴᠡᠭ

【出处】《蒙医疗术》《五疗》。

【定位】在足背,位于踇趾端上 3 寸处,左右两侧对称,共 2 穴(图 3-25)。

【局部解剖】皮肤,皮下组织,第一跖骨。分布有腓深神经的趾背神经和趾背动、静脉。

【主治】腹内沉重感及睾丸肿胀等症。

【操作】选用 I 号蒙医银针,直刺 0.2~0.5 寸,温针给予针柄加热,温度 38~42℃,15~20min。

可单针刺不加热,留针 15~20min。

可单灸,直接灸 1~5 炷或间接灸 5~20min。

小儿慎刺。

踇趾第二穴 ᠭᠣᠣᠵᠢᠢᠨ ᠬᠣᠶᠠᠳᠤᠭᠠᠷ ᠴᠡᠭ

【出处】《蒙医疗术》《五疗》。

【定位】在足背,踇趾、次趾夹缝处,左右两侧对称,共 2 穴(图 3-25)。

【局部解剖】皮肤,皮下组织,第 1、2 近节趾骨间。分布有腓深神经的趾背神经和趾背动、静脉。

【主治】头痛及尿频等症。

【操作】选用 I 号蒙医银针,直刺 0.3~0.5 寸,温针给予针柄加热,温度 38~42℃,15~20min。

火针或单针刺不加热,留针 15～20min。

可单灸,直接灸 1～5 炷或间接灸 5～20min。

小儿慎刺。

姆趾第三穴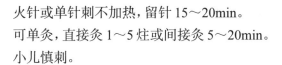

【出处】《蒙医疗术》(《五疗》)。

【定位】在足背,姆趾甲上缘直上一横指处(足姆趾背侧长毛发处正中),左右两侧对称,共2穴(图3-25)。

【局部解剖】皮肤,皮下组织,甲根。分布有腓深神经的背外侧神经和趾背动、静脉。

【主治】目赤、颈项强直伴活动受限、口吐泡沫、舌旁发疹等症。

【操作】选用 I 号蒙医银针,直刺 0.2～0.3 寸,温针给予针柄加热,温度 38～42℃,15～20min。

火针或单针刺不加热,留针 15～20min。

可单灸,直接灸 1～5 炷或间接灸 5～20min。

小儿慎刺。

参 考 文 献

[1] SI L G, WANG Y H, WUYUN G, et al. The effect of Mongolian medical acupuncture on cytokines and neurotransmitters in the brain tissue of insomniac rats[J]. Eur J Integr Med, 2015, 7(5): 492-498.

[2] 木日根吉雅, 阿古拉, 王月洪, 等. 蒙医温针对失眠大鼠脑组织多巴胺含量的影响 [J]. 中国民族医药杂志, 2014, 20(7): 50-51.

[3] 木日根吉雅, 阿古拉. 蒙医温针对失眠大鼠海马中 Glu、GABA、ACh 含量的影响 [J]. 中国民族医药杂志, 2014, 20(6): 43-44.

[4] 王月洪, 阿古拉, 斯楞格, 等. 蒙医温针对大鼠睡眠时间和自主活动的影响 [J]. 上海针灸杂志, 2014, 33(5): 472-475.

[5] 包乌恩奇, 阿古拉, 萨仁图雅, 等. 治疗失眠症体会 [J]. 中国蒙医药, 2012, 7(2): 95-98.

[6] 何福龙, 李艳飞. 蒙医温针疗法治疗失眠 [J]. 中国民族民间医药, 2011(1): 6.

[7] 阿古拉, 苏朝鲁门, 张朝鲁门, 等. 蒙医温针对慢性疲劳大鼠行为学及下丘脑脑组织中单胺类神经递质含量的影响 [J]. 世界科学技术: 中医药现代化, 2008, 10(1): 129-132.

[8] 阿古拉, 卢峻, 陈英松, 等. 蒙医温针对疲劳大鼠作用的神经内分泌机制研究 [J]. 北京中医药大学学报, 2008, 31(9): 643-646.

[9] 陈英松,卢峻,苏·朝鲁门,等.蒙医温针对疲劳大鼠血清肿瘤坏死因子 -α、促肾上腺皮质激素和皮质酮含量的影响 [J].针刺研究,2008,33(4):258-261.

[10] 阿古拉,陈英松.蒙医温针疗法治疗慢性疲劳综合征的临床研究 [J].辽宁中医药大学学报,2006,8(5):116-117.

[11] 李玉棠,萨仁图雅,白金荣,等.蒙医温针疗法对单纯性肥胖症的临床疗效研究 [J].中国民族医药杂志,2014,20(11):5-7.

[12] 斯琴,王朝鲁.蒙医温针结合芒针治疗腰椎间盘脱出症 50 例临床疗效观察 [J].包头医学院学报,2014,30(3):66-67.

[13] 其那日图.蒙医温针疗法治疗腰椎间盘突出症 60 例疗效观察 [J].中国民族医药杂志,2014,20(9):26.

[14] 阿拉腾其木格.蒙医温针疗法对慢性期腰椎间盘突出症的疗效研究 [J].内蒙古民族大学学报,2011,2(17):83-84.

[15] 诺敏,布日乐吉.蒙医温针治疗坐骨神经痛的临床观察 [J].中国民族民间医药,2011(24):2.

[16] 陈平,郭文奇.蒙医温针配合康复训练治疗膝关节骨性关节炎临床观察 [J].中国民族医药杂志,2006,12(3):30-31.

[17] 张宏华.蒙医温针加康复训练治疗膝关节骨性关节炎 21 例临床疗效观察 [J].中国民族民间医药,2014(17):7-9.

[18] 齐宏伟.蒙医温针治疗膝关节骨质增生 [J].中国民族医药杂志,2012,18(5):13.

[19] 姚哈斯,洪玉光.蒙医温针疗法治疗膝骨性关节炎的临床观察 [J].中国民族医药杂志,2015,21(4):7-9.

第四章

蒙医温针火针疗法的选穴

一、蒙医温针火针疗法的选穴原则

人体是一个矛盾的统一体,各部位之间在生理上保持着密切的联系,在发病以后,局部病变必然会影响到其他部位和整体;而整体变化又必然会对局部造成影响。所以蒙医药学中"辨证施治"的理论,就是整体观点在诊断治疗上的具体应用。

"辨证施治"也叫"辨证论治",是从患者的整体出发,依据其各方面的反应,既重视病因,又注意疾病发展的阶段性;既重视病症,又注意患者体质的差异性。蒙医通过"三诊"全面地收集临床资料进行综合分析得出辨证施治的依据。

蒙医温针火针疗法的选穴原则是以蒙医"辨证施治"学说为指导,根据不同疾病的病因病机,并结合白脉分布、疼痛点、病变部位等具体情况辨证取穴。蒙医温针火针疗法辨证取穴方法多来源于临床经验,用穴少而精,疗效确切,临床上经常可以达到一针即验的疗效。蒙医温针火针疗法常用穴位是指根据文献记载及临床经验,总结出的适应病症范围相对明确且疗效确切的固定穴位。这些固定穴位的主治功效在长期的临床实践中得到反复验证,本书上一章重点介绍了 260 个蒙医温针火针疗法常用穴位的定位、主治等内容。临床上蒙医温针治疗某种疾病时,在根据疾病的症状及病因病机等情况进行辨证分析的基础上,从蒙医温针火针疗法常用穴位中选取相应主治功效的一个或几个穴位。有时候也可以根据临床需要,结合医生临床经验选取非固定穴位。这类非固定穴位一般都随病而定,没有固定的位置和名称,主要以局部压痛、或快感、或有特殊感应及适合针刺之处等来定穴位。因此,蒙医穴位广义上包括常用固定穴位和随病而取的非固定穴位。蒙医穴位数量因此较多,蒙医疗术铜人全身共标记有 611 个穴位孔。

蒙医温针火针疗法的选穴基本方法可以归纳为穴位主治取穴、白脉分布取穴、痛点取穴、病变部位取穴 4 种。

1. 穴位主治取穴 穴位主治取穴是指从蒙医温针火针疗法常用固定穴位中选取相应主治功效的穴位的方法。如对不消化病，取火衰穴温针施治等。

2. 白脉分布取穴 白脉分布取穴是指根据内白脉和外白脉分布情况，在相应的区域选取穴位的方法，可以选取固定穴位，也可以选取非固定穴位。如对下肢麻木，可在患侧管脉分布区域取髋穴或附近其他非固定穴位温针施治等。

3. 痛点取穴 痛点取穴是指寻找最明显的压痛点选取穴位的方法，可以选取固定穴位，也可以选取非固定穴位。如对颈椎病进行蒙医温针治疗时，可在颈项部寻找最有压痛的赫依穴或其他非固定穴位施治等。

4. 病变部位取穴 病变部位取穴是指在病变部位寻找最适合刺激的位置选取穴位的方法，可以选取固定穴位，也可以选取非固定穴位。如蒙医温针治疗膝关节炎时，可选取膝眼穴或髌骨外上方等其他合适的非固定穴位施治等。

二、蒙医多媒体人体穴位模型

蒙医多媒体人体穴位模型是根据蒙医传统疗法理论将蒙医穴位标记于人体上的医学多媒体穴位模型（图4-1）。

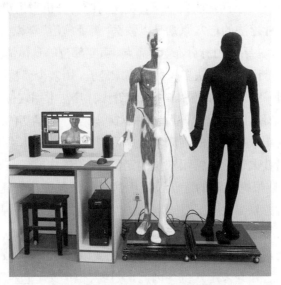

图4-1 蒙医多媒体人体穴位模型

（一）研制成果

"蒙医多媒体人体穴位模型的研究"属内蒙古医科大学蒙医药学院立项研

发项目，编号 NYM2006HZ001，笔者为主持人，课题组成员有乌勒彩拉、陈英松、郑耀勇、张玉兰、朱奇烨、陈塔娜、乌云格日乐，起止年月为 2006 年 12 月至 2007 年 12 月。蒙医多媒体人体穴位模型是查阅大量蒙医文献及结合临床实践，组织蒙医学专家对蒙医穴位的相关内容进行分析、归纳、总结，对蒙医传统疗法常用固定穴位名称、部位、位置、常用疗法、适应证和操作方法等进行规范，并结合现代物理学、电子技术、计算机技术和多媒体技术等相关知识研制而成的国内首例蒙医疗术电子穴位模型。

（二）结构

蒙医多媒体人体穴位模型由蒙医多媒体人体穴位光电模型，蒙医多媒体人体穴位按摩模型，计算机软件系统 3 个部分组成。

1. 模型外形

（1）模型身高为 170cm，真人比例，下面设有木板底座。

（2）蒙医多媒体人体穴位光电模型相应产品型号为 MAW-170E，右半身突出显示解剖，附带光电笔；模型人体表面穴位定位为蒙医穴位，穴位的名称以蒙文和汉文标注；穴位个数 115 个；模型上分布的穴位点数有 168 个，其中头部 13 个、胸腹部 46 个、后背部 54 个、上肢部 20 个、下肢部 35 个。

（3）蒙医多媒体人体穴位按摩模型相应产品型号为 MAW-170A，穿黑色紧身外套；模型人体表面穴位定位为蒙医穴位，穴位个数 112 个；模型上分布的穴位按压点数有 135 个，其中头部 13 个、胸腹部 45 个、后背部 32 个、上肢部 15 个、下肢部 30 个。

2. 计算机软件系统 蒙医多媒体人体穴位模型教学软件内容为蒙医，软件界面文字是汉文简体；由主界面和穴位声像界面组成，主界面连接模型；穴位声像界面上设置穴位搜索功能、范围搜索功能、穴位信息界面、图像显示、语音声响功能等。多媒体语音为普通话，内容包含穴位名称、部位名称、位置、白脉名称、适应疗法、灸疗法实施方法及适应证、针刺疗法实施方法及适应证；穴位搜索有按拼音搜索和按穴位名称搜索两种；图像有体表图像和深层解剖图像两种。

（三）穴位内容

蒙医多媒体人体穴位模型共标记常用穴位 115 个，分布的穴位点有 168 个，具体分布位置见图 4-2、图 4-3。

头部穴位：囟门穴、前额穴、眉穴、顶会穴、前顶会穴、后顶会穴、顶会左穴、顶会右穴、枕会穴、耳前穴、唇上穴、唇下穴。

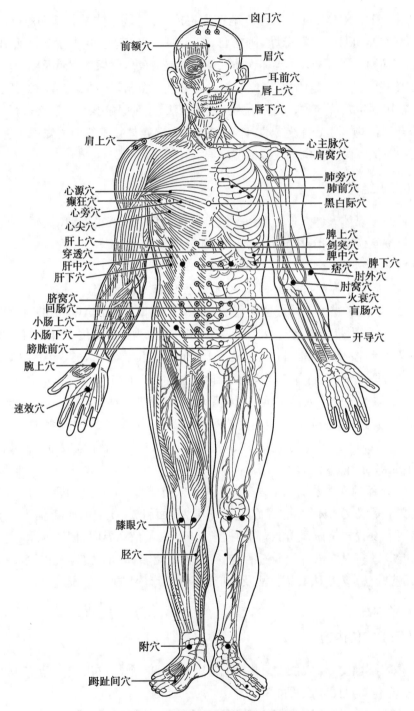

图 4-2 蒙医疗术人体穴位正面图

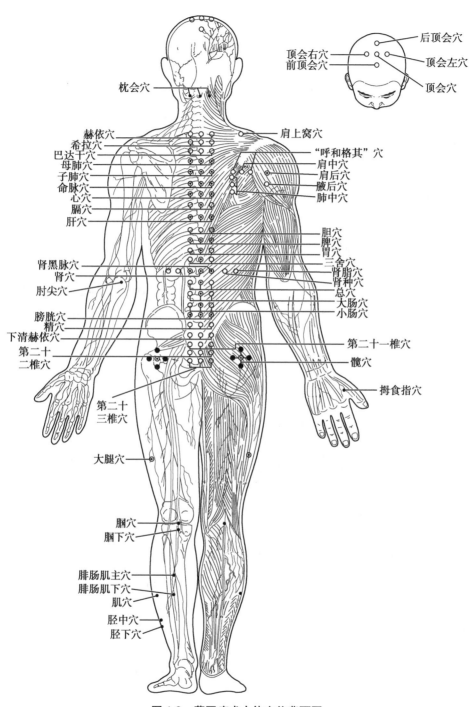

图 4-3 蒙医疗术人体穴位背面图

后背部穴位：赫依穴、希拉穴、巴达干穴、母肺穴、子肺穴、命脉穴、心穴、膈穴、肝穴、胆穴、脾穴、胃穴、三舍穴、肾穴、总穴、大肠穴、小肠穴、膀胱穴、精穴、下清赫依穴、第二十一椎穴、第二十二椎穴、第二十三椎穴、肺中穴、"呼和格其"穴、肩中穴、肾黑脉穴、肾种穴、肾脂穴。

胸腹部穴位：心主脉穴、黑白际穴、剑突穴、痞穴、火衰穴、脐窝穴、盲肠穴、回肠穴、小肠上穴、小肠下穴、膀胱前穴、子宫前穴、心源穴、癫狂穴、心尖穴、大分位穴、小分位穴、肺旁穴、肺前穴、肩上窝穴、心旁穴、心肺会穴、第八肋骨穴、锁骨下窝穴、肝上穴、肝中穴、肝下穴、脾上穴、脾中穴、脾下穴、穿透穴、开导穴、边缘穴、会阴穴。

上肢部穴位：肩窝穴、肩前穴、肩后穴、肩上穴、腋后穴、肘外穴、肘窝穴、肘尖穴、腕上穴、速效穴、拇食指穴、小指无名指穴、十指尖穴、无名指穴、拇指穴、腕背穴。

下肢部穴位：髋穴、髋突穴、长皱纹穴、大腿穴、大腿内穴、膝眼穴、髌鼻穴、胫穴、腘穴、腘下穴、腓肠肌主穴、腓肠肌下穴、肌穴、胫中穴、胫下穴、附穴、跟上穴、蹞趾间穴、副穴、蹞趾第一穴、蹞趾第二穴、蹞趾第三穴、足十趾尖穴、跟间穴。

（四）操作方法

蒙医多媒体人体穴位模型操作简便，容易掌握。其步骤如下：

1. 将光电模型、按摩模型、电脑和播放器等连接上电源。

2. 打开蒙医多媒体人体穴位模型界面，连接光电模型和按摩模型后进入穴位声像界面，见图4-4、图4-5。

3. 选定播放内容，如穴位名称、部位等，见图4-6。

4. 选择在界面上显示的形式，如穴位蒙文名称或汉语名称、体表图像或解剖图像等，见图4-7、图4-8。

5. 搜索穴位：①按拼音搜索穴位输入穴位名称拼音首字母即可，如搜索"眉穴"就写"mx"搜索，如图4-9所示；②按名称搜索就直接输入穴位名称搜索，见图4-10。

6. 光电模型是用光电笔操作，若想了解某一个穴位的相应内容，就用光电笔在模型上点那个穴位点，便会在电脑界面上显示和播放其穴位相应的信息，见图4-11。

7. 模拟模型上进行点穴训练，用手指准确按压穴位点后，其相应的信息会在电脑界面上显示和播放，同时光电模型上的相应穴位也会闪亮，见图4-12。

8. 操作结束后，点击"返回"至主界面，再点击"退出"，见图4-13。

9. 关闭电脑，断开电源。

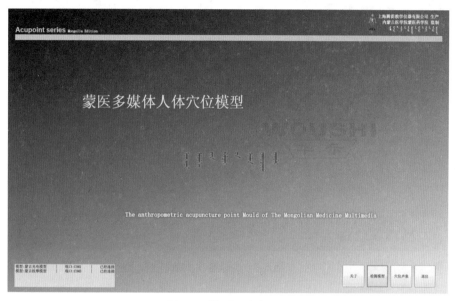

图4-4　模型系统主界面

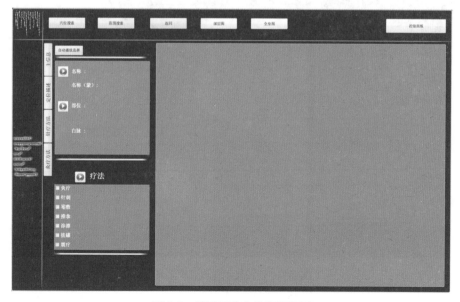

图4-5　模型系统穴位声像界面

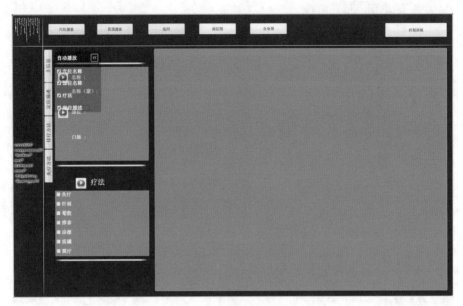

图 4-6 选择播放内容

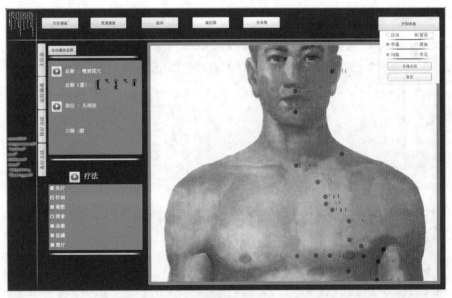

图 4-7 选择显示穴位蒙文名称

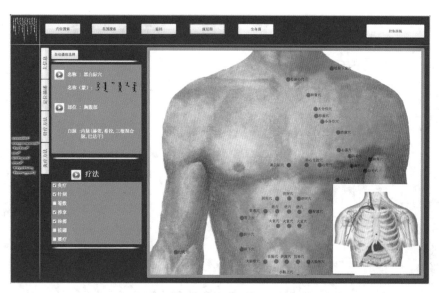

图 4-8　显示穴位体表和解剖位置图片

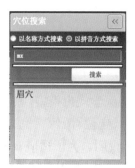

图 4-9　按拼音搜索穴位

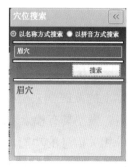

图 4-10　按穴位名称搜索穴位

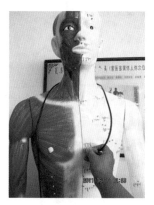

图 4-11　在光电模型上用光电笔操作

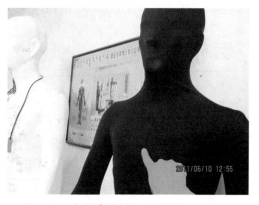

图 4-12　在按摩模型上用手指按压穴位点

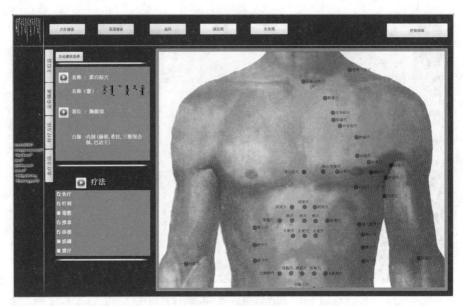

图 4-13　返回主界面

（五）特色和意义

蒙医多媒体人体穴位模型是国内首例根据蒙医传统疗法理论将蒙医穴位标记于人体上的蒙医学穴位模型，从根本上有别于其他医学穴位模型，具有国际先进水平。模型具有检索蒙医传统疗法穴位蒙汉名称、定位、图像、针法、灸法、适应证等相关信息的功能，并用文字和相应图谱显示说明。为了适应双语教学模式，系统设置了中文语音播放系统及蒙文文字注释系统，并配置了深层解剖结构显示系统，便于学生掌握穴位相关内容，练习点穴及操作实践。该模型引进到本科实验教学、研究生课题及临床实践，收到了良好的效果。

三、蒙医疗术铜人

蒙医疗术铜人是标记蒙医温针火针疗法等各种传统外治疗法穴位的铜人模型（图 4-14），现收藏于内蒙古医科大学所属蒙医药博物馆。该蒙医疗术铜人的体腔实，两足与鞋可以脱离。主体为黄铜铸造而成，鞋为紫铜皮焊接而成。

1. 蒙医疗术铜人的各部尺寸　总重量为 21kg，身高 61cm，莲花底座高 7cm。其中头部：头顶长 12.5cm，头围 28.5cm，面长 6.8cm，面宽 7cm，眉长 2.1cm，眼长 2cm，鼻长 2.5cm，鼻高 0.7cm，口长 2.1cm，耳长 4.6cm。项部：项高 2.5cm，项

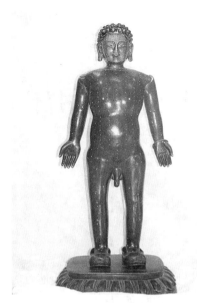

图 4-14 蒙医疗术铜人

围 15.5cm。躯干部：躯干长 25cm，胸围（平乳）42cm，两乳距 7cm，腹围（平脐）40cm，两髂距 16cm，阴茎长 5cm，阴茎粗 5cm。上肢部：上肢长（从肩峰至中指尖）25cm，肩宽 21.5cm，肱长 9cm，臂长 7.5cm，掌指长 7.5cm，肘围 12.2cm，手腕围 9.5cm。下肢部：下肢长（从髂至足底）30cm，股长 14cm，小腿（从膝至踝）长 16cm，足长 9.8cm，足宽 4.5cm，股部最粗部分 19.5cm，膝关节围 17cm。底座部：呈上部方形比下部方形窄的梯子形，上部的长度 25.5cm、宽度 19cm、高度 1.6cm，下部的长度 30cm、宽度 24cm、高度 1cm，两个方形中间距离 4.4cm，刻有 25 瓣莲花。两个鞋底长度 11cm，最宽处 5.5cm，最细处 4.8cm。颈部的裂缝长度 7.5cm，在颈部向下 1.5cm 处。

2. 蒙医疗术铜人的穴位数和分布情况 此蒙医疗术铜人没有经脉，只有孔穴，但均未记录穴名。铜人全身共有孔穴 611 个，除发际、掌、跖部无穴外，其他部位均有孔穴分布，每个孔穴均为直径 0.2～0.3 mm（小米粒大小）的圆形凹陷。左右侧对称穴 257 对，单穴 97 个，其中位于正中线上的单穴 62 个，35 个穴位没有标出其左右侧对称的穴位。铜人全身孔穴的分布统计如下：头部 110 穴（面部：9 列、75 穴，枕侧：9 列、35 穴）；颈部 7 穴；躯干部 257 穴（胸腹部：9 列、143 穴，背部：5 列、114 穴）；上肢部 119 穴（肱臂部：7 列、81 穴，手部：38 穴）；下肢部 118 穴（腿部：4 行、72 穴，足部：46 穴）。

第五章

蒙医温针火针疗法操作技术

一、基本练习

（一）针刺练习

蒙医温针火针疗法，其针刺操作需要经常不断地练习才能达到熟能生巧的程度。操作熟练后，不但动作敏捷，而且刺破皮肤时不痛或不太痛。如果操作不熟练，则不能得心应手地工作，进针费力而使患者疼痛加倍。由于操作运用不协调而引起患者不满，会直接影响治疗效果，因此，毫不懈怠地练习针刺技巧是很重要的。蒙医温针疗法主要选用银针，针身柔软，术者如不适当用力，很难直接刺入皮内并进行捻转，所以需要反复练习各种针刺技巧。可以先在纸上进行穿刺练习，将精纸和粗纸折成宽 7~8cm、厚 2cm 方块，用棉线紧紧缠绕后，先用短针，后用长针反复练习穿刺。方法是左手拿住纸块，右手拇、食、中指持针柄，边捻转边加大力度逐渐刺透纸块。捻针时尽量使针身保持垂直，逐渐加大指力。第二步可以在棉团上针刺练习，将棉团（直径 6~7cm）用线缠绕（内松外紧），再用一层布包住。然后用细针捻转穿刺并按要求练习各种针刺手法。在掌握了一定的技巧后就可以在自己身上试刺，试刺时要细心观察了解针刺技巧与刺激的关系，针尖达到不同组织构造时的手感等。针刺操作要达到无痛、熟练、指力均衡的程度，不使针身弯曲，且能随心捻转，持针的手要敏捷，针感迅速。

（二）加热练习

加热是蒙医温针疗法操作技术的关键环节，针刺后在针柄上加热，使温热刺激通过针体传入体内。应严格掌握加热程度和加热时间，一般给予针柄加热温度在 38~42℃，持续加热时间为 15~20 分钟。所以，主要反复练习在针柄上加热的各种技巧。临床常用的方法有：在针体装裹白山蓟绒（或艾绒），或用白山蓟卷（或艾卷）剪成长约 2cm 一段，从针尾插入到针柄部，点火加热；或直接在针柄上用蜡烛或酒精灯火焰加热；或用特制蒙医温针仪等设备加热。可以自己捏住针尖，在针柄上进行加热练习，细心感受传热情况及加热刺激的程度等。为了防止白山蓟（艾）灰脱落烫伤皮肤或损坏患者衣物，针柄上的白山蓟绒（艾绒）团必须捻紧，针旁可放置弯盘，也可以预先用硬纸剪成圆形纸片，并在中心剪出小缺口，置于针下穴区，加热时要嘱咐患者不要任意移动肢体，以防灼伤。如果用蒙医温针仪等专用设备加热，应遵循使用说明及注意事项的要求，认真练习操作方法，正确选择适合的参数，保证最佳加热刺激效果。

（三）烧针练习

烧针练习是指用火将针尖烧到红热的方法，是蒙医火针疗法操作技术的关键环节。在练习过程中，让针尖部位处于火的外焰，因外焰的温度最高，可使针尖部迅速红透；同时要仔细观察烧针过程中针尖部颜色的变化，一般针尖部通红并开始发白时温度达到最高，应反复练习如何使颜色达到此要求。

此时的火针进针时针不弯，入皮时没有明显疼痛，出针时不粘针，不滞针，轻快滑利，无痛感。出针后，针孔与周围皮肤基本平整无突起，局部微红，仅有短暂的微痒，甚至不痒。烧得红透的针尖在接触人体皮肤的一瞬间热量足，穿透力较强，刺进穴位阻力非常小。

二、针具

1. 针的构造 针分针尖、针身、针根、针柄、针顶五个部分。针的主要部分叫针身；针身的尖锐部分叫针尖；针身的终止部位叫针根；为了便于把持，用金属细丝螺旋状包缠制作的部分叫针柄；针柄的终止部分叫针顶。

2. 针的制作 针刺疗法主要使用金属特制的器械，有金针、银针、青铜针、铜针、铁针、骨针等。目前在临床上主要用银针。针质量的好坏，与其制作材料有关。质量好的针尖，光滑而无豁口，犹如松树的针叶。针尖的锥度适当而刺入时阻力小。针身光滑而直，圆而平，结实而富有弹性。针根没有生锈腐蚀。针柄的缠丝结实，把持舒适，这样的针便于操作，利于捻转。针顶稍凸起便于观察针的捻转度及方向，并且在针柄上缠绕的灸炷不易脱落。

3. 形状和规格 针的形状有多种：如大麦头针、蛙头针、矛头针、荞麦头针等。要根据病患部位和病情决定使用何种针。如大麦头针尖细而中段粗，主要用于医治心、肺、肾及关节的疾病；矛头针用于针刺排出关节黄水或脓液；荞麦头针用于刮除眼翳（图5-1）。

按照现代临床蒙医诊疗技术规范要求，我们对蒙医温针火针疗法针具等进行了规范化研究（笔者主持完成内蒙古自然科学基金项目《蒙医温针疗法操作技术及器械的规范化研究》，编号 200508010918），制定了蒙医温针疗法的针具规格（表5-1），本书即采用此标准。

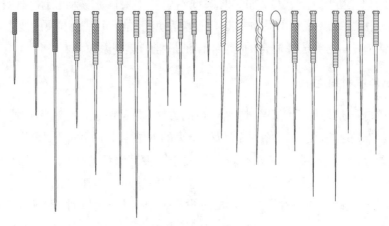

图 5-1 针的形状

表 5-1 蒙医温针银针规格

银针规格	Ⅰ号	Ⅱ号	Ⅲ号	Ⅳ号	Ⅴ号
针长 /cm	3	5	8	11	13
针身长 /cm	2	3	5	7	8
针柄长 /cm	1	2	3	4	5
针身直径 /mm	0.3	0.8	0.8	0.8	0.9

三、常用加热材料及器具

（一）常用加热材料

1. 白山蓟 白山蓟具有易于点燃，火力温柔而持久，灰烬不散的特点。并具有改善赫依血运行，祛除巴达干赫依之邪的功能，是较理想的灸材。生长成熟的白山蓟在秋季采集，除去杂质，阴干后用木棒或其他器具反复捶捣成棉花样白山蓟绒。将加工好的白山蓟绒装裹在针柄上，点火加热；或将白山蓟绒做成白山蓟卷（条），再剪成长 0.5～1cm 一段，从针尾插入到针柄加热部位，点火加热；或将白山蓟卷（条）的一端点燃，对准针体加热部位，进行熏烤。

在蒙医临床中，对穴位单灸时也可选用白山蓟绒，称白山蓟灸法。白山蓟灸又分直接灸和间接灸两种。直接灸是将白山蓟绒制灸炷直接放在穴位上施灸。间接灸是在灸炷和穴位表皮之间另放其他物质再施灸，如隔姜灸、隔蒜灸等。或将白山蓟制成灸条点燃一头，置于距穴位表皮约1寸空间处施灸。一般灸1～5炷或间接灸5～20分钟。

2. 艾绒 由菊科植物艾蒿的干叶制成。其色泽灰白，柔软如绒，易燃而不起火焰，气味芳香，适合灸用。根据加工程度的不同有粗细之分，粗者多用于温针或制作艾条，细者多用于制作艾炷。质地以陈年者为佳。将加工好的艾绒装裹在针柄上，点火加热；或将艾绒制作成艾条，再剪成长0.5～1cm一段，从针尾插入到针柄加热部位，点火加热；或将艾条的一端点燃，对准针体加热部位，进行熏烤。

蒙医临床中，对穴位单灸时经常选用艾绒，称艾灸法。艾灸又分直接灸和间接灸两种。直接灸是将艾绒制灸炷直接放在穴位上施灸。间接灸是在灸炷和穴位表皮之间另放其他物质再施灸，如隔姜灸、隔蒜灸等。或将艾条点燃一头，置于距穴位表皮约1寸空间处施灸。一般灸1～5炷或间接灸5～20分钟。

3. 酒精灯 酒精灯是以酒精为燃料的加热工具，用于加热物体。酒精灯由灯体、灯芯管和灯帽组成。蒙医温针火针疗法用酒精灯加热时，直接将酒精灯火焰靠近针柄加热部位，进行加热。酒精量不超过酒精灯容积的2/3，也不能少于1/4。用完酒精灯，火焰必须用灯帽盖灭，不可用嘴吹灭，以免引起灯内酒精燃烧，发生危险。

4. 蜡烛 蜡烛是一种日常照明工具，主要用石蜡制成，在古代，通常由动物油脂制造。蒙医温针疗法用蜡烛加热时，直接将点燃蜡烛的火焰靠近针柄加热部位，进行加热。

（二）MLY-I型蒙医疗术温针仪

MLY-I型蒙医疗术温针仪是一种蒙医温针疗法加热专用新型医疗器械。根据蒙医温针疗法的性能特征及临床应用情况，运用现代电能转换为热能的原理，结合温针刺激及药物导入等方面的最新研究成果，对蒙医传统温针疗法的器具及操作方法进行革新，以减少副作用、提高疗效为切入点，对器械的制作及设计进行反复验证，最终研制成功的具有蒙医疗术特色的新型医疗器械。2005年10月制定注册产品标准，并经内蒙古自治区产品质量检验研究院检验，各项指标均达到了合格标准。该项研究核心技术-电热温针器已获国家实用新型专利授权（电热温针器，国家知识产权局，专利号 ZL201120058078.0）。

MLY-Ⅰ型蒙医疗术温针仪由温针仪主机和多个温灸器组成。主机包括变压器、整流器、指示仪表和功率调节装置，变压器的输出端与整流器的输入端连接，整流器输出端上依次串联指示仪表、功率调节装置和温灸器的电热丝，并组成一个闭合的回路；温灸器由圆桶装的温灸器壳体、发热体、电热丝、绝缘隔热层组成，温灸器壳体底部的中心有壳体针孔，发热体置于温灸器壳体内，发热体为T形结构，在发热体的竖杆内设有发热针孔，在发热体的竖杆外壁上装有电热丝，发热体的竖杆与温灸器壳体内壁之间装有绝缘隔热层，发热体针孔与发热器壳体针孔连通。该器械在继承蒙医传统温针疗法的特色与优点的同时，克服了蒙医传统温针疗法加热时火力不均、针眼易感染、有烟等不足，从而更加适应现代医疗市场要求。具有操作简单、易于掌握、无污染且可量化等优点，已在临床中广泛应用。同时也为蒙医温针疗法开展动物实验研究等方面提供了方便。

1. 主要特点　①利用电能将银针或毫针加热，具有较好的加热传热作用；②利用电能加温白山蓟绒或艾绒等，使热能最有效地作用于白山蓟绒或艾绒上，加强热能和白山蓟绒或艾绒等的穿透皮肤的能力，提高了蒙医温针疗法的有效性与安全性；③根据不同的病症及刺激程度要求，可灵活选用白山蓟绒或艾绒等不同材料。

2. 技术指标　①额定电压：220V±22V，输出功率≤20W，工作电流：0～30mA；②额定频率：（50±1）Hz；③输出电机：四路；④热灸温度：30～60℃范围内稳定可调；⑤工作条件：环境温度0～30℃；相对湿度不高于85%；⑥外形尺寸：13.3cm×35.3cm×27.5cm；⑦重量：2.5kg。

3. 操作方法　①在使用前将输出旋钮转到零位，按下电源开关接通电源，指示灯发光，显示电源工作正常；②输出线的输出插头插入输出孔，工作指示灯亮，一般使用前预热5分钟为宜；③温灸器壳体内围绕发热体的竖杆装好白山蓟绒或艾绒或其他药物，也可以根据不同疾病，自行配伍相应灸药；④按下与其相对应的电流测量键，调节温控旋钮，顺时针旋转为增高，反之为降低，调节增加电流量时应视患者的身体情况，以调到患者能承受的适当量，并视病情等灵活调节时间；⑤患者需多穴位治疗时，可将另一个（或多个）输出线接在相应输出孔，工作指示灯亮之后，按病情调温即可；⑥治疗完毕，首先将输出调节旋钮按逆时针方向旋回零位，然后关闭电源。

4. 注意事项　①使用本机治疗时必须在医生的指导下进行；②每个穴位治疗时间不能过长，一般不超过20分钟，避免烫伤；③本机避免敲打、碰撞，防止受潮热，贮存温度10～30℃为宜。

四、操作方法

（一）操作前准备

1. 针具的选用 蒙医温针火针治疗前必须细致检查针具情况,针具生锈弯曲或不符合要求时,需要更换。挑选针具应注意以下几点。

（1）检查针尖:主要检查针尖是否有弯曲和倒钩。用拇、食、中指抓住针柄,一边捻转一边用无名指腹轻触针尖边缘,可判断是否有钩。

（2）检查针身:细致检查针身是否粗糙、有斑点、生锈剥蚀、弯曲等。将针放在光滑干净的桌子上,使其轻轻翻滚,弯曲部分不能紧贴桌面。如果有微小斑点及生锈剥蚀时,可用放大镜详细检查针根。

（3）检查针柄:一手抓住针柄,另一手紧紧捏住针身向相反方向牵拉,或交错牵拉、捻转。

2. 加热材料准备 蒙医温针火针治疗前必须选好并认真准备加热材料及器具、温针仪等。

3. 穴位的确定和消毒

（1）穴位的确定:根据患者情况,制定施疗方案,按施疗方案确定选穴。为了明确穴位,可用手指按压穴位并观察患者的反应。正确的穴位用手指按压时患者应有明显的麻木感。

（2）术前消毒:主要包括器械的消毒,术者手的消毒,针刺部位的消毒等。

1）器械的消毒:消毒方法有多种,其中高压灭菌法最佳。将针等器械用布包好,以 1.0～1.5kPa 压强,115～123℃温度,煮沸 30 分钟以上才能达到无菌的要求。也有药液浸泡消毒法,如把器械放置在 75% 的酒精里浸泡 30～60 分钟后擦干使用。还可使用器械消毒液,如在 0.1% 新洁尔灭加 0.5% 亚硝酸钠溶液里浸泡消毒等。消毒过的针及其他器械放在专用针盘里用消毒纱布覆盖。

2）术者手的消毒:施疗前用肥皂水洗手或用酒精棉擦手后方可操作。

3）针刺部位的消毒:将针刺部位的皮肤用 75% 的酒精棉由内向外环行擦拭消毒。或在穴位处先涂 2% 的碘酒,待干后再用 75% 的酒精擦掉碘酒。

（二）刺法

1. 患者体位 患者体位对确定穴位和施术都有直接影响。体位的选择应以术者能正确找到穴位,操作方便,患者感觉舒适为原则。对体弱病重和易晕针患者最好采用卧位。为避免弯针、断针或加重疼痛，在蒙医温针火针治疗针刺和加热时都不要改变患者体位。临床上常采用以下几种体位：

（1）仰卧位：适合于针刺身体前面的穴位。

（2）俯卧位：适合于针刺背、腰、臀以及下肢后面的穴位。

（3）侧卧位：适合于针刺身体侧面的穴位。

（4）后仰坐位：适合于针刺头、面部、颈项前部、胸部、肩、前臂、膝部和胫、踝等的穴位。

（5）前俯坐位：适合于针刺头顶、枕部及颈项后部及肩、背部穴位。

（6）偏斜坐位：适合于针刺头顶、颞、腮部穴位。

（7）屈肘掌侧位：适合于针刺肩、上臂、前臂屈侧及掌部穴位。

（8）屈肘手背位：适合于针刺肩、上臂、前臂伸侧及手背部穴位。

（9）屈肘掌外侧位：适合于针刺肩、上臂、前臂外侧及腕、掌部穴位。

2. 针刺的总方法 明确穴位后，用右手拇指和食指在针尖以上 0.5 寸处持针，迅速地刺破皮肤，逐渐深刺。此时必须集中注意力，严格掌握针刺方向和深度，注意患者施术部位麻木等感觉，同时注意患者的面部表情。

3. 针刺的具体方法 正确掌握针刺的角度、方向及深度，对增强针感，促进痊愈及防止发生异常现象等颇为重要。正确的穴位，不单指皮肤表面的穴位位置，还包括正确的针刺角度、方向及深度。进针的方向、角度和深度不同时，即使针刺同一穴位，针尖达到的组织结构及针感、功效等都有差别。根据医疗需要及患者体质强弱、胖瘦等具体情况，针刺的具体方法有横刺、直刺、下刺、上刺、十字形刺、外翻刺、避开脏腑刺、避开要害部位刺等 8 种（图 5-2）。

（1）横刺：将针横向刺入，针身与皮肤呈 15°～25° 角。此法用于肌肉较薄部位及肝、脾、肾等重要脏腑对应的体表穴位。将两穴互相穿透时亦可用此法。

（2）直刺：针身与皮肤呈 90° 的直角，针尖垂直而下，适用于肌肉丰满部位和脊椎关节、下腹部等处。

（3）斜刺：包括下刺和上刺。下刺指针尖向下，针身与皮肤呈近 45° 的斜角，适用于不能深刺部位的穴位或针刺肺与心穴、剑突穴等；上刺指针尖向上，针身与皮肤呈近 45° 的斜角，此法适用于不能深刺部位的穴位及肺、心等重要脏腑对应的体表穴位。

（4）十字形刺：针身与皮肤呈 90° 的直角直刺下去穿透皮肤之后，针尖向四方旋动，适用于肌肉丰满部位的穴位，胃痞块及脓液等。

（5）外翻刺：针尖刺入后向外翻，由一穴位向另一穴位穿透，适用于胃部穴位、膝眼及大腿下部诸穴位。

（6）避开脏腑刺：在胸部及腹部针刺时，必须注意不要伤及五脏六腑而准确地针刺所需之穴位。

（7）避开要害刺：病在要害部位而进行针刺疗法施治时，要注意不伤及要害部位，如眼病、心脏积水、肝痞、肾痞及排脓等。

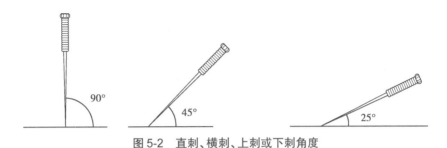

图 5-2　直刺、横刺、上刺或下刺角度

4. 针刺手法　有单手针刺、双手针刺、管针针刺 3 种。

（1）单手针刺：用一手拇指和食指持针，中指尖触到穴位、指腹支住针身下端，以拇指和食指之力将针沿中指刺入皮肤。

（2）双手针刺：两手配合针刺，有如下几种常用方法。

1）嵌刺：这是在临床上最多用的刺法。用左手拇指或食指指甲嵌于穴位，右手持针使针尖沿指甲刺入皮肤。

2）抓刺：用左手拇指和食指抓住针身下端，右手拇指和食指抓住针柄，针尖对准穴位，用两手平衡力量把针迅速刺入皮肤。此法主要在用 3 寸以上的长针针刺时应用。

3）抻刺：左手五指伸直，用食指和中指抻开穴位的皮肤，右手持针，从左手食指和中指间刺入皮肤。当捻针时，为避免弯针，以食指和中指夹住针身。此法主要在长针深刺时使用。在皮肤松弛或褶皱部位针刺时，用拇指和食指或食指和中指抻开皮肤，如针刺腹部诸穴位等。

4）捏刺：用左手拇指与食指捏住穴位的皮肤，右手持针，在捏起处的正中针刺。此法用于肌肉较薄的部位，特别是面部穴位的针刺。

（3）管针针刺：用左手将特制的金属或其他安全材料制作的套管放置于针刺的穴位上，右手持针沿套管内刺入皮肤。视针刺穴位选好长或短针及金属套管，套管要比针短 0.3～0.5 寸。将套管对准穴位放置，然后先将针放进套管中，用左手食指指腹叩击露出的针柄针刺，然后取下套管，刺入适当深度。

5. 针刺度　针刺度指进针的深浅度。

（1）总针刺度：针刺进针时刺皮肤较硬，到肌肉软而顺畅，到骨骼则受阻。

因此要根据针刺的穴位及该部位的特点、肌肉的厚薄以及病情等灵活制定针刺度。针刺过程中要详细观察患者面部表情的变化，并询问是否出现眩晕等症状，以防发生意外。在脏腑器官及要害处等不能深刺。在头部及胸部穴位要浅而斜刺或横刺。刺皮肤时似有干涩感，在肌肉柔软处进针快，触及骨头时受阻而不能进。针尖达到针刺的深度时将针向外稍拔出一点放置。

（2）具体针刺度：当针尖接近五脏时，患者出现神志紊乱，身体颤抖、眼睛倒翻，针身颤动。针尖接近其他要害部位时亦有类似表现。触及主脉时，针旁出现搏动；触及肺叶时，患者鼻孔煽动，微有咳嗽；触及肝、脾时，恶心、流涎；触及肾时，肾脏剧痛，肾脉欲裂。脏器进针，脏器收缩似被吸引，肝、脾、肾三者无此现象；针刺胃时，感觉较硬，此时肝有翻搅感，易转化为肝病，应格外谨慎；触及痞块时，有坚硬之感，伴刺痛致使患者难以忍受而失声。痞块初期要围绕针刺，陈旧后可频频进针，水肿的郁气等可以直接针刺排出；头部及四肢关节可以刺入关节间隙或刺及骨头，针刺肌肉可视其厚度进针半寸。

总而言之，针刺手法以既给以适当的刺激又不伤及主要脏腑及器官为原则。每个穴位的针刺度要视患者的具体情况、年龄、体力、脉道之深浅、疾病的不同时期等灵活掌握。如形体消瘦者、身体虚弱者要浅刺，身体强壮者可以适当深刺；老年人、小儿则都不能深刺；头面部及胸腹部位的穴位应浅刺；四肢及臀部穴位可适当深刺；肘部及髋部穴位白脉运行较深，所以针刺可以稍深；手指、足趾白脉运行较浅，所以进针应稍浅；当疾病分布于皮肤或扩散于肌肉之际，应浅刺；渗于骨骼或窜行于脉道时，稍深刺；降于脏、落于腑而趋于陈旧时，可适当深刺。针刺深度与角度及方向是相互关联的。深刺法多用于直刺，浅刺法则主要用于横刺或上刺及下刺。头、脊椎、眼部、胸部前后部的穴位，都位于主要脏器附近，更要严格掌握针刺的深度、角度及方向，以防发生医疗事故。

（三）加热

1. 加热方法

（1）熏烤加热法：将加热材料裹在针柄上，点燃加热的方法。此方法用于蒙医温针疗法。多用白山蓟绒或艾绒加热，将加工好的白山蓟绒（艾绒）装裹在针柄上，点火加热；或将白山蓟（艾绒）做成白山蓟卷条（艾条），再剪成长0.5～1cm一段，从针尾插入到针柄加热部位，点火加热；或将白山蓟卷条（艾条）的一端点燃，对准针体加热部位，进行熏烤。

（2）火焰加热法：直接将加热材料燃烧的火焰靠近针柄加热部位进行加热的方法。蒙医温针疗法多用酒精灯或蜡烛加热，直接将酒精灯或蜡烛火焰靠近针柄加热部位,进行加热。蒙医火针疗法用酒精灯或蜡烛加热,直接将针尖在酒精灯或蜡烛火焰上烧红,迅速进行针刺。

(3)温针仪加热法:用蒙医温针疗法专用温针仪加热的方法。只用于蒙医温针疗法。

2. 加热温度 根据不同穴位及病情等,灵活掌握加热温度。蒙医温针疗法给予针柄加热温度为38～42℃。蒙医火针疗法需烧至针尖变红后,方可针刺。

3. 加热时间 根据不同穴位及病情等,灵活掌握蒙医温针疗法加热时间,如面部眼睛周围穴位可加热 3～5 分钟;胸腹部穴位可加热 10～15 分钟;背部及四肢穴位可加热 15～20 分钟等。蒙医火针疗法针刺之后不再进行加热,留针 1～3 分钟即可。

(四)拔针

拔针是蒙医温针火针疗法的最后一步。拔针时先用左手拇指和食指拿住消毒棉按住针刺处周围的皮肤,右手拇指和食指抓住针柄缓慢地边捻边拔,至皮下时迅速拔出。蒙医温针治疗后,皮肤上可能有局部充血或是有红、热、痛及轻微的水肿现象,拔针后做好针刺部位的消毒,以防感染。

五、疗程与间隔时间

急性疾患每天或隔日 1 次,一般每天针刺主治功效相近的不同穴位,3 次为 1 个疗程;慢性疾患 3～7 天 1 次,一般每次针刺主治功效相近的不同穴位,3～5 次为 1 个疗程。2 个疗程之间应该有 1～2 周的休息。

视频 1　常用材料及器具		视频 3　加热	
视频 2　针刺的总方法		视频 4　拔针	

第六章

蒙医温针火针疗法意外的防治

一、晕针

晕针是指在针刺过程中，患者突然出现脸色苍白、头晕目眩、心慌气短、冷汗淋漓、烦躁干呕、疲乏无力、脉象沉而细等症状，重者可出现四肢发凉、神志不清、二便失禁等症状。这些多由患者体弱、精神过于紧张或疲劳过度、出汗过多、饥饿、腹泻、大出血、体位不当或术者操作手法过于粗暴等原因所致。患者有晕针情况时当立即停止针刺并拔针，令患者卧床。症状轻者静卧片刻，喝热水或热奶茶就可苏醒；重者可在上述处理后，针刺人中穴、二十指趾尖、胫穴或在顶会穴、小肠上穴、膀胱前穴等施以间接灸，必要时亦可采取其他抢救措施。

为了防止出现上述晕针现象，应先了解患者的体质及对刺激的耐力。对初次接受针刺治疗而有紧张表现的患者，应做好解释安慰，解除其顾虑，最好使患者取卧位或舒适而能持久的体位，一次针刺的穴位不可过多，刺激量不应过重。对过于疲劳或饥饿的患者，应在休息或用餐后再行针刺。要时刻注意观察患者的情况，如有面色苍白、发呆、紧张、作呕等症状出现时要及早采取措施。

二、滞针

滞针是指进针后出现的捻针及拔针困难。这主要由于进针不当，过于突然用力，或将针刺入肌腱，捻转过甚或单向捻转，致使肌纤维缠绕针身，或由于患者惧怕和疼痛而精神紧张，局部肌肉强烈收缩等所致。若由于患者体位变更而致滞针时，要及时纠正其体位。由于患者精神紧张或局部肌肉收缩所致者，令患者放松紧张状态，用手指揉摩针刺穴位周围，可使肌肉放松。如由于单向捻转所致者，反向捻转及左右捻转即可。对初次受针刺治疗和惧怕针刺的患者，应事先进行安慰，解除其顾虑，针刺时要避开肌腱，刺针的捻转度不可过大或过快，特别是禁止持续性单向捻转。滞针时切不可用力拔出。

三、弯针

弯针是指进针后针身弯曲，导致针柄的方向和角度与进针前有所变异而导致捻针及拔针困难的现象。这是由于术者的针刺技术不熟练，持针指用力过度，或针尖触及坚硬组织，或进针后患者体位变动压迫针柄所致。如果针身稍微弯曲，则反复捻转徐徐拔出即可；如弯度较大，则轻轻捻动、把针沿弯曲之方向拔出；如针身不止一处弯曲，应视针柄倾斜方向，分段徐徐拔出。为了避免断针，不可骤然拔针。如由于患者体位变动所致，令其恢复原体位，使局部肌肉放松后拔针。术者必须练习针刺技术，熟能生巧，治疗时使患者取舒适的体位，留针时尽量避免变动体位，并注意避免碰压针柄。弯针时不可硬刺下去或用力拔出。

四、断针

断针是指拔针时针身折断，或残端留在患者体内。主要由于针质欠佳，针身或针根腐蚀，或针刺时操作不当，如过度用力捻针，导致肌肉收缩，或患者体位变动，压迫针刺部位及针柄，或滞针、弯针后没有及时处理等原因所致。处理方法是嘱患者不要紧张，不要乱动，以防断端向肌肉深层陷入，如断端还在体外，可用镊子取出；如断端陷入肌肉层内，先看该部位是否在重要脏腑旁边或是否阻碍活动，避免过度活动导致断端深入，应用 X 线明确其位置，外科手术取出。为避免断针，在针刺前要详细检查针具。针刺时不可将针身完全刺入体内，应保持部分针身露于体外。

五、肿胀

肿胀是指拔针后，针孔出现发紫、肿胀、疼痛等症状。当针刺时不慎伤及细小血管，尤其针尖弯曲成钩时易发生此类现象。皮肤轻微发紫者会自然消退。如发紫、肿胀较严重并妨碍活动时，先冷敷止血，后施热敷；或轻揉该部位以散瘀血。

操作前详细检查针具，明确解剖位置，针刺时避开血脉。持针之手要敏捷，针刺要害部位的穴位时更要谨慎从事。

六、后遗刺激

后遗刺激是指拔针之后，在针孔部位出现酸痛、胀痛、麻木等刺激性症状。多由术者操作手法过重或留针时间过长所致。轻者在该部位轻揉症状即可消失；重者除在局部轻揉外可用艾团施间接灸。通常在拔针之后轻揉可防止出现后遗刺激。

七、刺伤重要器官

指由于针刺过深而刺伤脏腑及要害部位。

1. 创伤性气胸　前后胸部和锁骨附近穴位针刺过深时，极易刺伤肺脏而导致创伤性气胸。此时，患者突然出现胸痛、气短、心颤、冷汗淋漓、神志昏迷、血压下降、昏厥等现象。听诊呼吸运动减弱，闻及过清音，肺泡音减低或消失，重者气管向健侧移位，借助 X 线检查可进一步确诊。有的患者在针刺后并无任何表现，数小时后逐渐出现胸痛、气急等症状，应予注意。为预防气胸，当施针刺疗法时，要集中注意力，令患者取适当的体位，视其胖瘦决定针刺深度。另外，在进针后不可过度捻转。对前后胸部的穴位，要用斜刺、横刺法，留针时间不宜过长。少量出气会自然吸收，如出现咳嗽等表现则必须详细检查后及时处理。如有气急、发紫、昏厥等表现则应当立即采取急救措施，如胸腔闭式引流术等。

2. 刺伤心、肝、脾、肾　在心、肝、脾、肾等脏区，针刺过深时，会造成严重后果，因此，对心脏扩大、肝脾肿胀的患者施术时，应格外注意。

刺伤肝、脾导致出血时，肝区或脾区发生疼痛，有时向后背放射痛。继续出血刺激腹膜时可有腹痛、腹肌僵硬伴压痛等表现。刺伤肾脏时出现腰痛，肾区压痛，叩痛及血尿等症状。如大出血则导致血压下降、昏厥等全身性症状。五脏轻微损伤经休息可自然恢复。如考虑出血，应详细检查，注意病情和血压的变化，必要时使用止血药或局部冷罨止血。如损伤重而引起休克时，必须立即采取急救措施。

此外，由于肿胀、尿闭、肠粘连等原因，胆、膀胱、胃、肠等六腑亦有被刺伤的可能。如刺伤大血管引起大出血，要格外留心。

3. 刺伤脑、脊髓　针刺颈项部正中及其两侧的穴位，如不严格限制进针的角度、方向及深度则易误伤延髓，引起严重后果。在背部正中线第 1 腰椎以上的穴位针刺，如进针过深，易伤脊髓。此时，患者有电击的感觉并向四肢放射，刺激严重可留后遗症。过强的刺激会使四肢短暂瘫痪,刺伤血管可引起血肿。因此,在这些部位针刺时,必须加倍注意针感,禁忌胡乱捻转针身。轻者稍休息即可恢复,如出现头痛、恶心、呕吐等表现或昏迷时应立即抢救。

4. 刺伤神经干 刺伤神经干及神经元时,受伤神经感觉和活动均受影响,患者有灼痛、反射性肌抽搐或痉挛等表现。

八、转化为热证

主要由于将热证误诊为寒证而施温针或痞病由于血、希拉之邪而转化为热证所致。常在温针治疗后1~3天内有反应,针孔红肿、跳痛、全身灼热感、头剧痛及某些部位的淋巴结肿痛等。同时,脉象及尿象均出现热证。为此,在针刺施治前,对患者务必全面诊察,特别要详查是否有潜伏热,操作要谨慎而熟练,嘱咐做好饮食起居方面的护理。

九、转化为寒证

主要由扩散之赫依引起,通常针刺后立即出现反应,表现为疼痛、颤抖、干呕等。有时由于刺破水痞,其水扩散于六腑造成全身浮肿。因此,在针刺施疗之前,要注意诱发赫依之因素,适当应用抑制赫依之药物,如有水痞则应更加谨慎。

中篇

临床应用

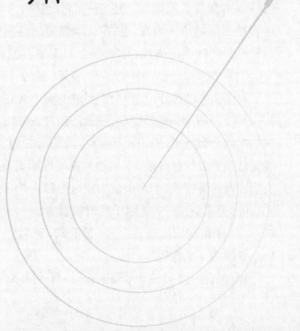

第七章

蒙医疗术科疾病

一、神经性头痛

神经性头痛主要是指紧张性头痛、功能性头痛及血管神经性头痛，多由精神紧张、生气引起，主要症状为持续性的头部闷痛、压迫感、沉重感，有的患者自诉为头部有"紧箍"感。大部分患者为两侧头痛，多为两颞侧、后枕部及头顶部或全头部。蒙医学称之为"赫依性头痛病"等。

【病因】神经性头痛源于头部肌肉紧张收缩，吸烟饮酒过度时会加剧。生活不规律、烟酒无度、睡眠不足等均为诱因。

【临床表现】头痛性质为钝痛、胀痛，伴压迫感、麻木感和束带样紧箍感。头痛的强度为轻度至中度，很少因头痛而卧床不起或影响日常生活。有的患者可有长年累月的持续性头痛，有的患者的症状甚至可回溯10～20年。患者可以整天头痛，头痛的时间要多于不痛的时间。因为激动、生气、失眠、焦虑或抑郁等因素常使头痛加剧。还有一部分患者，不仅具有紧张性头痛的特点，还有血管性头痛的临床表现，主诉双颞侧搏动性头痛。这种既有紧张性头痛，又有血管性头痛的临床表现，称为混合型头痛。患者多伴有头晕、烦躁易怒、焦虑不安、心慌、气短、恐惧、耳鸣、失眠多梦、腰酸背痛、颈部僵硬等症状。

对于头痛的诊疗，进行全面系统的病史询问及相应的辅助检查是十分必要的。2004年2月国际头痛学会(International Headache Society，HIS)颁布了第2版《国际头痛疾病分类》(ICHD-Ⅱ)。该标准将头痛分为3大部分14类，包括原发性头痛、继发性头痛及颅神经痛、中枢性和原发性面痛及其他头痛。蒙医传统疗法对各类头痛皆有显著疗效，但目前认为蒙医温针火针疗法主要对神经性头痛作用显著。

【治疗】方法一：适用于病情较轻者。

穴位：每次依次选顶会穴、顶前穴、顶后穴、顶右穴、顶左穴中1个，隔2日1次，5次为1个疗程。

操作：选用Ⅰ号或Ⅱ号蒙医银针，平刺0.5～1寸。温针给予针柄加热，温度

38～42℃，15～20分钟；或火针留针15～20分钟。

方法二：适用于病情较重者。

穴位：首次选顶会穴，并配中间赫依穴；第二次开始每次依次选顶前穴、顶后穴、顶右穴、顶左穴中1个，隔2日1次，5次为1个疗程。

操作：选用Ⅰ号或Ⅱ号蒙医银针，顶会穴平刺0.5～1寸，中间赫依穴直刺0.5～1寸，给予针柄加热，温度38～42℃，15～20分钟。

【按语】①保持身心愉快，避免情绪激动。②清淡饮食，忌刺激性食物。③劳逸结合，注意休息。

二、面神经瘫痪

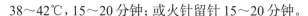

面神经瘫痪，简称面瘫，学名面神经麻痹，也称面神经炎、贝尔麻痹、亨特综合征。蒙医学称之为"面萨病"。是以面部表情肌群运动功能障碍为主要特征的一种常见病，一般症状是口眼㖞斜。它是一种常见病、多发病，不受年龄和性别限制，患者往往连最基本的抬眉、闭眼、鼓腮、努嘴等动作都无法完成。

【病因】临床上根据损害发生部位可分为中枢性面神经炎和周围性面神经炎两种。中枢性面神经炎病变位于面神经核以上至大脑皮层之间的皮质延髓束，通常由脑血管病、颅内肿瘤、脑外伤、炎症等引起。周围性面神经炎病损发生于面神经核和面神经。

【临床表现】多数患者往往在清晨洗脸、漱口时突然发现一侧面颊动作不灵、嘴巴㖞斜。病侧面部表情肌完全瘫痪者，前额纹消失、眼裂扩大、鼻唇沟平坦、口角下垂，露齿时口角向健侧偏㖞。病侧不能做皱额、蹙眉、闭目、鼓气和噘嘴等动作。鼓腮和吹口哨时，因患侧口唇不能闭合而漏气。进食时，食物残渣常滞留于病侧的齿颊间隙内，并常有口水自该侧淌下。由于泪点随下睑外翻，使泪液外溢而流泪。

蒙医温针火针疗法主要对周围性面神经炎作用显著。

【治疗】方法一：适用于病情较轻者。

穴位：每次依次选耳后穴、颊穴、眉上穴中1个，隔2日1次，3次为1个疗程。

操作：选用Ⅰ号或Ⅱ号蒙医银针，平耳后穴刺0.5～1寸，颊穴向外上方平刺0.5～1寸，眉上穴平刺0.3～0.5寸。温针给予针柄加热，温度38～42℃，15～20分钟；或火针留针15～20分钟。

方法二：适用于病情较重者。

穴位：每次依次选耳后穴、颊穴、眉上穴、唇上穴、唇下穴、眉穴中1个，隔日 1 次,6 次为 1 个疗程。

操作:选用 I 号或 II 号蒙医银针,平耳后穴刺 0.5~1 寸,颊穴向外上方平刺 0.5~1 寸,眉上穴平刺 0.3~0.5 寸,唇上穴向上斜刺 0.3~0.5 寸,唇下穴直刺 0.3~0.5 寸或斜刺 0.5~1 寸,眉穴向上或左、右平刺 0.3~0.5 寸。温针给予针柄加热,温度 38~42℃,15~20 分钟;或火针留针 15~20 分钟。

【按语】①保持心情舒畅。②保护面部,避免受寒。③注意眼睛和口腔卫生,防止感染。④适当热敷,并做面部运动锻炼。

三、三叉神经痛

三叉神经痛是最常见的脑神经疾病,以一侧面部三叉神经分布区内反复发作的阵发性剧烈痛为主要表现,女略多于男,发病率可随年龄而增长。三叉神经痛多发生于中老年人,右侧多于左侧。蒙医学认为,三叉神经痛属"亚玛"病。

【病因】三叉神经痛的病因及发病机制,至今尚无明确的定论,各学说均无法解释其临床症状。目前为大家所支持的是三叉神经微血管压迫导致神经脱髓鞘学说及癫痫样神经痛学说。

【临床表现】在头面部三叉神经分布区域内,骤发、骤停,呈闪电样、刀割样、烧灼样难以忍受的剧烈性疼痛,病情顽固。说话、洗脸、刷牙或微风拂面,甚至走路时都会突然发作。疼痛历时数秒或数分钟,呈周期性发作,发作间歇期同常人。

对继发性三叉神经痛一定要查明原因,针对原发病可以采取蒙医温针疗法等治疗措施。

【治疗】穴位:每次依次选顶会穴、患侧颞穴和前额穴中 1 个,每日 1 次,3 次为 1 个疗程。

操作:选用 I 号或 II 号蒙医银针,顶会穴向前平刺 0.5~1 寸,颞穴直刺 0.3~0.5 寸,前额穴向上平刺 0.5~1 寸。温针给予针柄加热,温度 38~42℃左右,15~20 分钟;或火针留针 15~20 分钟。

【按语】①充分休息,不宜过度劳累,减少冷热刺激。②严重者需要手术治疗等其他更有效的方法。

四、面肌痉挛

面肌痉挛,又称面肌抽搐,表现为一侧面部不自主抽搐。抽搐呈阵发性且

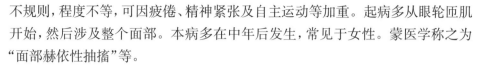

不规则，程度不等，可因疲倦、精神紧张及自主运动等加重。起病多从眼轮匝肌开始，然后涉及整个面部。本病多在中年后发生，常见于女性。蒙医学称之为"面部赫依性抽搐"等。

【病因】面肌痉挛是由颅内血管压迫面神经引起面神经兴奋性增高，至于为什么会出现血管压迫神经，原因尚不清楚；脑桥小脑角的非血管占位性病变，如肉芽肿、肿瘤和囊肿等因素亦可致面肌痉挛等。

【临床表现】初期多为一侧眼轮匝肌阵发性不自主抽搐，逐渐缓慢扩展至一侧面部的其他面肌，口角肌肉的抽搐最易为人注意，严重者甚至可累及同侧的颈阔肌，但额肌较少累及。抽搐的程度轻重不等，为阵发性、快速、不规律的抽搐。严重者呈强直性，致病侧眼不能睁开，口角向同侧㖞斜，无法说话，常因疲倦、精神紧张、自主运动而加剧，但不能自行模仿或控制其发作。少数患者于抽搐时伴有面部轻度疼痛，个别病例可伴有同侧头痛、耳鸣。

面肌痉挛可以分为两种，一种是原发性面肌痉挛，一种是继发性面肌痉挛，即面瘫后遗症产生的面肌痉挛。两种类型可以从症状上区分出来。原发性面肌痉挛在静止状态下也可发生，痉挛数分钟后缓解，不受控制；面瘫后遗症产生的面肌痉挛，只在做眨眼、抬眉等动作时发生。

【治疗】穴位：每次依次选顶会穴、患侧颞穴和前额穴中1个，每日1次，3次为1个疗程。

操作：选用Ⅰ号或Ⅱ号蒙医银针，顶会穴向前平刺0.5～1寸，颞穴直刺0.3～0.5寸，前额穴向上平刺0.5～1寸。温针给予针柄加热，温度38～42℃，15～20分钟；或火针留针15～20分钟。

【按语】①需要保持心情舒畅，防止精神紧张及急躁。②自我热敷，适当进行面部运动锻炼。③严重者需要手术治疗等其他更有效的方法。

五、颈椎病

颈椎病又称颈椎综合征，是颈椎骨关节炎、增生性颈椎炎、颈神经根综合征、颈椎间盘脱出症的总称，是一种以退行性病理改变为基础的疾患。主要由于颈椎长期劳损、骨质增生，或椎间盘脱出、韧带增厚，致使颈椎脊髓、神经根或椎动脉受压，出现一系列功能障碍的临床综合征。表现为椎节失稳、松动，髓核突出或脱出，骨刺形成，韧带肥厚和继发的椎管狭窄等，刺激或压迫了邻近的神经根、脊髓、椎动脉及颈部交感神经等组织，引起一系列症状和体征。蒙医学称之为"躯干乎杨病""颈部乎杨病"等。

【病因】由于颈椎的退行性变及慢性劳损,或发育性颈椎椎管狭窄,或颈椎的先天性畸形等原因刺激或压迫了邻近的神经根、脊髓、椎动脉及颈部交感神经等,出现一系列功能障碍的临床表现。

【临床表现】颈部疼痛,活动受限,常累及肩背部并放射至上肢乃至手指。疼痛可为钝痛、烧灼痛或放射痛,疼痛也可深达肌肉、骨骼、关节等,后期可出现相应部位的感觉减退或消失,伴头晕。

颈椎病的常用试验检查(物理检查):有前屈旋颈试验、椎间孔挤压试验(压顶试验)、臂丛牵拉试验、上肢后伸试验等。

1. X线检查

(1)正位:观察有无寰枢关节脱位、齿状突骨折或缺失。第7颈椎横突有无过长,有无颈肋。钩椎关节及椎间隙有无增宽或变窄。

(2)侧位:①曲度的改变,颈椎变直、生理前突消失或反弯曲。②异常活动度,在颈椎过伸过屈侧位X线片中,可以见到椎间盘的弹性有改变。③椎体前后接近椎间盘的部位均可产生骨赘及韧带钙化。④椎间盘可以因为髓核突出,椎间盘含水量减少发生纤维变性而变薄,表现在X线片上为椎间隙变窄。⑤半脱位及椎间孔变小,椎间盘变性以后,椎体间的稳定性低下,椎体往往发生半脱位,或者称之为滑椎。⑥项韧带钙化。

(3)斜位:主要观察椎间孔的大小以及钩椎关节骨质增生的情况。

2. CT检查 可在X线诊断的基础上进一步观察后纵韧带骨化、椎管狭窄、脊髓肿瘤等所致的椎管扩大或骨质破坏,测量骨质密度以估计骨质疏松的程度。此外,由于横断层图像可以清晰地见到硬膜鞘内外的软组织和蛛网膜下腔,故能正确地诊断椎间盘突出症、神经纤维瘤、脊髓或延髓的空洞症,对于颈椎病的诊断及鉴别诊断具有一定的价值。

3. 肌电图检查 可提示神经根长期受压而发生变性,从而失去对所支配肌肉的抑制作用。

【治疗】方法一:适用于脊髓型、交感神经型颈椎病。

穴位:首次选中间赫依穴,第二次选患侧或两侧赫依穴,隔2日1次,2次为1个疗程。

操作:选用Ⅰ号或Ⅱ号蒙医银针,赫依中间穴直刺0.5寸,赫依两侧穴位斜刺0.5~1寸。温针给予针柄加热,温度38~42℃,15~20分钟;或火针留针15~20分钟。

方法二:适用于椎动脉型颈椎病。

穴位:首次选中间赫依穴,第二次选患侧或两侧赫依穴,第三次选患侧或两

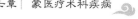

侧枕会穴,隔2日1次,3次为1个疗程。

操作:选用Ⅰ号或Ⅱ号蒙医银针,中间赫依穴直刺0.5寸,两侧赫依穴斜刺0.5~1寸,两侧枕会穴向下颌方向斜刺0.5~1寸。温针给予针柄加热,温度38~42℃,15~20分钟;或火针留针15~20分钟。

方法三:适用于神经根型颈椎病。

穴位:首次选中间赫依穴,第二次选患侧或两侧赫依穴,第三次选患侧两侧肩上穴,隔2日1次,3次为1个疗程。

操作:选用Ⅰ号或Ⅱ号蒙医银针,中间赫依穴直刺0.5寸,两侧赫依穴斜刺0.5~1寸;选用Ⅲ号或Ⅳ号蒙医银针,两侧肩上穴直刺0.5~0.8寸。温针给予针柄加热,温度38~42℃,15~20分钟;或火针留针15~20分钟。

【按语】①低头位工作不宜太久,需坚持做颈保健操。②注意颈肩部保暖,预防着凉。③睡眠时枕头高低和软硬要适宜。④神经根型颈椎病炎性反应重者,可配合消炎脱水药物治疗。⑤对脊髓型颈椎病,如治疗效果不佳或进行性加重趋势者,应考虑手术治疗。

六、落枕

落枕是一种常见病,好发于青壮年,以冬春季多见。患者通常入睡前无任何症状,晨起后却感到项背部明显酸痛,颈部活动受限。这说明病起于睡眠之后,与睡枕及睡眠姿势有密切关系。

【病因】肌肉扭伤,如夜间睡眠姿势不良,头颈长时间处于过度偏转的位置,使头颈处于过伸或过屈状态,致颈部一侧肌肉紧张,使颈椎小关节紊乱,时间较长即可发生静力性损伤,使伤处肌筋强硬不和,气血循行不畅,局部疼痛不适,活动明显受限等;感受风寒,如睡眠时受寒,使颈背部气血凝滞,筋络痹阻,以致僵硬疼痛,活动不利。

【临床表现】一般表现为起床后感觉颈后部、上背部疼痛不适,以一侧为多,或有两侧俱痛者,或一侧重,一侧轻;当身体由平躺改为直立,颈部肌群力量改变,可引起进行性加重,甚至累及肩部及胸背部。多数患者可回想到昨夜睡眠位置欠佳,检查时颈部肌肉有触痛。由于疼痛,使颈项活动不利,不能自由旋转,严重者俯仰困难,甚至头颈强直于异常位置,使头偏向病侧。检查时颈部肌肉有触痛,浅层肌肉有痉挛、僵硬,触之有"条索感"。有颈椎病等颈肩部疾病的患者,稍感风寒或睡姿不良,即可引发本病,甚至可反复"落枕"。

【治疗】穴位:首次选中间赫依穴,第二次选两侧赫依穴,隔2日1次,2次为 1 个疗程。

操作：选用Ⅰ号或Ⅱ号蒙医银针，中间赫依穴直刺 0.5 寸，赫依两侧穴位斜刺 0.5～1 寸。温针给予针柄加热，温度 38～42℃，15～20 分钟；或火针留针 15～20 分钟。

【按语】①睡眠时枕头不能过高、过低、过硬。②避免颈部外感风寒。

七、肩周炎

肩周炎又称肩关节周围炎。以肩部逐渐产生疼痛，夜间为甚，逐渐加重，肩关节活动功能受限而且日益加重，达到某种程度后逐渐缓解，直至最后完全复原为主要表现的肩关节囊及其周围韧带、肌腱和滑囊的慢性特异性炎症。肩周炎是以肩关节疼痛和活动不便为主要症状的常见病症。本病的好发年龄在 50 岁左右，女性发病率略高于男性，多见于体力劳动者。如得不到有效的治疗，有可能严重影响肩关节的功能活动。肩关节可有广泛压痛，并向颈部及肘部放射，还可出现不同程度的三角肌的萎缩。

【病因】软组织退行性病变，对各种外力的承受能力减弱；长期过度活动，姿势不良等所产生的慢性致伤力；上肢外伤后肩部固定过久，肩周组织继发萎缩、粘连；肩部急性挫伤、牵拉伤后治疗不当等。

【临床表现】多数为慢性发作，起初肩部呈阵发性疼痛，以后疼痛逐渐加剧，呈钝痛，或刀割样痛，且呈持续性，气候变化或劳累后常使疼痛加重，疼痛可向颈项及上肢（特别是肘部）扩散，当肩部偶然受到碰撞或牵拉时，常可引起撕裂样剧痛。肩痛昼轻夜重为本病一大特点，若因受寒而致痛者，则对气候变化特别敏感。肩关节向各方向活动均可受限，以外展、上举、内旋、外旋更为明显，随着病情进展，由于长期失用引起肩关节囊及肩周软组织的粘连，肌力逐渐下降，加上喙肱韧带固定于缩短的内旋位等因素，使肩关节各方向的主动和被动活动均受限，严重时肘关节功能也可受影响，屈肘时手不能摸到同侧肩部，尤其在手臂后伸时不能完成屈肘动作。患者肩部怕冷，即使在暑天，肩部也不敢吹风。多数患者在肩关节周围可触到明显的压痛点，压痛点多在肱二头肌长头肌腱沟、肩峰下滑囊、喙突、冈上肌附着点等处。三角肌、冈上肌等肩周围肌肉早期可出现痉挛，晚期可发生失用性肌萎缩，出现肩峰突起，上举不便、后伸不能等典型症状，此时疼痛症状反而减轻。

X 线检查：早期，肩部软组织充血水肿时，X 线片上软组织对比度下降，肩峰下脂肪线模糊变形乃至消失；中晚期，肩部软组织钙化，X 线片可见关节囊、滑液囊、冈上肌腱、肱二头肌长头腱等处有密度淡而不均的钙化斑影；病程晚期，X线片可见钙化影致密锐利，部分病例可见大结节骨质增生和骨赘形成等。此外，在肩锁关节可见骨质疏松、关节端增生或形成骨赘或关节间隙变窄等。

MRI检查：肩关节MRI检查可以确定肩关节周围结构信号是否正常，是否存在炎症，可以作为确定病变部位和鉴别诊断的有效方法。

【治疗】方法一：适用于病情较轻者。

穴位：首次选肩穴，第二次选肩中穴，隔2日1次，2次为1个疗程。

操作：肩穴，选用Ⅲ号或Ⅳ号蒙医银针，直刺或向下斜刺0.8~1.5寸；肩中穴，选用Ⅰ号或Ⅱ号蒙医银针，直刺或斜刺0.5~1寸。温针给予针柄加热，温度38~42℃，15~20分钟；或火针留针15~20分钟。

方法二：适用于病情较重者。

穴位：首次选肩穴，第二次选肩中穴，第三次选肩前穴，隔2日1次，3次为1个疗程。

操作：肩穴、肩中穴，刺法同上。肩前穴：选用Ⅱ号或Ⅲ号蒙医银针，直刺0.5~1寸。温针给予针柄加热，温度38~42℃，15~20分钟；或火针留针15~20分钟。

方法三：适用于病情较重者。

穴位：首次选肩穴，第二次选肩中穴，第三次选肩前穴，第四次选肩上穴，隔2日1次，4次为1个疗程。

操作：肩穴、肩中穴、肩前穴，刺法同上。肩上穴：选用Ⅲ号或Ⅳ号蒙医银针，直刺0.5~0.8寸。温针给予针柄加热，温度38~42℃，15~20分钟；或火针留针15~20分钟。

【按语】①注意肩部的保暖，避免着凉。②治疗前排除肩关节结核、肿瘤等疾患。③治疗期间避免肩部受外伤，以防新的损伤造成出血粘连而不利于恢复。④坚持适当的功能锻炼，自主锻炼、被动锻炼，以利于肩部各种功能的恢复。

八、臂丛神经痛

臂丛由颈5至胸1的脊神经前支组成，有时胸2亦参与。主要支配肩及上肢的感觉和运动。组成臂丛神经的各部受损时，产生其支配范围内的疼痛，总称为臂丛神经痛。蒙医学称之为"上肢白脉病"。

【病因】臂丛神经痛可分原发性和继发性两类，以后者多见。原发性臂丛神经痛病因不明，可能是变态反应性疾病，偶有家族性病例，可见于轻度外伤、注射、轻度系统性感染。继发性臂丛神经痛臂丛邻近病变压迫，即神经根压迫和神经干压迫等所致。

【临床表现】40～50岁居多，女性多于男性，右侧多于左侧，常无明显诱因，症状逐渐发生。常发生于凌晨，使患者痛醒。上肢疼痛和麻木，由肩胛区向臂内侧及手掌尺侧放射。呈刺痛、钻痛、灼痛，伴有麻木。久坐、上肢伸展、举物、提物等均可使疼痛加剧，臂内收、屈肘，症状可减轻。

体检检查可出现手、前臂尺侧感觉减退及感觉过敏。可有手部肌力减弱及肌肉轻度萎缩。锁骨下动脉受压可出现手部皮肤发冷、肤色苍白、青紫等。

【治疗】穴位：首次选中间赫依穴和患侧肩穴，第二次选患侧赫依穴和肘外穴，或肘外穴周围压痛最明显点，第三次选患侧肩前穴和腕上穴，隔日1次，3次为1个疗程。

操作：中间赫依穴，选用I号或II号蒙医银针，直刺0.5寸；两侧赫依穴位，选用I号或II号蒙医银针，斜刺0.5～1寸；肩穴，选用III号或IV号蒙医银针，直刺或向下斜刺0.8～1.5寸；肩前穴，选用II号或III号蒙医银针，直刺0.5～1寸；肘外穴和肘外穴周围压痛最明显点，选用II号或III号蒙医银针，直刺0.8～1.2寸；腕上穴，选用I号或II号蒙医银针，直刺0.5～1寸。温针给予针柄加热，温度38～42℃，15～20分钟；或火针留针15～20分钟。

【按语】①继发性臂丛神经痛要针对原发病治疗。②急性期患者要注意休息，避免提重物。③平时要注意保暖，避免着凉。

九、肱骨外上髁炎

肱骨外上髁炎在临床上十分多见。打网球者经常反手挥拍击球，若不得法常引发本病，因此俗称为网球肘。蒙医学称之为"肘关节黄水病"。

【病因】因职业需反复用力伸腕活动，如乒乓球、网球中的"反拍"击球。泥瓦工、理发员、会计，以及偶然从事单纯收缩臂力活动工作的人，都会引起附着于肱骨外上髁部肌腱、筋膜的慢性劳损。

【临床表现】主要表现为肘关节外髁处局限性疼痛，并向前臂放射，尤其是在内旋时。患者常主诉持物无力，偶尔可因剧痛而使持物掉落。静息后再活动或遇寒冷时疼痛加重。

临床检查时可发现肱骨外上髁处有压痛点；腕伸肌紧张试验阳性，即屈腕并在前臂旋前位伸肘时可诱发疼痛。此外，抗阻力后旋前臂亦可引起疼痛。

【治疗】穴位：选肘窝穴、肘尖穴，每次1穴，隔2日1次，2次为1个疗程。

操作：选用Ⅰ号、Ⅱ号或Ⅲ号蒙医银针，直刺0.5～1寸。温针给予针柄加热，温度38～42℃，15～20分钟；或火针留针15～20分钟。

【按语】①注意肩部保暖，避免着凉。②治疗期间尽量减少腕部背伸运动，避免肘部过度用力。急性发作者应绝对避免肘关节运动。③坚持适当的功能锻炼，前臂在内旋的同时屈肘，然后伸直肘关节。

十、手腕腱鞘囊肿

手腕腱鞘囊肿是指发生于关节囊或腱鞘附近的一种内含胶冻状黏液的良性肿块，其多为单房性，也可为多房性。手腕腱鞘囊肿症状很明显，发病部位会有轻微酸痛感，囊液变多时就会变硬而且有压痛的感觉。如果患处在手腕处，就会伴有腕部无力，不适或酸痛、放射性痛，严重的话可能伴有一定的功能障碍。

【病因】发病原因不明。目前主要认为与关节囊、韧带、腱鞘上的结缔组织因局部营养不良，发生退行性黏液性变性或局部慢性劳损有关。

【临床表现】手腕背侧或掌侧出现局部肿块隆起，生长缓慢，很少有疼痛或不适。个别发生于腕管或掌部小鱼际者，可压迫正中神经或尺神经，出现相应的感觉和运动障碍；肿块呈半球形，豌豆至拇指头大小，一般不超过2cm，表面光滑饱满，与皮肤无粘连，触之坚硬，有弹性，可有囊性感，基底固定，压之有酸胀或痛感；手腕腱鞘囊肿的患者在每日起床后会感到明显的晨僵。

【治疗】穴位：囊中最高点。

操作：选用Ⅰ号或Ⅱ号蒙医银针，直刺0.3～0.5寸。温针给予针柄加热，温度38～42℃，15～20分钟；或火针留针15～20分钟。拔针后，按压使囊肿内容物外溢或向四周流散。术后按常规护理，加压包扎3天。

【按语】①避免局部过度活动，尽量减少劳损筋膜间的摩擦。②局部治疗后，宜保持清洁，预防感染。③注意休息，做柔软操或局部按摩。

十一、腰肌劳损

腰肌劳损是指腰部肌肉及其附着点筋膜或骨膜的慢性损伤性炎症，是腰痛的常见原因之一，主要症状是腰或腰骶部胀痛、酸痛，反复发作，疼痛可随气候变化或劳累程度而变化，如日间劳累则加重，休息后可减轻，时轻时重，为临床常见病，多发病，发病因素较多。其日积月累，可使肌纤维变性，甚而少量撕裂，形成瘢痕、纤维条索或粘连，遗留长期慢性腰背痛。

【病因】腰部外伤后治疗不及时或处理方法不当，长期反复的过度腰部运动及过度负荷，以及劳损、受凉等因素均可致病。慢性腰肌劳损与气候、环境条件也有一定关系，气温过低或湿度太大都可促发或加重腰肌劳损。

【临床表现】腰部酸痛或胀痛，部分呈刺痛或灼痛。适当活动和经常改变体位时减轻，活动过度又加重；不能坚持弯腰工作，常被迫时时伸腰或以拳头叩击腰部以缓解疼痛；腰部有压痛点，多在骶棘肌处，髂骨后棘部、骶骨后骶棘肌止点处或腰椎横突处；腰部外形及活动多无异常，也无明显腰肌痉挛，少数患者腰部活动稍受限。

X线检查：多无异常，少数或可有骨质增生或脊柱畸形。

【治疗】方法一：适用于病情较轻者。

穴位：首次选两侧肾穴，第二次选两侧肾黑脉穴，隔2日1次，2次为1个疗程。

操作：选用Ⅰ号或Ⅱ号蒙医银针，肾穴斜刺0.5～1寸，肾黑脉穴直刺0.5～0.8寸。温针给予针柄加热，温度38～42℃，15～20分钟；或火针留针15～20分钟。

方法二：适用于病情较重者。

穴位：首次选两侧肾穴，第二次选两侧肾黑脉穴，第三次选两侧总穴，隔2日1次，3次为1个疗程。

操作：选用Ⅰ号或Ⅱ号蒙医银针，肾穴、总穴均斜刺0.5～1寸，肾黑脉穴直刺0.5～0.8寸。温针给予针柄加热，温度38～42℃，15～20分钟；或火针留针15～20分钟。

【按语】①加强腰背肌锻炼。②在工作、劳动中尽可能变换姿势，注意纠正习惯性不良姿势。③避免受寒着凉。

十二、急性腰扭伤

急性腰扭伤是腰部肌肉、筋膜、韧带等软组织因外力作用突然受到过度牵拉而引起的急性撕裂伤，常发生于搬抬重物、腰部肌肉强力收缩时。急性腰扭伤可使腰骶部肌肉的附着点、骨膜、筋膜和韧带等组织撕裂。

【病因】损伤较轻的是因行走滑倒、跳跃、闪扭身躯、跑步而引起，多为肌肉、韧带遭受牵制所致；损伤较重的是因用力过猛或姿势不正、配合不当，造成腰部的肌肉筋膜、韧带、椎间小关节与关节囊的损伤和撕裂。

【临床表现】患者损伤后立即出现腰部疼痛，呈持续性剧痛，次日可因局部出血、肿胀，腰痛更为严重；也有的只是轻微扭转一下腰部，当时并无明显痛感，但次日感到腰部疼痛。腰部活动受限，不能挺直，俯、仰、扭转均感困难，咳嗽、喷嚏、大小便时可使疼痛加剧。站立时往往用手扶住腰部，坐位时用双手撑于椅子，以减轻疼痛。腰肌扭伤后一侧或两侧当即发生疼痛；有时可在受伤后半天或隔夜才出现疼痛、腰部活动受限，静止时疼痛稍轻、活动或咳嗽时疼痛较甚。检查时局部肌肉紧张、压痛及牵引痛明显，但无瘀血现象。

X 线检查：一般韧带损伤多无异常发现，或见腰生理前突消失。棘上、棘间韧带断裂者，侧位片表现棘突间距离增大或合并棘突、关节突骨折。

【治疗】穴位：首次选两侧肾穴，第二次选两侧总穴，隔 2 日 1 次，2 次为 1 个疗程。

操作：选用 I 号或 II 号蒙医银针，斜刺 0.5～1 寸。温针给予针柄加热，温度 38～42℃，15～20 分钟；或火针留针 15～20 分钟。

【按语】①避免受寒着凉。②应及时诊断，积极治疗，以免延误而转为慢性。

十三、坐骨神经痛

坐骨神经痛是以坐骨神经通路及分布区域疼痛为主的综合征。蒙医学称之为"下肢白脉病""腰腿痛"等。

【病因】病因多种多样。绝大多数患者的坐骨神经痛是继发于坐骨神经局部及周围结构的病变对坐骨神经的刺激压迫与损害，称为继发性坐骨神经痛，如腰椎间盘突出、腰椎骨性关节病、腰骶椎先天畸形、骶髂关节炎等疾病引起坐骨神经痛。少数系原发性，即坐骨神经炎，常伴随各种类型的感染及全身性疾病发生，如上呼吸道感染，多为单侧，不伴有腰、背痛，疼痛一般为持续性。

【临床表现】疼痛主要限于坐骨神经分布区，大腿后部、小腿后外侧和足部，疼痛剧烈的患者可呈特有的姿势。肌力减退的程度可因病因、病变部位、损害程度不同差异很大，可有坐骨神经支配肌肉全部或部分肌力减弱或瘫痪。有坐骨神经牵拉征，拉塞格征及其等位征阳性，此征的存在常与疼痛程度相平行；跟腱反射减退或消失，膝反射可因刺激而增高；可有坐骨神经支配区域的各种感觉的减退或消失，包括外踝的振动觉减退，亦可有极轻的感觉障碍。

影像学检查：包括腰骶椎、骶髂关节 X 线片，脊柱 MRI，CT 脊髓造影，除临床的盆腔物理检查外，可做盆腔的 CT 或 MRI。

【治疗】方法一：适用于原发性坐骨神经痛或由腰 4/5 椎间盘突出等病变引起的继发性坐骨神经痛。

穴位：首次选患侧或两侧小肠穴，第二次选患侧髋穴，第三次选患侧腘穴，第四次选患侧腓肠肌主穴，隔日1次，4次为1个疗程。

操作：小肠穴，选用Ⅰ号或Ⅱ号蒙医银针，斜刺0.5～1寸；髋穴，选用Ⅳ号或Ⅴ号蒙医银针，直刺1.5～3寸；腘穴、腓肠肌主穴，选用Ⅲ号或Ⅳ号蒙医银针，直刺1～1.5寸。温针给予针柄加热，温度38～42℃，15～20分钟；或火针留针15～20分钟。

方法二：适用于原发性坐骨神经痛或由腰骶椎间盘突出等病变引起的继发性坐骨神经痛。

穴位：首次选患侧或两侧膀胱穴，第二次选患侧髋穴，第三次选患侧腘穴，第四次选患侧腓肠肌主穴，隔日1次，4次为一个疗程。

操作：膀胱穴，选用Ⅰ号或Ⅱ号蒙医银针，斜刺0.5～1寸；髋穴、腘穴、腓肠肌主穴，刺法同上。温针给予针柄加热，温度38～42℃，15～20分钟；或火针留针15～20分钟。

【按语】①急性期卧床休息，腰椎间盘突出症者应睡硬板床。②平时注意保暖，劳动或锻炼应注意正确姿势。

十四、梨状肌综合征

腓总神经高位分支自梨状肌肌束间穿出，坐骨神经从梨状肌肌腹中穿出，当梨状肌受到损伤，发生充血、水肿、痉挛、粘连和挛缩时，该肌间隙或该肌上、下孔变狭窄，挤压其间穿出的神经、血管，因此而出现的一系列临床症状和体征称为梨状肌综合征。

【病因】臀部外伤出血、粘连、瘢痕形成；注射药物使梨状肌变性、纤维挛缩；髋臼后上部骨折移位、骨痂过大均可使坐骨神经在梨状肌处受压。此外，少数患者因坐骨神经出骨盆时行径变异，穿行于梨状肌内，但髋外旋时肌肉强力收缩，可使坐骨神经受到过大压力，长此以往可产生坐骨神经慢性损伤。

【临床表现】疼痛是本病的主要表现，以臀部为主，并可向下肢放射，严重时不能行走或行走一段距离后疼痛剧烈，需休息片刻后才能继续行走。患者感觉疼痛位置较深，主要向同侧下肢的后面或后外侧放射，有的还会伴有小腿外侧麻木、会阴部不适等。严重时臀部呈现"刀割样"或"灼烧样"疼痛，双腿屈曲困难，双膝跪卧，夜间睡眠困难。大小便、咳嗽、打喷嚏时因腹压增加而使患侧肢体的窜痛感加重。

直腿抬高试验：直腿抬高在60°以前出现疼痛为试验阳性；梨状肌紧张试

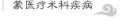

验：患者仰卧位于检查床上，将患肢伸直，做内收内旋动作，如坐骨神经有放射性疼痛，再迅速将患肢外展外旋，疼痛随即缓解，即为梨状肌紧张试验阳性。

【治疗】穴位：首次选患侧髋穴，第二次选患侧髋穴周围压痛最明显点，隔日1次，2次为1个疗程。

操作：选用Ⅳ号或Ⅴ号蒙医银针，直刺1.5～3寸。温针给予针柄加热，温度38～42℃，15～20分钟；或火针留针15～20分钟。

【按语】①治疗期间注意休息，避免造成新的损伤。②注意局部保暖，避免受凉。

十五、膝关节炎

膝关节炎是一种以退行性病理改变为基础的疾患。多发生于中老年人群，其症状多表现为膝盖红肿痛、上下楼梯痛、坐起立行时膝部酸痛不适等。也有表现为肿胀、弹响、积液等，如不及时治疗，则会引起关节畸形、残废。膝关节部位还常患有膝关节滑膜炎、韧带损伤、半月板损伤、膝关节游离体、腘窝囊肿、髌骨软化、鹅足滑囊炎、膝内/外翻等关节疾病。蒙医学称之为"膝关节黄水病"等。

【病因】膝关节炎的发生一般由膝关节退行性病变、外伤、过度劳累等因素引起。膝关节炎多发于中老年人，是引起老年人腿疼的主要原因。另外，体重过重、不正确的走路姿势、长时间下蹲、膝关节的受凉受寒也是导致膝关节炎的原因。

【临床表现】多数膝关节炎患者初期症状较轻，若不接受治疗病情会逐渐加重。主要症状有膝部酸痛、膝关节肿胀、膝关节弹响等。膝关节僵硬、发冷也是膝关节炎的症状，劳累、受凉或轻微外伤后症状加剧，严重者会发生活动受限。

X线检查：用来判断骨骼间隙宽窄、骨折等骨骼受损情况；MRI核磁共振：可以检查关节内软骨、韧带、半月板、滑膜、滑液囊等病变及骨髓病变。还可以检查出膝盖内是否有积液产生。

【治疗】穴位：首次选患侧压痛重的膝眼穴，第二次选患侧另一个膝眼穴，隔2日1次，2次为1个疗程。

操作：内侧膝眼穴，选用Ⅱ号或Ⅲ号蒙医银针，从前向后外与额状面成45°角斜刺0.5～1寸；外侧膝眼穴，选用Ⅲ号或Ⅳ号蒙医银针，向后内斜刺0.8～1.5寸。温针给予针柄加热，温度38～42℃，15～20分钟；或火针留针15～20分钟。

【按语】①治疗期间注意休息，尽量减少病变膝关节活动。②注意局部保暖，避免受凉。

第八章

蒙医内科疾病

一、头晕

头晕是一种常见的脑部功能性障碍，也是临床常见的症状之一。表现为头昏、头涨、头重脚轻、脑内摇晃、眼花等。头晕可单独出现，但常与头痛并发。头晕伴有平衡觉障碍或空间觉定向障碍时，患者感到外周环境或自身旋转、移动或摇晃。偶尔头晕或体位改变而头晕不会有太大的问题，如果长时间头晕，可能是重病的先兆，应引起重视。本病归属于蒙医学"赫依病"的范畴。

【病因】头晕可由多种原因引起，最常见于发热性疾病、高血压病、脑动脉硬化、颅脑外伤综合征、神经症等。此外，还见于贫血、心律失常、心力衰竭、低血压、药物中毒、尿毒症、哮喘等。抑郁症早期也常有头晕症状。头晕又称为眩晕，是一种主观的感觉异常，可分为两类：一为旋转性眩晕，多由前庭神经系统及小脑的功能障碍所致，以倾倒的感觉为主，感到自身晃动或视物旋转；二为一般性眩晕，多由某些全身性疾病引起，以头昏的感觉为主，感到头重脚轻。

【临床表现】轻者表现为头晕、眼花、头重脚轻；重者如坐船，旋转不定，不能站立，或伴有恶心、呕吐、耳鸣、眼花、汗出、面色苍白、上肢或单肢麻木等症状，严重者可能会突然仆倒。

【治疗】穴位：首次选顶会穴和中间赫依穴，第二次选顶会前穴和两侧赫依穴，第三次选顶会后穴和中间心穴，隔日1次，3次为1个疗程。

操作：选用Ⅰ号或Ⅱ号蒙医银针，顶会穴、顶会前穴、顶会后穴向后平刺0.5~1寸，中间赫依穴和中间心穴直刺0.5寸，两侧赫依穴斜刺0.5~1寸。温针给予针柄加热，温度38~42℃，15~20分钟；或火针留针15~20分钟。

【按语】①合理膳食，戒烟戒酒。②注意休息，适当运动。③控制情绪，心态保持平衡。

二、萨病

萨病是蒙医内科常见病，又称"嘎热格病""诺乐病""影病"等。萨病即是半身不遂，指一侧上下肢、面肌和舌肌下部的运动障碍，它是急性脑血管病的一个常见症状。轻度偏瘫患者虽然尚能活动，但走起路来，往往上肢屈曲，下肢伸直，瘫痪的下肢走一步划半个圈，这种特殊的走路姿势，叫偏瘫步态。

【病因】中老年人群中多见，通常骤然发病。因长期多摄锐性食品或油脂类食品而恶血和希拉偏盛者猛然发怒、用力过度等原因导致脑血管受阻或破裂出血、脑髓受损；或体质虚弱、劳累过度、兴奋至极等诱因，引起巴达干赫依偏盛，巴达干黏液堵塞脑血管所致。

【临床表现】常见症状为半身肢体不遂、口眼㖞斜、语言障碍、口角流涎、吞咽困难等。患者应该及时就诊，以免延误了治疗的最佳时期，蒙医采用蒙西医结合治疗，以蒙药和传统外治疗法为主。

【治疗】穴位：首次选顶会穴、患侧赫依穴和总穴，第二次选中间枕会穴、患侧膀胱穴、肩穴和中髋穴，第三次选患侧枕会穴、患侧精穴、肘外穴和大腿穴，第四次选患侧肩前穴、上髋穴、腕上穴和胫中穴，第五次选患侧腋后穴、后髋穴、拇食指穴和足背穴，隔日1次，5次为1个疗程。

操作：选用Ⅰ号～Ⅴ号蒙医银针中适合长度的银针，顶会穴向后平刺0.5～1寸，患侧赫依穴和总穴斜刺0.5～1寸，中间枕会穴向下颌方向直刺0.5～1寸，患侧枕会穴向下颌方向斜刺0.5～1寸，患侧膀胱穴和精穴斜刺0.5～0.8寸，肩穴向下斜刺0.8～1.5寸，中、上、后髋穴向下斜刺1.5～3寸，肘外穴直刺0.8～1.2寸，大腿穴直刺1～2寸，肩前穴、腕上穴、足背穴直刺0.5～1寸，胫中穴直刺1～1.5寸，腋后穴直刺0.8～1.2寸，拇食指穴斜刺0.5～0.8寸。温针给予针柄加热，温度38～42℃，15～20分钟；或火针留针15～20分钟。

【按语】①蒙医温针火针治疗多用于萨病恢复期，身体虚弱者慎用。②临床常将蒙医温针火针疗法与其他蒙医外治疗法结合应用于本病的治疗，放血、普通针刺等疗法治疗效果也较好。③治疗期间，应经常按摩患肢，并进行主动或被动运动，有利于康复。

三、癫痫

癫痫是由于脑或神经受损，出现突发性昏厥、全身抽搐等症状，并以反复发作为特征的一种短暂脑功能失调综合征。又称"乌额德格"病。

【病因】主要由各种热病遗留或痧毒、黏毒等侵入脑白脉，阻塞感能中枢之道而发病。诱因有炽热、搏热、黏脑刺痛等热邪残留，脑部震动受损或外伤、脑痧瘤和脑巴达干热时用力过猛以及过度劳累或惊恐，过度摄食锐、腻、热饮食等。

【临床表现】一般情况下，发作前有先兆症状，比如胃不适、心悸、头晕目眩、恶心、闻到异味等。有些患者有恐惧感，感觉悬在空中。然后昏厥骤然发作，做出无意识的头部或心前区的动作。

【治疗】穴位：首次选顶会穴和中间赫依穴，第二次选顶会前穴和中间巴达干穴，第三次选顶会后穴和中间心穴，隔日 1 次，3 次为 1 个疗程。

操作：选用Ⅰ号或Ⅱ号蒙医银针，顶会穴、顶会前穴、顶会后穴向后平刺0.5～1 寸，中间赫依穴、巴达干穴和中间心穴直刺 0.5 寸。温针给予针柄加热，温度 38～42℃左右，15～20 分钟；或火针留针 15～20 分钟。

【按语】①对继发性癫痫，应重视原发病的诊断与治疗。②在治疗过程中，应避免精神刺激、过度劳累，注意饮食起居。

四、老年痴呆症

老年痴呆症，又称阿尔茨海默病。是一种起病隐匿的进行性发展的神经系统退行性疾病。临床上以记忆障碍、失语、失用、失认、视空间技能损害、执行功能障碍以及人格和行为改变等全面性痴呆表现为特征。65 岁以前发病者，称早老性痴呆；65 岁以后发病者，称老年性痴呆。蒙医学称之为健忘症。

【病因】病因迄今未明，可能是一组异质性疾病，在多种因素（包括生物和社会心理因素）的作用下才发病。从目前研究来看，该病的可能因素和假说多达 30 余种，如家族史、女性、头部外伤、低教育水平、甲状腺病、母育龄过高或过低、病毒感染等。

【临床表现】该病起病缓慢或隐匿，患者及家人常说不清何时起病。少数患者在躯体疾病、骨折或精神受到刺激后症状迅速明朗化。女性较男性多。主要表现为认知功能下降、精神症状和行为障碍、日常生活能力的逐渐下降。

【治疗】穴位：首次选顶会穴和中间赫依穴，第二次选顶会前穴和中间希拉穴，第三次选顶会后穴和中间巴达干穴，第四次选心穴，隔日 1 次，4 次为 1 个疗程。

操作：选用Ⅰ号或Ⅱ号蒙医银针，顶会穴、顶会前穴、顶会后穴向后平刺0.5～1 寸，中间赫依穴、希拉穴、巴达干穴和中间心穴直刺 0.5 寸，两侧心穴斜刺

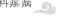

0.5~1 寸。温针给予针柄加热，温度 38~42℃，15~20 分钟；或火针留针 15~20 分钟。

【按语】①在治疗期间应戒酒，慎用安眠镇静的药物。②要注意精神调摄与智能训练，在日常生活中保持健康生活习惯，勤动手、动脑。

五、癔症

癔症是主要表现为多疑的精神思维紊乱症，又称"相思病""伤感性癫狂"等。

【病因】随着三根七素平衡失调，赫依增多与血相搏，脉窍闭塞，感能运行受阻所引起。诱因主要有过度惊恐、愤怒、多疑、厌倦、重欲、羞涩等引起心理活动失调，或失血过多、过度劳累等。

【临床表现】在青壮年和女性人群中的发病率相对较高。在发病、发作和演变过程中出现不同程度的失眠、心悸等赫依偏盛性心神损伤症状。在人类的各种疾病中，几乎可以说癔症的症状最为繁多。它可以表现出人体各系统和各部位的症状，癔症的发生与心理因素、社会文化因素、个体性格特征有密切关系，故多是功能性的。常在精神刺激后急骤起病，如号啕痛哭或时而大笑，大吵大闹或声嘶力竭吐露愤懑，甚至抓头发、撕衣服、捶胸顿足、以头撞墙、地上打滚等，发作时间长短不一。癔症患者具有高度情感性，他们的情感反应强烈且极不稳定，变化多端，如片刻前还是满面春风，转眼间已阴云密布，情绪时高时低，变化常在瞬息之间。

临床上结合详细的躯体和神经系统检查及脑电图、头颅 CT 等辅助检查结果，与癫痫发作、反应性精神病、精神分裂症及脑器质性疾病进行鉴别。

【治疗】穴位：首次选顶会穴，第二次选中间赫依穴，第三次选中间心穴，隔日 1 次，3 次为 1 个疗程。

操作：选用Ⅰ号或Ⅱ号蒙医银针，顶会穴向后平刺 0.5~1 寸，中间赫依穴和中间心穴直刺 0.5 寸。温针给予针柄加热，温度 38~42℃，15~20 分钟；或火针留针 15~20 分钟。

【按语】①对患者加以开导，使其心情舒畅，解除疑虑，建立治愈的信心。②改善环境条件，注意精神调节，利于病情的恢复。

六、癫狂病

蒙医癫狂病指精神和思维严重错乱，以智能和行为异常为主要症状的一种心神病,又称"癫狂邪魔症"。临床表现与现代医学精神分裂症、躁狂抑郁症类似。

【病因】因赫依偏盛,与巴达干希拉相搏入感能,致使心神之道受阻而发病。

【临床表现】可有家族史。多发于中青年,女性发病偏多;以情感过度高涨与低落、躁狂状态与抑郁状态交替出现为基本特点。躁狂状态表现为情绪高涨,联想迅速,动作增多,甚至兴奋躁动,打人毁物等;抑郁状态表现为情绪低落,联想迟钝,动作减少,睡眠障碍,甚至有欲自杀行为等;躁狂与抑郁状态可间歇交替发生,而缓解期精神状态可完全正常。

【治疗】穴位:首次选顶会穴和中间赫依穴,第二次选中间命脉穴和中间心穴,第三次选黑白际穴和癫狂穴,隔日1次,3次为1个疗程。

操作:选用Ⅰ～Ⅲ号蒙医银针,顶会穴向后平刺0.5～1寸,中间赫依穴、命脉穴和心穴直刺0.5寸,黑白际穴直刺0.3～0.5寸,癫狂穴直刺0.5～0.8寸。温针给予针柄加热,温度38～42℃,15～20分钟;或火针留针15～20分钟。

【按语】①在治疗过程中,要对患者进行严密监护,并结合心理疗法。②癫狂病易复发,尤其是春季或受到精神刺激时经常复发。因此,病情缓解后亦应继续治疗,以巩固疗效。

七、失眠症

失眠症简称失眠,是指无法入睡或无法保持睡眠状态,导致睡眠不足。又称入睡和维持睡眠障碍,为各种原因引起入睡困难、睡眠深度或频度过短、早醒及睡眠时间不足或睡眠质量差等。蒙医认为赫依偏盛紊乱是失眠症基本原因,又称其"不能入睡""少眠""易醒""睡眠不佳"等。

【病因】很多因素都可以造成失眠,精神因素、机体疾病、文化程度、生活习惯、工作环境以及睡眠条件等因素与失眠的形成有着密切的关系。心理因素造成的失眠被人们所重视,如情绪不稳定、心情抑郁、过于兴奋、生气愤怒等均可引起失眠。

【临床表现】主要症状是对白天活动表现的影响,例如感觉疲劳、烦躁、情绪失调、注意力不集中和记忆力差等。患者一般进入睡眠的潜伏期延长,睡眠时间缩短,在入睡过程中生理性觉醒增多。失眠症的病程差异较大,如果是心理性或医疗性应激事件引起,病程可以是有限的。最常见的情形是,最初阶段的进行性失眠加重,持续数周到数月,随之较稳定的慢性睡眠困难持续数年。有的患者虽只经历过一次,但在以后遇到某些生活事件会出现睡眠的明显波动。

【治疗】穴位:首次选顶会穴,第二次选中间及两侧赫依穴,第三次选中间及两侧心穴,隔日 1 次,3 次为 1 个疗程。

操作:选用Ⅰ号或Ⅱ号蒙医银针,顶会穴向后平刺 0.5～1 寸,中间赫依穴和中间心穴直刺 0.5 寸,两侧赫依穴和两侧心穴斜刺 0.5～1 寸。温针给予针柄加热,温度 38～42℃,15～20 分钟;或火针留针 15～20 分钟。

【按语】①蒙医温针治疗失眠症多配合应用镇赫依类蒙药,以提高疗效。②其他疾病引起失眠者,应同时治疗原发病。

八、哮喘

哮喘又名支气管哮喘,是由多种细胞及细胞组分参与的慢性气道炎症,此种炎症常引起气道反应性增高,导致反复发作的喘息、气促、胸闷、咳嗽等症状,多在夜间或凌晨发生,此类症状常伴有广泛而多变的气流阻塞,可以自行或通过治疗而逆转。

【病因】哮喘是一种复杂的,具有多基因遗传倾向的疾病。最重要的诱发因素可能是吸入变应原。

【临床表现】哮喘表现为发作性咳嗽、胸闷及呼吸困难。部分患者咳痰,多于发作趋于缓解时痰多,如无合并感染,常为白黏痰,质韧,有时呈米粒状或黏液柱状。发作时的严重程度和持续时间个体差异很大,轻者仅有胸部紧迫感,持续数分钟,重者极度呼吸困难,持续数周或更长时间。症状的特点是可逆性,即经治疗后可在较短时间内缓解,部分自然缓解,当然,少部分不缓解而呈持续状态。发作常有一定的诱发因素,不少患者发作有明显的生物规律,每天凌晨 2—6 时发作或加重,一般好发于春夏交接时或冬天,部分女性在月经前或月经期间哮喘发作或加重。要注意非典型哮喘患者,有的患者常以发作性咳嗽作为唯一的症状,临床上常易误诊为支气管炎;有的青少年患者则以运动时出现胸闷、气紧为临床表现。

【治疗】穴位:首次选中间及两侧母肺穴,第二次选中间及两侧子肺穴,隔 3 日 1 次,2 次为 1 个疗程。

操作:选用Ⅰ号或Ⅱ号蒙医银针,中间母肺穴和子肺穴直刺 0.5 寸,两侧母肺穴和子肺穴 0.5～1 寸。温针给予针柄加热,温度 38～42℃,15～20 分钟;或火针留针 15～20 分钟。

【按语】①哮喘应积极治疗原发疾病。②发作严重或哮喘持续状态应配合药物治疗。③气候变化时应注意保暖。④过敏体质者,注意避免接触变应原或进食致过敏食物。

九、呃逆

呃逆由横膈肌痉挛引起。健康人也可发生一过性呃逆,多与饮食有关,特别是饮食过快、过饱,摄入很热或很冷的食物饮料、饮酒等,外界温度变化和过度吸烟亦可引起。呃逆频繁或持续 24 小时以上,称为难治性呃逆,多发生于某些疾病。

【病因】呃逆是因为膈肌收缩,空气被迅速吸进肺内,两条声带之中的裂隙骤然收窄,引起奇怪的声响。蒙医认为,主要因巴达干赫依偏盛,如膈肌和胃,阻碍上行赫依之道,或血希拉偏盛伤及膈肌和肝,体质衰弱,气滞血瘀等所致。

【临床表现】呃逆为膈肌痉挛引起的收缩运动,吸气时声门突然关闭发出一种短促的声音。可发于单侧或双侧的膈肌。正常健康者可因吞咽过快、突然吞气或腹内压骤然增高而引起呃逆。有的可持续较长时间而成为顽固性呃逆。

发作时胸部透视可判断膈肌痉挛为一侧性或两侧性,必要时做胸部 CT 检查,排除膈神经受刺激的疾病,做心电图判断有无心包炎和心肌梗死;疑中枢神经病变时可做头部 CT、磁共振、脑电图等检查;疑有消化系统病变时,进行腹部 X 线检查、B 型超声、胃肠造影,必要时做腹部 CT 和肝胰功能检查,为排除中毒与代谢性疾病可做临床生化检查。

【治疗】穴位:首次选中间及两侧膈穴,第二次选中间及两侧胃穴,隔日 1 次,2 次为 1 个疗程。

操作:选用 I 号或 II 号蒙医银针,中间膈穴和胃穴直刺 0.5 寸,两侧膈穴和胃穴 0.5～1 寸。温针给予针柄加热,温度 38～42℃,15～20 分钟;或火针留针 15～20 分钟。

【按语】①呃逆停止后,应积极治疗引起呃逆的原发病。②急重症患者出现呃逆,可能是病情转重之象,宜加以注意。

十、消化不良

消化不良是由胃动力障碍所引起的疾病,也包括胃轻瘫和食管反流病。消化不良主要分为功能性消化不良和器质性消化不良。蒙医所称胃消化不良症,指在饮食消化过程中,由于三根失调,胃火衰败,消化力减弱而形成消化不良诸症的总称。又称"糟粕不消化症""浊瘤疾症"等。

【病因】引起消化不良的原因很多,包括胃和十二指肠部位的慢性炎症,使食管、胃、十二指肠的正常蠕动功能失调。患者的精神不愉快、长期闷闷不乐或突然受到猛烈的刺激等均可引起。胃轻瘫则是由糖尿病、原发性神经性厌食和胃切除术所致。

【临床表现】反复发作上腹部不适或疼痛、饱胀、烧心（反酸）、嗳气等。常因胸闷、早饱感、腹胀等不适而不愿进食或尽量少进食，夜里也不易安睡，睡后常有噩梦。

除胃镜下能见到轻型胃炎外，其他检查如 B 超、X 线造影及血液生化检查等，一般都无异常表现。

【治疗】穴位：首次选痞穴，第二次选火衰穴，第三次选中间和两侧胃穴，隔日 1 次，3 次为 1 个疗程。

操作：选用 I～III 号蒙医银针，痞穴和火衰穴直刺 0.5～1 寸；中间胃穴直刺 0.5 寸，两侧胃穴 0.5～1 寸。温针给予针柄加热，温度 38～42℃，15～20 分钟；或火针留针 15～20 分钟。

【按语】①生活要规律，消除思想顾虑，注意控制情绪，心胸宽阔。②避免食用有刺激性的辛辣食物及生冷食物。

十一、胃下垂

胃下垂是由于膈肌悬力不足，支持内脏器官的韧带松弛，或腹内压降低，腹肌松弛，导致站立时胃大弯抵达盆腔，胃小弯弧线最低点降到髂嵴连线以下。常伴有十二指肠球部位置的改变。正常人的胃在腹腔的左上方，直立时的最低点不应超过脐下两横指，其位置相对固定，对于维持胃的正常功能有一定作用。胃下垂属于蒙医"胃衰病"范畴。

【病因】凡能造成膈肌位置下降的因素，如膈肌活动力降低，腹腔压力降低，腹肌收缩力减弱，胃膈韧带、肝胃韧带、胃脾韧带、胃结肠韧带过于松弛等，均可导致下垂。

【临床表现】轻度下垂者一般无症状，下垂明显者可以出现如下症状：腹胀及上腹不适、腹痛、恶心、呕吐、便秘等。

胃肠钡餐造影，依据站立位胃小弯弧线最低点与两侧髂嵴连线的位置分为 3 度：①轻度，指胃小弯弧线最低点位于髂嵴连线下 1～5cm；②中度，指胃小弯弧线最低点位于髂嵴连线下 5～10cm；③重度，指胃小弯弧线最低点位于髂嵴连线下 10cm 以上。

【治疗】穴位：首次选火衰穴，第二次选中间和两侧脾穴，第三次选中间和两侧胃穴,隔日1次,3次为1个疗程。

操作:选用Ⅰ~Ⅲ号蒙医银针,火衰穴直刺0.5~1寸,中间脾穴和胃穴直刺0.5寸,两侧脾穴和胃穴0.5~1寸。温针给予针柄加热,温度38~42℃,15~20分钟;或火针留针15~20分钟。

【按语】①应养成良好的饮食习惯,定时定量,对体瘦者,应增加营养。②积极参加体育锻炼有助于防止胃下垂继续发展,还可因体力和肌力增强而增强胃张力、胃蠕动,改善症状。

十二、慢性结肠炎

各种原因引起的结肠慢性炎症均可称为慢性结肠炎,是一种慢性、反复性、多发性,由各种致病原因导致的肠道炎性水肿、溃疡、出血病变。慢性结肠炎属于蒙医"肠痼疾"范畴。

【病因】慢性结肠炎的病因复杂,最常见的病因是非特异性结肠炎,如肠易激综合征、炎症性肠病、肠菌群失调、小肠吸收不良等。一般认为和感染、免疫遗传、环境、食物过敏、防御功能障碍及精神因素有关。

【临床表现】病程长,慢性反复发作,以腹痛、腹泻为主要特征,黏液便,便秘或泄泻交替性发生,时好时坏,缠绵不断,可见于任何年龄,但以20~30岁青壮年多见。

做结肠镜、钡餐灌肠、X线检查及血检、粪检等进一步确诊。

【治疗】穴位:首次选两侧脐旁穴,第二次选两侧脐旁外穴,第三次选中间和两侧总穴,第四次选中间和两侧大肠穴,隔日1次,4次为1个疗程。

操作:选用Ⅰ~Ⅲ号蒙医银针,脐旁穴和脐旁外穴直刺0.5~1寸,中间总穴和大肠穴直刺0.5寸,两侧总穴和大肠穴0.5~1寸。温针给予针柄加热,温度38~42℃,15~20分钟;或火针留针15~20分钟。

【按语】①注意劳逸结合,不可太过劳累,保持良好睡眠,解除各种精神压力。②注意衣着,保持冷暖适宜。适当进行体育锻炼以增强体质。③一般进食相对清淡、柔软、易消化、富有营养和足够热量的食物。忌烟酒、辛辣食物等。④注意食品卫生,避免肠道感染诱发或加重本病。

第九章

其他疾病

一、慢性疲劳综合征

慢性疲劳综合征是一种身体出现慢性疲劳症状的病症,具体定义是长期(连续 6 个月以上)原因不明的严重疲劳感觉或身体不适。

【病因】目前医界认为慢性疲劳综合征可能是由病毒感染、免疫系统问题、神经系统问题、精神疾病等多重因素造成。临床及流行病学研究对该病与环境及其他风险因素的关系仍未能达成一致的看法。

【临床表现】发热、咽痛、淋巴结肿大、极度疲劳、失去食欲、复发性上呼吸道感染、小肠不适、黄疸、焦虑、抑郁、烦躁及情绪不稳、睡眠中断、对光及热敏感、暂时失去记忆力、无法集中注意力、头痛、痉挛、肌肉与关节痛。这些症状与感冒及其他病毒感染相似,因此容易误判。

【治疗】穴位:首次选顶会穴,第二次选中间及两侧赫依穴,第三次选中间及两侧巴达干穴,第四次选中间及两侧心穴,第五次选中间及两侧命脉穴,第六次选中间及两侧肾穴,隔日 1 次,6 次为 1 个疗程。

操作:选用Ⅰ号或Ⅱ号蒙医银针,顶会穴向后平刺 0.5~1 寸,中间赫依穴、巴达干穴、心穴、命脉穴、肾穴直刺 0.5 寸,两侧赫依穴、巴达干穴、心穴、命脉穴、肾穴斜刺 0.5~1 寸。温针给予针柄加热,温度 38~42℃,15~20 分钟;或火针留针 15~20 分钟。

【按语】①蒙医温针火针治疗本病可较好地缓解病情,疗效满意。②保持情绪乐观,避免精神刺激,劳逸结合。

二、痛经

痛经为最常见的妇科症状之一,指行经前后或月经期出现下腹部疼痛、坠胀,伴有腰酸或其他不适,症状严重者影响生活质量。痛经分为原发性和继发性两类,原发性痛经指生殖器官无器质性病变的痛经,占痛经 90% 以上;继发性痛经指由盆腔器质性疾病引起的痛经。

【病因】原发性痛经的发生主要与月经时子宫内膜前列腺素、血管加压素、内源性缩宫素、β- 内啡肽等物质的含量增高有关。也有由精神、神经因素所致者。

【临床表现】原发性痛经在青春期多见,常在初潮后 1~2 年内发病。疼痛多自月经来潮后开始,最早出现在经前 12 小时,以行经第 1 日疼痛最剧烈,持续 2~3 日后缓解。疼痛常呈痉挛性,位于下腹部耻骨上,可放射至腰骶部和大腿内侧;可伴有恶心、呕吐、腹泻、头晕、乏力等症状,严重时面色发白、出冷汗。

妇科检查无异常发现。

【治疗】穴位:首次选中间总穴,第二次选两侧总穴,隔 3 日 1 次,2 次为 1 个疗程。

操作:选用Ⅰ~Ⅱ号蒙医银针,中间总穴直刺 0.5 寸,两侧总穴斜刺 0.5~1 寸。温针给予针柄加热,温度 38~42℃,15~20 分钟;或火针留针 15~20 分钟。

【按语】①重视心理治疗,消除紧张和顾虑。②足够的休息和睡眠,规律而适度地锻炼。③疼痛不能忍受时辅以药物治疗。④对继发性痛经,应重视原发病的诊断与治疗。

三、遗精

遗精指不因性生活而精液遗泄的病症。其中因梦而遗精者称"梦遗";梦而遗精,甚至清醒时精液流出的谓"滑精"。必须指出,凡成年未婚男子,或婚后夫妻分居等长期无性生活者,1 个月发生遗精 1~2 次属生理现象。如遗精次数过多,每周 2 次以上或清醒时遗精,并伴有头昏、精神萎靡、腰腿酸软、失眠等症,则属病态。

【病因】多因劳倦过度,用心太过,恣情纵欲,感触见闻,饮食辛辣等因素诱发。

【临床表现】不因性生活而精液频繁遗泄,每周 2 次以上,或在睡中有梦而遗,或在睡中无梦而遗,或有少量精液随尿而外流,甚者可在清醒时自行流出,常伴有头晕、耳鸣、健忘、心悸、失眠、腰酸膝软、精神萎靡,或尿时不爽,小腹及阴部作胀不适等症状。

【治疗】穴位:首次选中间精穴,第二次选两侧精穴,隔 3 日 1 次,2 次为 1 个疗程。

操作:选用Ⅰ号或Ⅱ号蒙医银针,中间精穴直刺 0.3 寸,两侧精穴斜刺 0.5~

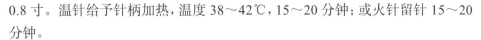

0.8 寸。温针给予针柄加热,温度 38～42℃,15～20 分钟;或火针留针 15～20 分钟。

【按语】①保持心情舒畅,积极参加健康的体育活动以排除杂念,节制性欲,戒除频繁手淫,防止过度疲劳及精神紧张。②睡眠时,养成侧卧习惯,被子不要盖得太厚太暖,内裤不宜过紧。③少食辛辣刺激性食物,宜戒烟、酒、咖啡等。

四、变应性鼻炎

变应性鼻炎即过敏性鼻炎,是指特应性个体接触变应原后,主要由 IgE 介导的介质(主要是组胺)释放,并有多种免疫活性细胞和细胞因子参与的鼻黏膜非感染性炎性疾病。其发生的必要条件有 3 个:特异性抗原,即引起机体免疫反应的物质;特应性个体,即所谓过敏体质;特异性抗原与特应性个体二者相遇。变应性鼻炎是一个全球性健康问题,可导致许多疾病和劳动力丧失。

【病因】变应性鼻炎是一种由基因与环境互相作用而诱发的多因素疾病。变应性鼻炎的危险因素可能存在于所有年龄段。

【临床表现】变应性鼻炎的典型症状主要是阵发性喷嚏、清水样鼻涕、鼻塞和鼻痒。部分伴有嗅觉减退。

【治疗】穴位:首次选中间及两侧母肺穴,第二次选中间及两侧子肺穴,隔3 日 1 次,2 次为 1 个疗程。

操作:选用Ⅰ号或Ⅱ号蒙医银针,中间母肺穴和子肺穴直刺 0.5 寸,两侧母肺穴和子肺穴 0.5～1 寸。温针给予针柄加热,温度 38～42℃,15～20 分钟;或火针留针 15～20 分钟。

【按语】①鼻过敏者须避开变应原,如花粉、尘螨、动物皮屑等。②平时少食用冰凉食品或较寒性食物,如冷饮、冰激凌、可乐、冰凉水果、苦瓜等。

五、神经性耳鸣

神经性耳鸣又称感音神经性耳鸣,其强调的是患者的主观感受。指人们在没有任何外界刺激条件下所产生的异常声音感觉。如感觉耳内有蝉鸣声、嗡嗡声、嘶嘶声等单调或混杂的响声,如果是持续性耳鸣,还可能伴有耳聋、眩晕、头痛等其他症状。可分为感音性(源于耳蜗)、周围神经性(源于听神经)及中枢神经性耳鸣。

【病因】多为老年性耳聋、耳毒性药物性听力损失、噪声性听力损失、梅尼埃病、迟发性膜迷路积水等引起,此外,还可见于外淋巴瘘、内耳感染、耳硬化症等疾病。

【临床表现】在没有任何外界刺激条件下产生异常声音感觉,如感觉耳内有蝉鸣声、嗡嗡声、嘶嘶声等单调或混杂的响声,实际上周围环境中并无相应的声音,也就是说耳鸣只是一种主观感觉。耳鸣可以短暂或持续性存在。严重的耳鸣可以扰得人一刻不得安宁,令人十分紧张。如果是短暂性的耳鸣,一般是生理现象,不必过分紧张。

【治疗】穴位:首次选顶会穴和中间赫依穴,第二次选两侧或患侧后枕窝穴,第三次选两侧或患侧耳后凹陷穴,隔3日1次,2次为1个疗程。

操作:选用Ⅰ号或Ⅱ号蒙医银针,顶会穴平刺0.5~1寸,中间赫依穴直刺0.5~1寸,后枕窝穴平刺0.3~0.5寸,耳后凹陷穴直刺0.5~1寸。温针给予针柄加热,温度为38~42℃,15~20分钟;或火针留针15~20分钟。

【按语】①注意休息,避免劳倦,保持心情舒畅。②应查明病因,必要时配合原发病治疗。

下篇

机制研究

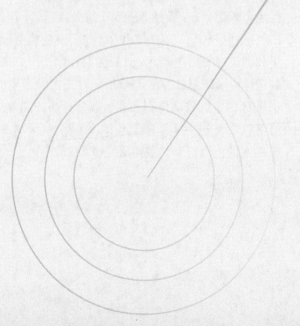

第十章

蒙医温针调节疲劳大鼠细胞因子和神经递质复杂机制研究

本项研究是笔者主持的 2006—2008 年国家自然科学基金项目：蒙医温针调节疲劳大鼠细胞因子和神经递质复杂机制研究（编号 30572462）。

慢性疲劳综合征（chronic fatigue syndrome，CFS）属蒙医"巴达干、赫依"性疾病范畴，以原因不明的、难以恢复的疲劳感为主要特征的综合征，可伴有长期低热、咽痛、头痛、肌肉关节肿痛、抑郁、健忘、失眠或嗜睡等症状。西医采取的对症处理的治疗方法，疗效不确切；而蒙医以整体观念为指导，辨证论治，在临床上显出了优势，但其作用机制却不够明了，对这种疾病的病因病理的探究亦未见公认的结果[1]。蒙医文献记载与现代临床试验证明，蒙医温针疗法对 CFS 的疗效更显著[2]。

本课题研究认为 CFS 是人类精神心理活动异常状态的延续，在这种长期的异常状态中，机体一直处于一种慢性应激状态，尤其体内的免疫系统常处于慢性免疫激活状态，导致细胞因子释放紊乱，干扰神经递质的功能，从而引起 CFS 的一系列症状[3]。前期工作中，我们发现疲劳模型大鼠脑中某些部位的细胞因子和神经递质出现紊乱，而蒙医温针疗法可以调整这种紊乱的状态。因而本课题选择以蒙医温针疗法调节细胞因子神经递质的状态为切入点，从蛋白基因水平研究 CFS 的致病机制和蒙医温针疗法的调节机制，希望能将蒙医温针疗法的宏观效果与微观探索结合起来，以期能从生物学角度初步阐明蒙医温针疗法治疗 CFS 的作用机制。主要研究成果如下。

一、蒙医温针疗法对大鼠疲劳模型肝脏 MDA、GSH、GSH-Px 和 SOD 含量的影响的研究

表 10-1　蒙医温针疗法对各组大鼠肝脏 MDA、GSH、GSH-Px 和 SOD 含量的影响($\bar{x} \pm s$)

组别	例数	MDA/ ($nmol \cdot mg^{-1} \cdot Pro^{-1}$)	GSH/ ($mg \cdot g^{-1} \cdot Pro^{-1}$)	GSH-Px/U	SOD/ ($U \cdot mg^{-1} \cdot Pro^{-1}$)
正常对照组	10	0.65 ± 0.18	55.23 ± 10.34	52.93 ± 6.15	213.20 ± 20.31
模型组	10	0.79 ± 0.15	$39.79 \pm 5.36^{**}$	$41.68 \pm 5.55^{**}$	$186.10 \pm 27.30^{*}$
模型+温针组	10	0.68 ± 0.13	$51.92 \pm 10.72^{\#}$	$47.59 \pm 4.99^{\#}$	$227.62 \pm 24.26^{\#\#}$

注：与正常组比，$^{*}P<0.05$，$^{**}P<0.01$；与模型组比，$^{\#}P<0.05$，$^{\#\#}P<0.01$。

本实验采用的是力竭游泳所致大鼠运动性疲劳模型[4]。适度的游泳训练可维持机体自由基代谢正常进行，而过度训练的力竭游泳则可导致机体自由基代谢失衡，造成对机体组织器官的损伤，产生运动性疲劳[5]。抑制和消除运动性内源自由基和脂质过氧化，对运动性疲劳恢复有重要作用。针灸治疗运动性疲劳对自由基的影响已有相关的实验研究报道[6]。有人针刺小鼠"足三里"穴，发现针刺组小鼠 SOD、GSH-Px 活性高于对照组，而 MDA 水平低于对照组，表明针刺能提高小鼠体内抗氧化酶活性，降低脂质过氧化反应，从而保护细胞免受运动性损伤，延缓运动性疲劳的发生[7]。

本课题研究结果见表 10-1：①与正常对照组相比，模型组丙二醛（MDA）含量有增高的趋势，但是无显著性差异（$P>0.05$）；与模型组相比，温针组 MDA 含量有下降的趋势，但是无显著性差异（$P>0.05$）。②与正常对照组相比，模型组谷胱甘肽（GSH）含量降低，有显著性差异（$P<0.01$）；与模型组相比，温针组 GSH 含量增高，有显著性差异（$P<0.05$）。③与正常对照组相比，模型组谷胱甘肽过氧化物酶（GSH-Px）含量降低，有显著性差异（$P<0.01$）；与模型组相比，温针组 GSH-Px 含量增高，有显著性差异（$P<0.05$）。④与正常对照组相比，模型组超氧化物歧化酶（SOD）含量降低，有显著性差异（$P<0.05$）；与模型组相比，温针组 SOD 含量增高，有显著性差异（$P<0.01$）。

肝脏是机体物质代谢的重要器官，其中的自由基代谢及抗氧化酶变化较为明显。肝脏和骨骼肌线粒体呼吸链电子传递中电子漏形成的超氧自由基是运动性内源自由基的主要来源，氧自由基生成增多及脂质过氧化反应增强，导致了对细胞结构和功能的一系列损害[8]。例如，细胞膜的流动性、完整性和通透性下

降；线粒体结构和功能受损伤，继而影响电子的传递和偶联磷酸化的进行；电子漏引起质子漏从而影响线粒体电子的传递和氧化磷酸化的进行等。MDA 是脂质过氧化的代谢产物，是造成细胞膜损伤的物质基础，其含量可以反映机体内脂质过氧化的程度，间接反映氧自由基对细胞的损伤程度。SOD 则是体内重要的防御自由基毒害的抗氧化酶，分解过氧化氢和脂质过氧化物，阻断脂质过氧化反应，保护细胞免受损伤。GSH-Px 是体内催化过氧化氢分解的重要酶，它特异催化 GSH 对过氧化氢的还原反应，可以起到保护细胞膜结构和功能完整的作用。GSH 是一种低分子清除剂，其量的多少是衡量机体抗氧化能力的重要因素 [9]。

　　蒙医理论认为疲劳与巴达干、赫依的功能失调有关。巴达干失调的症状有嗜睡、身重、头晕、健忘等。赫依失调的症状有头晕、耳鸣、寒战、不定位疼痛、失眠、骨骼关节疼痛等。本实验所取蒙医"顶会"穴，主治赫依性喑哑症、神志不清、癫狂、视力减退、头晕、头痛等；"心穴"主治心悸，癫狂，巴达干、赫依性心病，失眠，神志昏迷等症。以上穴位调节巴达干、赫依紊乱有较好效果。

　　蒙医温针疗法是一种行之有效的治疗疲劳的方法，结合现代电子技术研制而成的温针仪，可以达到传统蒙医温针的作用，同时为蒙医传统疗法操作技术的规范及器械的革新奠定了基础。该方法治疗运动性疲劳的机制研究尚未见报道。本实验观察到，疲劳模型组动物肝脏的 SOD、GSH、GSH-Px 均比正常对照组降低，提示模型组体内的抗氧化酶活性降低；而温针组 SOD、GSH、GSH-Px 均比模型组升高，提示蒙医温针疗法能提高疲劳大鼠肝脏的抗氧化酶活性，以增加对自由基损伤的抵抗力和对自由基的清除，阻断脂质过氧化反应，保护细胞免受损伤，从而促进疲劳的恢复。但是蒙医温针疗法对 MDA 的影响不甚明显，具体原因还有待进一步研究。

二、艾灸对疲劳模型大鼠血清 IL-6 和 IL-10 的影响的研究

表 10-2　艾灸法对各组大鼠血清 IL-6 和 IL-10 含量的影响（$\bar{x} \pm s$）

组别	例数	IL-6/(pg·ml^{-1})	IL-10/(pg·ml^{-1})
正常组	10	53.69±20.43	38.92±17.30
模型组	10	105.76±32.09**	84.35±21.71**
艾灸组	10	69.03±10.79#	62.21±18.80*##

注：与正常组比，*$P<0.05$，**$P<0.01$；与模型组比，#$P<0.05$，##$P<0.01$。

　　从表 10-2 可见：①与正常组相比，模型组 IL-6 含量降低，有显著性差异

（$P < 0.01$）；与模型组相比，艾灸组 IL-6 含量增高，有显著性差异（$P < 0.05$）。②与正常组相比，模型组 IL-10 含量降低，有显著性差异（$P < 0.01$）；与模型组相比，艾灸组 IL-10 含量增高，有显著性差异（$P < 0.05$）。

IL-6 是一种多功能细胞因子，既可由淋巴细胞产生，也能由非淋巴细胞合成。在体内免疫反应调节、血细胞的增生、防御机制和急性期反应中起重要作用。IL-6 是一种糖蛋白，它既可诱导急性期时相关蛋白的产生，也是 β 细胞终末分化并分泌抗体的必需因子，在免疫调节中发挥重要作用[10]。IL-10 是主要由 Th2 细胞所产生的一种细胞因子，活化的 B 细胞、单核巨噬细胞和库普弗（Kupffer）细胞等也可产生 IL-10。它是以抑制 Th 细胞克隆细胞因子合成为特点的多效免疫调节因子。IL-10 是维护细胞因子网络平衡的重要负调节因子。其作用机制可能是降低抗原递呈细胞 MHC Ⅱ类抗原表达，或诱导抗原递呈细胞产生另一种细胞因子，改变细胞内信号传递途径，从而选择性抑制某些细胞因子 mRNA 转录，并与 Th2 细胞产生的 IL-4、IL-5 有协同作用[10]。

近年来研究结果分析，运动对 IL 影响研究较多的主要有 IL-1、IL-2 和 IL-6，并且其分泌异常是运动性疲劳产生的机制之一[11-12]。因而调节免疫功能，对运动性疲劳恢复有重要作用。艾灸治疗运动性疲劳对细胞因子的影响已有相关的研究报道[13]。有人艾灸强壮穴观察对慢性疲劳综合征患者免疫功能的影响，结果表明，艾灸后患者免疫功能改善，说明艾灸强壮穴能有效提高患者免疫功能[14-15]。也有人研究发现，艾灸膈俞后体内 IL-2 显著升高，表明艾灸通过调节细胞因子水平而起到增强免疫功能的作用。

本实验结果显示，运动性疲劳大鼠模型[4-5]血清中的 IL-6、IL-10 含量均明显高于正常组（$P < 0.05$）。说明运动性疲劳大鼠与 IL-6、IL-10 有密切关系。IL-6、IL-10 水平的增高是免疫功能激活的标志之一，这些细胞因子可能通过扰乱神经递质的功能，而引起以疲劳为主症，伴随不明原因的周身疲乏无力、肌肉关节酸痛、发热等一系列症状的慢性疲劳的发生[16-17]。艾灸组可使升高的 IL-6、IL-10 含量趋于正常，说明艾灸法可能通过对细胞因子的影响，起到调整神经免疫网络，缓解疲劳、周身疲乏无力、肌肉关节酸痛、发热等症状的作用，从而达到治疗慢性疲劳的目的[18]。

综上所述，细胞因子不仅可以激活免疫系统，而且对神经和内分泌系统也有重要的调节作用。在本实验中，疲劳模型大鼠血清中的 IL-6、IL-10 有异常的增高，这些免疫学的变化可能是运动性疲劳发生的病理机制之一。经过艾灸法治疗的疲劳模型组 IL-6、IL-10 趋于正常，起到调整神经免疫网络的作用，从而发挥抗疲劳作用。

三、蒙医温针对运动性疲劳大鼠血清TNF-α、ACTH和皮质
酮含量的影响的研究

1. 对大鼠力竭游泳时间和悬尾不动时间的影响　在造模第21天温针组力竭游泳时间与模型组相比明显延长,有显著性差异($P<0.05$),如表10-3所示。在造模第21天模型组悬尾不动时间与对照组相比明显延长,有显著性差异($P<0.05$);温针组悬尾不动时间与模型组相比明显缩短,有显著性差异($P<0.05$),如表10-4所示。

表10-3　模型组和温针组的力竭游泳时间比较($\bar{x}\pm s$)

组别	例数	力竭游泳时间/s
模型组	19	679.65±256.55
温针组	19	875.84±200.60#

注:与模型组比,#$P<0.05$。

表10-4　各组悬尾不动时间的比较($\bar{x}\pm s$)

组别	例数	悬尾不动时间/s
对照组	20	32.01±20.9
模型组	19	58.74±43.63*
温针组	19	32.04±20.73#

注:与对照组相比,*$P<0.05$;与模型组比,#$P<0.05$。

2. 对大鼠血清TNF-α、ACTH和皮质酮含量的影响　模型组与对照组相比,TNF-α、促肾上腺皮质激素(ACTH)和皮质酮含量均升高,有显著性差异($P<0.01$)。温针组与模型组相比,TNF-α、ACTH和皮质酮含量降低,有显著性差异($P<0.01$,$P<0.05$,$P<0.01$),如表10-5所示。

表10-5　各组血清TNF-α、ACTH和皮质酮含量的比较($\bar{x}\pm s$)

组别	例数	TNF-α/(pg·ml^{-1})	ACTH/(pg·ml^{-1})	皮质酮/(pg·ml^{-1})
对照组	10	41.30±7.77	20.85±9.18	10.59±2.06
模型组	10	63.79±13.27**	49.78±11.23**	25.14±5.41**
温针组	10	45.32±7.03##	38.19±8.29#	15.57±4.78##

注:与对照组相比,**$P<0.01$;与模型组比,#$P<0.05$,##$P<0.01$。

本实验采用的力竭游泳运动性疲劳模型，反映了疲劳长期积累而引起机体功能紊乱的一种病理状态[4]。力竭游泳时间是反映大鼠体力及疲劳状况的经典指标，悬尾实验中的不动时间也可以在一定程度上反映大鼠的体力及疲劳状况[19]。本实验从力竭游泳时间和悬尾不动时间的改善，显示了蒙医温针的抗疲劳效果。

有研究表明，力竭游泳可引起下丘脑 - 垂体 - 肾上腺轴（HPA 轴）功能亢进，ACTH 含量明显增加。多种细胞因子如 IL-1、IL-6 和 TNF-α 作用于 HPA 轴，刺激皮质激素的合成[20-21]。TNF-α 是由被激活的巨噬细胞和单核细胞产生的多肽类介质，在体内具有广泛的生物学作用。研究表明，TNF 参与了多种疾病的病理过程，在免疫调节、抗病毒、炎症、内毒性休克以及某些慢性病、恶病质性消瘦和营养不良综合征等细胞反应中具有重要作用[22]。而运动性疲劳时，TNF 明显增高，并且通过激活 HPA 轴，促进 ACTH 和皮质酮的释放[23-24]。有人观察到针刺具有改善运动能力，调节下丘脑 - 垂体 - 性腺轴功能紊乱的作用[25-27]。另外，有研究表明，针灸可以提高疲劳大鼠血清 TNF-α 的含量而起到抗疲劳作用[15]。

本实验结果表明：21 天模型组大鼠血清 ACTH 和皮质酮与正常组比较明显升高（$P < 0.01$），而温针组血清 ACTH 和皮质酮与模型组比较明显降低（$P < 0.05$），说明蒙医温针可以抑制皮质酮过度释放，调节运动性疲劳大鼠的免疫功能。另外，模型组 TNF-α 的含量比正常组显著升高（$P < 0.01$），而温针组显著下降（$P < 0.05$）。这支持大强度运动训练后 TNF 含量明显增加引起运动性疲劳的观点。蒙医温针有效地调节运动性疲劳大鼠 TNF-α 的含量而起到免疫调节作用。

本实验所取蒙医顶会穴、心穴，对调节巴达干、赫依紊乱有较好效果。

以上研究表明蒙医温针可能通过降低运动性疲劳大鼠血清 TNF-α、ACTH 和皮质酮的含量，调节内分泌和免疫功能，发挥抗疲劳的作用。是否还有其他细胞因子参与蒙医温针抗疲劳的作用，还有待进一步研究。

四、蒙医温针对疲劳大鼠行为学与血清皮质酮、睾酮及皮质酮与睾酮比值的影响的研究

本研究采用 21 天力竭游泳制备大鼠运动性疲劳模型[5]。力竭是疲劳长期积累而引起机体功能紊乱的一种病理状态[4]。我们在此模型上初步观察蒙医温针抗疲劳的效应和机制。

1. 对大鼠力竭游泳时间的影响　力竭游泳时间是反映大鼠体力及疲劳状

况的经典指标。在造模第 7 天,温针组的力竭游泳时间与模型组相比明显延长且有显著性差异($P < 0.05$),显示了抗疲劳效果(见表 10-6);这种效果在造模第 14 天、21 天持续存在,而以第 14 天的抗疲劳效果最为显著($P < 0.01$)。吴立红报道了第 1～10 天中经皮穴位电刺激大鼠"足三里"对力竭游泳时间的影响[28]。发现从力竭游泳第 6 天开始,治疗组力竭游泳时间比模型组明显延长,至第 10 天仍有效。另外,研究报道显示力竭游泳第 7 天,经皮穴位电刺激治疗组的力竭游泳时间比模型组明显延长[26]。这些提示第 6 天或第 7 天可能是经皮穴位电刺激治疗力竭游泳疲劳大鼠起效的时间。本实验结果显示温针组在第 7 天与模型组有明显差异,与上述经皮穴位电刺激的报道接近。

表 10-6　模型组和温针组大鼠力竭游泳时间的比较($\bar{x} \pm s$)

组别	例数	第 7 天 /s	第 14 天 /s	第 21 天 /s
模型组	19	459.45±212.20	495.79±89.97	679.65±256.55
温针组	19	771.74±490.51[#]	1 105.84±333.31[##]	875.84±200.60[#]

注:与模型组比,[#]$P < 0.05$,[##]$P < 0.01$。

2. 对大鼠体重的影响　在造模第 7 天、14 天、21 天,各组体重未见显著性差异($P > 0.05$),提示本研究中大鼠的疲劳状况与体重等因素没有直接关系(见表 10-7)。

表 10-7　各组大鼠体重的比较($\bar{x} \pm s$)

组别	例数	第 7 天 /g	第 14 天 /g	第 21 天 /g
对照组	20	225.9±14.8	252.9±16.8	263.6±21.9
模型组	19	233.7±9.2	252.4±9.8	265.2±11.3
温针组	19	231.9±8.9	245.6±14.9	261.9±15.6

3. 对大鼠悬尾实验行为的影响　悬尾实验也可以在一定程度上反映大鼠的体力及疲劳状况。

(1)不动时间:在造模第 7 天、14 天、21 天,温针组与对照组、模型组相比,不动时间均明显缩短且有显著性差异($P < 0.05$,$P < 0.01$,$P < 0.05$),显示了抗疲劳效果;以第 14 天的效果最为显著($P < 0.01$)。

(2)挣扎次数:在造模第 7 天,各组挣扎次数无显著性差异($P > 0.05$)。在第 14 天,模型组、温针组分别与对照组相比,挣扎次数增加,有显著性差异($P < 0.01$,$P < 0.01$)。在第 21 天,模型组、温针组与对照组相比,挣扎次数减少,有显著性

差异（$P<0.01$，$P<0.05$）。结果见表 10-8。我们未观察到温针组和模型组在挣扎次数上有显著差异。这种不动时间和挣扎次数变化的不一致，是否因不动时间受温针影响较敏感所致，尚有待探讨。

表 10-8　各组大鼠悬尾不动时间和挣扎次数的比较（$\bar{x}\pm s$）

项目	组别	例数	第 7 天	第 14 天	第 21 天
不动时间 /s	对照组	20	60.0±29.35	46.26±19.01	32.01±20.9
	模型组	19	65.71±28.86	47.46±16.70	58.74±43.63[*]
	温针组	19	38.33±16.51[*#]	20.85±13.20[**##]	32.04±20.73[#]
挣扎次数	对照组	20	10.2±3.9	7±3.4	11.3±5.1
	模型组	19	9.1±5.0	12.4±4.0[**]	7.2±3.5[**]
	温针组	19	9.3±3.9	11.3±4.1[**]	8.1±3.2[*]

注：与正常对照组比，[*]$P<0.05$，[**]$P<0.01$；与模型组比，[#]$P<0.05$，[##]$P<0.01$。

4. 对大鼠血清皮质酮（C）和睾酮（T）的影响　与对照组相比，模型组皮质酮明显升高并有显著性差异（$P<0.01$，$P<0.01$）。与模型组相比，温针组皮质酮明显下降并有显著性差异（$P<0.05$，$P<0.01$）。模型组与温针组的睾酮均比对照组明显升高且有显著性差异（$P<0.05$，$P<0.05$）。模型组的 T/C 比值比对照组明显降低且有显著性差异（$P<0.05$），温针组的 T/C 比值比模型组明显降低且有显著性差异（$P<0.05$）（见表 10-9）。

表 10-9　各组大鼠血清皮质酮、睾酮和 T/C 的比较（$\bar{x}\pm s$）

组别	例数	皮质酮 /(nmol·L^{-1})	睾酮 /(ng·ml^{-1})	T/C
对照组	11	10.59±2.0	30.93±10.78	3.11±1.47
模型组	10	25.14±5.41[**]	51.71±9.58[**]	2.00±0.40[*]
温针组	10	15.57±4.78[##]	58.44±13.45[**]	3.61±1.12[#]

注：与正常对照组比，[*]$P<0.05$，[**]$P<0.01$；与模型组比，[#]$P<0.05$，[##]$P<0.01$。

皮质酮与睾酮是两种代表性的类固醇激素。在对蛋白质代谢的作用上，皮质酮促进蛋白质分解代谢；睾酮促进蛋白质合成，并与人体运动能力、肌力及疲劳恢复关系密切[29]。T/C 比值可以反映机体分解和合成代谢的平衡状况，是判断过度运动的一个指标。一般情况下，机体的皮质酮与睾酮代谢处于平衡状态。运动性疲劳使下丘脑 - 垂体 - 肾上腺皮质轴和下丘脑 - 垂体 - 性腺轴功能紊乱，引起皮质酮与睾酮分泌异常[30]。而运动性疲劳对皮质酮、睾酮的影响，文献报道不尽一致[31]。有报道在短时间大强度运动时，皮质酮与睾酮同步增长；而在长时间大强度力竭性运动后，皮质酮升高，睾酮出现衰竭。另有研究显示，大鼠6周大运动量游泳造成血皮质酮与睾酮明显降低。本研究结果显示，3周力竭游泳引起模型组血清皮质酮、睾酮升高，皮质酮与睾酮出现同步变化。未出现运动性血清睾酮降低，可能是由于力竭游泳时间仅有3周，属于短时间大强度运动，不及6周的长时间大强度力竭性运动。另外，模型组T/C比值较对照组明显降低，提示机体分解代谢大于合成代谢，机体处于以消耗为主的疲劳状态。而温针组T/C比值较模型组升高，提示机体合成代谢增强，抑制了分解状态，有利于疲劳的恢复。

蒙医温针具有取穴少、疗效快、针感强的特点[1]。本实验取蒙医顶会穴、心穴，对调节巴达干、赫依紊乱有较好效果。

综上所述，本研究结果初步显示，蒙医温针可能通过调节血清睾酮/皮质酮（T/C）比值，改善运动性疲劳大鼠的体能，发挥抗疲劳作用。由于睾酮分泌受到下丘脑-垂体-性腺轴调节，是否还有其他激素参与温针抗疲劳作用，还需要进一步深入研究。

五、蒙医温针对疲劳大鼠基因表达影响的研究

运动性中枢疲劳的发生和发展是一个复杂的过程，涉及多个基因表达调控网络的变化。因此，通过开展蒙医温针调节疲劳大鼠基因表达的研究，有望揭示蒙医温针治疗慢性疲劳综合征的分子机制。研究人员建立慢性疲劳综合征大鼠模型，并分为正常对照组、模型组、蒙医温针治疗组。断头处死后快速取各组大鼠脑组织，采用生物芯片北京国家工程研究中心27K大鼠全基因组寡核苷酸芯片，共有26 962条70mer长度的寡核苷酸，进行基因芯片杂交，进而分析大鼠脑组织基因表达谱的变化。研究结果显示，与正常对照组相比，疲劳大鼠脑组织有625个差异表达基因，其中上调基因105个，下调基因520个。进一步对差异表达基因进行功能富集分析后发现，多个信号通路与慢性疲劳综合征发展过程密切相关，包括代谢（例如糖和肌醇代谢）、肌动蛋白结合、细胞黏附、激酶活化、炎症反应、神经递质改变等多方面。将蒙医温针治疗组与模型组相比较发现，蒙医温针治疗能有效调节自由基代谢相关基因的表达，提示蒙医温针可能通过调节自由基代谢相关基因的表达发挥其治疗慢性疲劳综合征的作用。有关基因方面的研究需进一步深入探索。

参 考 文 献

[1] 阿古拉. 蒙医传统疗法大成 [M]. 赤峰：内蒙古科学技术出版社，2000：128.

[2] 戈毕，包华. 蒙医温针疗法治疗疲劳征的临床研究 [J]. 蒙医药（蒙文版），1998，1（1）：21-22.

[3] POWERS S K，DERUISSEAU K C，QUINDRY J，et al. Dietary antioxidants and exercise[J]. Journal of sports sciences，2004，22（1）：81-94.

[4] 侯莉娟，刘晓莉，乔德才. 大鼠游泳运动疲劳模型建立的研究 [J]. 实验动物科学与管理，2005，22（1）：1-3.

[5] 郑澜，陆爱云. 运动性疲劳动物模型的研究 [J]. 中国体育科技，2003，39（2）：20-23.

[6] 杨波，张钧. 氧自由基脂质过氧化反应致运动性疲劳产生的机制研究 [J]. 中国临床康复，2005，9（4）：188-190.

[7] 朱梅菊，高顺生，李红，等. 针刺足三里穴对运动小鼠体内自由基代谢的影响 [J]. 中国运动医学杂志，2001，20（3）：263-265.

[8] 王熙梅，王俊兰，郑师陵. 运动训练强度与大鼠肝脏自由基代谢之间的关系 [J]. 河北医学，2003，9（8）：733-734.

[9] VINA J，GIMENO A，SASTRE J，et al. Mechanism of free radical production in exhaustive exercise in humans and rats：role of xanthine oxidase and protection by allopurinol[J]. IUBMB life，2000，49（6）：539-544.

[10] 陈慰峰，金伯泉. 医学免疫学 [M]. 北京：人民卫生出版社，2005：64-67.

[11] Cannon J G，Angel J B，Ball R W，et al. Acute phase responses and cytokine secretion in chronic fatigue syndrome[J]. Journal of clinical immunology，1999，19（6）：414-421.

[12] MORASKA A，CAMPISI J，NGUYEN K T，et al. Elevated IL-1beta contributes to antibody suppression produced by stress[J]. Journal of Applied Physiology，2002，93（1）：207-215.

[13] 田华张，陈俊玲. 艾灸强壮穴对慢性疲劳综合征患者免疫功能的影响 [J]. 深圳中西医结合杂志，2006，8（4）：227.

[14] 崔瑾，申定珠，熊芳丽. 针灸膈俞对白细胞共同抗原及免疫功能的影响 [J]. 四川中医，2006（2）：101-102.

[15] 罗英华，陈敏聪，冯耀华，等. 针刺对慢性疲劳大鼠血清 IL-1 及 TNF-α 的影响 [J]. 天津中医药，2006，6（3）：206-208.

[16] 何伟. 运动与细胞因子的研究进展 [J]. 体育科学，2005，25（7）：63-67.

[17] 孙卫民，王惠琴. 细胞因子研究方法 [M]. 北京：人民卫生出版社，1997.

[18] 林文注，王佩. 实验针灸学 [M]. 上海：上海科学技术出版社，1999（9）：288-289.

[19] CHRO G P，吴卫平. 应激与应激系统紊乱的概念：概述身体的和行为的内环境稳定 [J]. 美国医学会杂志：中文版，1992，11（5）：290.

[20] DEMITRACK M A, CROFFORD L J. Evidence for and pathophysiologic implications of hypothalamic-pituitary-adrenal axis dysregulation in fibromyalgia and chronic fatigue syndrome[J]. Annals of the New York Academy of Sciences，1998，840（1）：684-697.

[21] 路翠艳，潘芳. 应激反应中 HPA 轴的中枢调控和免疫调节 [J]. 中国行为医学科学，2003，12（3）：353.

[22] 刘波，戴国钢，马建，等. 大强度运动和中医治疗对兔膝关节软骨 IL-1、TNF、PGE_2 的影响 [J]. 中国运动医学杂志，2004，5（3）：306.

[23] KAVELAARS A, KUIS W, KNOOK L, et al. Disturbed neuroendocrine-immune interactions in chronic fatigue syndrome[J]. The Journal of clinical endocrinology and metabolism，2000，85（2）：692-696.

[24] Pall M L. Elevated, sustained peroxynitrite levels as the cause of chronic fatigue syndrome[J]. Medical hypotheses，2000，54（1）：115-125.

[25] 阿古拉，陈英松. 蒙医温针疗法治疗慢性疲劳综合征的临床研究 [J]. 辽宁中医药大学学报，2006，8（5）：116-117.

[26] 王京京，孟宏，文娜，等. 电针"四关"穴对慢性疲劳大鼠模型的行为学影响 [J]. 针刺研究，2004，29（2）：130-134.

[27] 韦迪，王国祥，谢业琪，等. 针刺对人体血睾酮水平的影响 [J]. 上海针灸杂志，1995（增刊）：129-130.

[28] 吴立红，方剑乔，邵晓梅，等. 经皮穴位电刺激足三里对抗大鼠运动性疲劳 [J]. 中国临床康复，2005，9（40）：114-117.

[29] WONG C S, SENGUPTA S, TJANDRA J J, et al. The influence of specific luminal factors on the colonic epithelium: high-dose butyrate and physical changes suppress early carcinogenic events in rats[J]. Diseases of the colon and rectum，2005，48（3）：549-559.

[30] VERVOORN C, VERMULST L J, BOELENS-QUIST A M, et al. Seasonal changes in performance and free testosterone: cortisol ratio of elite female rowers[J]. European journal of applied physiology and occupational physiology，1992，64（1）：14-21.

[31] 胡红梅. 不同运动量训练对大鼠血睾酮及相关指标的影响 [J]. 体育学刊，2001，8（3）：63-67.

第十一章

蒙医温针对 PCPA 致失眠大鼠的催眠作用及其机制研究

本项研究是笔者主持的 2013—2016 年国家自然科学基金项目：蒙医温针对 PCPA 致失眠大鼠的催眠作用及其机制研究（编号 81260571）。

本课题以蒙医传统理论为基础 [1-3]，通过实验手段验证了蒙医温针法具有多途径、多靶向、多层次的治疗失眠的作用，坚持了蒙医整体观念、辨证论治的原则，初步探讨了温针改善睡眠的作用机制，为揭示温针治疗失眠症作用机制奠定了坚实的工作基础。

建立对氯苯丙氨酸（PCPA）致失眠大鼠模型 [4]，通过观察大鼠皮毛、昼夜节律、饮食情况、体重变化来评估模型。观察模型大鼠 10 天发现，连续 2 次腹腔注射 PCPA 即起效，自腹腔注射 PCPA 后 28～30 小时开始，动物出现昼夜节律消失、躁动、饮水进食减少，体重减轻；腹腔注射 PCPA 后第 3 天，动物睡眠觉醒百分比开始改变，第 6 天左右达高峰，第 7 天开始恢复，失眠时间持续 7～10 天，具有可逆性。造模实验结果表明：腹腔注射 PCPA 可使正常大鼠的睡眠 - 觉醒周期消失，是复制失眠大鼠模型的比较稳定的方法；腹腔注射 PCPA 后大鼠昼夜节律消失、躁动等行为改变与蒙医"三根失调，赫依偏盛"引起的癫狂、心悸、激荡、夜不能寐等临床表现吻合；失眠模型建立后第 3 天开始用蒙医温针连续刺激 7 天，第 8 天取材，符合 PCPA 致失眠大鼠模型的时间线，能够观察到温针对失眠大鼠的影响。本项研究主要研究进展及重要结果如下。

一、蒙医温针催眠作用研究

选用戊巴比妥钠诱导大鼠睡眠的模型，其意义在于观察蒙医温针与戊巴比妥钠的协同作用。通过前期实验对戊巴比妥钠的阈剂量进行了摸索，确定致大鼠睡眠的戊巴比妥钠阈剂量值为 45mg/kg。比较治疗组和空白对照组睡眠潜伏期和睡眠持续时间之间的差异,用 t 检验检验其显著性。实验结果(见表 11-1)发现,蒙医温针与戊巴比妥钠有协同作用,可延长戊巴比妥钠诱导大鼠睡眠的时间,与空白对照组比较差异有显著性($P < 0.01$),反映了蒙医温针镇静催眠的确定性。

表 11-1 两组戊巴比妥钠致眠大鼠的睡眠潜伏期及睡眠时间比较($\bar{x} \pm s$)

组别	例数	睡眠潜伏期 /min	睡眠时间 /min
空白组	15	15.99±9.26	50.35±17.17
温针组	15	16.25±7.91	75.50±28.84[*]

注:与对照组比较,[*]$P < 0.01$。

二、蒙医温针对失眠大鼠一般情况和行为学的影响

连续观察了失眠模型大鼠和温针治疗组大鼠的行为改变、体重变化,发现失眠后的大鼠饮食、能量消耗增加,体重下降,大鼠昼夜节律消失、倦怠、体毛蓬乱、无光泽[5-7]。温针治疗组的大鼠在给予温针刺激后第 2 天开始表现为安静、活动减少等现象,睡眠时间、饮水、进食、精神状态等均逐渐恢复,直至第 8 天(腹腔注射 PCPA 后第 7 天),体重与空白组无明显差异($P > 0.05$)。失眠模型组的大鼠从造模成功到造模第 8 天为止仍存在上述行为改变,与温针组比较,失眠模型组的大鼠体重增长率显著降低($P < 0.05$)。利用旷场实验方法,记录大鼠在 OFT-100 自发活动实验仪 5 分钟内的活动情况,观察蒙医温针对失眠大鼠行为学的影响。结果(见表 11-2):在水平活动上,各组大鼠失眠第 7 天,模型组在活动时间上明显高于空白对照($P < 0.01$);在垂直活动上,模型组站立次数明显高于对照组,有明显差异($P < 0.05$);蒙医温针组明显低于模型组($P < 0.05$)。旷场实验中水平运动参数、垂直运动参数和中央格停留时间分别反映动物的活

表 11-2 各组大鼠旷场实验水平活动和垂直活动参数比较($\bar{x} \pm s$)

组别	例数	运动时间 /s	中央格停留时间 /s	站立次数 / 次
空白组	15	16.28±10.65	0.50±1.59	1.21±1.67
模型组	15	30.27±17.79[**]	2.01±4.99	3.07±3.32[*]
温针组	15	14.56±10.26[△]	0.21±0.67	1.43±1.65[▲]
地西泮组	15	14.63±12.49[△]	0.83±2.28	0.36±1.08[△]

注:与对照组比较,[*]$P < 0.05$,[**]$P < 0.01$;与失眠模型组比较[▲]$P < 0.05$,[△]$P < 0.01$。

动度,对新鲜环境的好奇程度及焦虑样行为。实验结果表明,蒙医温针能够改善失眠所致大鼠焦虑样行为减少、探索行为增强的异常变化。行为学实验提示:蒙医温针有效调节失眠模型大鼠的精神情绪行为的异常,具有安神、镇静的作用。

三、蒙医温针对 PCPA 失眠大鼠的细胞因子的影响

为探讨蒙医温针促睡眠的作用机制,我们用酶联免疫吸附法检测了失眠模型大鼠血清、脑组织(下丘脑、海马、大脑皮层、脑干)的白细胞介素 IL-1β、IL-2、IL-6 和肿瘤坏死因子 -α(TNF-α)含量[8-9],进行统计。结果(见表 11-3~表 11-6),IL-1 含量:蒙医温针能显著降低下丘脑、大脑前额皮质异常增加的 IL-1 含量,与模型组比较有显著差异($P < 0.05$,$P < 0.01$);对海马 IL-1 含量略有降低作用,与模型组无明显差异($P > 0.05$)。IL-2 含量:蒙医温针能显著降低下丘脑、海马、大脑前额皮质异常增加的 IL-2 含量,与模型组比较有显著差异($P < 0.05$,$P < 0.05$,$P < 0.01$)。IL-6 含量:蒙医温针能显著降低下丘脑、海马、大脑皮层异常增加的 IL-6 含量,与模型组比较有显著差异($P < 0.05$,$P < 0.01$,$P < 0.01$);对脑干 IL-1β、IL-2、IL-6 含量均无影响,与模型组比较无明显差异($P > 0.05$,$P > 0.05$,$P > 0.05$)。TNF-α 含量:蒙医温针能显著降低下丘脑异常增加的 TNF-α 含量,与模型组比较有显著差异($P < 0.05$);对海马、大脑皮层、脑干 TNF-α 含量无影响,与模型组比较无明显差异($P > 0.05$,$P > 0.05$,$P > 0.05$)。蒙医温针能显著降低血清中异常增加的 IL-1、IL-2、IL-6 的含量,与模型组比较有显著差异($P < 0.05$,$P < 0.05$,$P < 0.05$)。结论:蒙医温针治疗失眠大鼠,可调节脑组织和血清内与睡眠相关细胞因子含量,揭示温针改善睡眠的机制与调节免疫功能、调节具有促眠作用的细胞因子含量有关。

表 11-3 大鼠脑组织内 IL-1β、TNF-α 含量($\bar{x} \pm s$)

组别	例数	IL-1β/(pg·mg^{-1})		TNF-α/(pg·mg^{-1})	
		下丘脑	海马	前额皮质	下丘脑
空白组	15	52.35±19.47	31.91±10.84	46.47±10.38	25.92±8.79
模型组	15	86.76±35.26*	68.91±22.48**	89.99±27.18**	32.97±14.16*
温针组	15	50.52±13.83▲	56.67±17.93*	66.68±19.60△	24.49±5.27△
地西泮组	15	44.53±13.12	45.47±10.86*▲	57.37±15.77*▲	20.79±10.81△

注:与对照组比较,*$P < 0.05$,**$P < 0.01$;与失眠模型组比较,▲$P < 0.05$,△$P < 0.01$。

表 11-4　大鼠脑组织内 IL-2 含量($\bar{x} \pm s$)

组别	例数	IL-2/(pg·mg⁻¹)		
		下丘脑	海马	前额皮质
空白组	15	40.58±15.46	22.96±5.37	29.00±9.14
模型组	15	59.72±19.66**	56.62±14.80**	61.84±13.10**
温针组	15	44.84±14.17▲	39.26±10.61**▲	43.77±10.46**▲
地西泮组	15	35.30±15.98△	41.22±13.36**▲	48.47±13.71**△

注: 与对照组比较,*P<0.05,**P<0.01;与失眠模型组比较,▲P<0.05,△P<0.01。

表 11-5　大鼠脑组织内 IL-6 含量($\bar{x} \pm s$)

组别	例数	IL-6/(pg·mg⁻¹)		
		下丘脑	海马	大脑皮层
空白组	15	106.59±49.21	96.42±24.86	95.91±29.78
模型组	15	139.09±57.40	153.29±40.15**	205.20±54.52**
温针组	15	101.46±47.29▲	109.52±29.68△	148.86±53.34**△
地西泮组	15	86.16±21.91△	99.29±31.45△	113.66±37.96△

注: 与对照组比较,*P<0.05,**P<0.01;与失眠模型组比较,▲P<0.05,△P<0.01。

表 11-6　大鼠血清 IL-1β、IL-2、IL-6 含量($\bar{x} \pm s$)

组别	例数	IL-1β/(pg·ml⁻¹)	IL-2/(pg·ml⁻¹)	IL-6/(pg·ml⁻¹)
空白组	15	28.90±6.39	33.50±6.20	76.41±11.20
模型组	15	61.07±13.84*	72.63±18.56*	160.41±36.16*
温针组	15	42.31±7.89▲	54.60±12.42*▲	100.91±23.46*△
地西泮组	15	44.28±10.97*△	55.77±12.67*▲	108.19±20.84*△

注: 与对照组比较,*P<0.05;与失眠模型组比较,▲P<0.05,△P<0.01。

四、蒙医温针对 PCPA 失眠大鼠脑组织单胺类神经递质的影响

检测失眠模型大鼠血清、脑组织(下丘脑、海马、大脑前额皮质、脑干)的 5-羟色胺(5-HT)、多巴胺(DA)、去甲肾上腺素(NE)含量[10-12],结果显示(表 11-7):蒙医温针可使失眠大鼠下丘脑、海马下降的 5-HT 含量明显升高,同时能够增高 5-HT 代谢产物 5-HIAA 含量,并可降低失眠大鼠脑海马内升高的 NE 含量,可降低失眠大鼠下丘脑内升高的 DA 含量,与模型组比较有显著性差异($P<0.05$,

$P < 0.05$，$P < 0.05$）。提示蒙医温针对失眠大鼠睡眠的作用机制是增加其下丘脑内 5-HT 合成与代谢，降低 NE、DA 含量，恢复 5-HT 通路与 NE 通路和 DA 通路间相互平衡和制约，进而恢复正常的睡眠 - 觉醒节律，达到治疗失眠症的目的[1, 13]。

表 11-7　大鼠脑组织内 5-HT、DA、NE 含量（$\bar{x} \pm s$）

组别	例数	5-HT/(ng·mg⁻¹)		DA/(pg·mg⁻¹)	NE/(pg·mg⁻¹)
		下丘脑	海马	下丘脑	海马
空白组	15	5.18±1.77	6.11±1.51	539.924±100.711	101.415±10.045
模型组	15	3.65±1.79*	3.67±0.84**	727.648±117.663*	111.157±18.127*
温针组	15	4.88±2.55	5.24±1.24△	640.474±96.929▲	89.227±15.671**▲
地西泮组	15	4.47±1.40	4.77±1.31▲	645.003±98.610▲	114.306±18.761**

注：与对照组比较，*$P < 0.05$，**$P < 0.01$；与失眠模型组比较，▲$P < 0.05$，△$P < 0.01$。

五、蒙医温针疗法对 PCPA 失眠大鼠氨基酸类神经递质的影响研究

　　蒙医温针对失眠大鼠海马谷氨酸（Glu）、γ- 氨基丁酸（GABA）、乙酰胆碱（ACh）的含量的影响研究结果显示（表 11-8、表 11-9）：蒙医温针可降低失眠大鼠下丘脑、海马、大脑前额皮质内升高的 Glu 含量，与模型组比较有显著差异（$P < 0.05$，$P < 0.05$，$P < 0.01$）；可升高失眠大鼠下丘脑、海马、大脑前额皮质的 GABA、ACh 含量，与模型组比较均有显著性差异（$P < 0.05$，$P < 0.05$，$P < 0.05$）。由此可推测，蒙医温针具有调节脑内 Glu、GABA 含量及 ACh 含量的多靶向综合作用，从而使大脑兴奋性降低，使神经功能的抑制作用占优势，实现增加睡

表 11-8　大鼠脑组织内 Glu、ACh 含量（$\bar{x} \pm s$）

组别	例数	Glu			ACh	
		下丘脑 /(ng·mg⁻¹)	前额皮质 /(ng·mg⁻¹)	海马 /(μmol·g⁻¹)	海马 /(μg·mg⁻¹)	前额皮质 /(ng·mg⁻¹)
空白组	15	0.423±0.220	0.466±0.252	2.095±0.599	194.607±59.203	0.757±0.225
模型组	15	0.723±0.277**	0.744±0.281**	4.131±1.187**	134.146±37.739**	0.475±0.243**
温针组	15	0.634±0.249**▲	0.595±0.261**△	3.112±0.816△	180.304±52.038▲	0.652±0.191▲
地西泮组	15	0.644±0.333**▲	0.704±0.305**	3.214±1.080▲	169.09±50.793	0.561±0.166

注：与对照组比较，*$P < 0.05$，**$P < 0.01$；与失眠模型组比较，▲$P < 0.05$，△$P < 0.01$。

眠、改善睡眠的治疗作用[11,13]。亦可认为，调节中枢神经递质 Glu、GABA 及 ACh 含量可能是蒙医温针治疗失眠的内在机制之一。

表 11-9　大鼠脑组织内 GABA 含量($\bar{x} \pm s$)

组别	例数	GABA		
		下丘脑/(ng•ml^{-1})	前额皮质/(ng•ml^{-1})	海马/(µmol•g^{-1})
空白组	15	0.691±0.228	0.628±0.209	14.846±5.028
模型组	15	0.420±0.161**	0.431±0.149**	8.956±2.736**
温针组	15	0.610±0.154△	0.600±0.219△	12.341±4.424▲
地西泮组	15	0.604±0.282△	0.575±0.162	10.967±2.572

注：与对照组比较，$^*P<0.05$，$^{**}P<0.01$；与失眠模型组比较，$^{▲}P<0.05$，$^{△}P<0.01$。

六、蒙医温针对失眠模型大鼠大脑 5- 羟色胺受体 5-TH$_1$ 和多巴胺 D$_1$ 受体的影响

为观察蒙医温针对失眠模型大鼠脑内神经递质受体的影响，我们采用放射性配体结合分析法，观察了失眠模型大鼠大脑海马、大脑皮层 5-HT$_1$ 受体和多巴胺 D$_1$ 受体的数量及结合活性，求出最大结合量（B$_{max}$），以及温针对其产生的影响作用。结果发现（见表 11-10），失眠模型大鼠大脑皮层、海马 5-HT$_1$ 受体的最大结合量，明显低于正常组（$P<0.01$，$P<0.01$），失眠大鼠大脑皮层多巴胺 D$_1$ 受体的最大结合量明显低于正常组（$P<0.01$）。温针可增加失眠大鼠大脑皮层、海马 5-HT$_1$ 受体的最大结合量，能显著增加失眠大鼠海马 DA 受体结合率。本研究表明，蒙医温针能调节 5-HT$_1$ 受体和多巴胺 D$_1$ 受体的含量，从而调控睡眠 - 觉醒节律，起到治疗失眠的作用。

表 11-10　温针对失眠大鼠脑组织内 5-HT$_1$、D$_1$ 受体的最大结合量（B$_{max}$）的影响($\bar{x} \pm s$)

组别	例数	5-HT$_1$/(fmol•mg^{-1}•Pro^{-1})		D$_1$/(fmol•mg^{-1}•Pro^{-1})	
		大脑皮层	海马	大脑皮层	海马
空白组	15	26.859±4.138	27.964±5.183	36.856±5.944	43.150±7.856
模型组	15	20.281±3.152**	20.086±2.981**	38.186±9.173	35.745±6.446**
温针组	15	24.628±6.167▲	23.853±4.755▲	34.271±4.572	41.375±5.064▲
地西泮组	15	24.503±3.986▲	24.548±5.025▲	32.040±5.979▲	40.945±7.038▲

注：与对照组比较，$^*P<0.05$，$^{**}P<0.01$；与失眠模型组比较，$^{▲}P<0.05$，$^{△}P<0.01$。

参 考 文 献

[1] 阿古拉, 苏朝鲁门, 张朝鲁门, 等. 蒙医温针对疲劳大鼠行为学及下丘脑脑组织中单胺类神经递质含量的影响 [J]. 世界科学技术: 中医药现代化, 2008, 10 (1): 129-132.

[2] 吴海波. 安神方治疗失眠症的疗效观察及相关机制研究 [D]. 广州: 南方医科大学, 2009.

[3] 何婷. 失眠相关因素研究系统性文献评价和针刺临床研究 [D]. 广州: 广州中医药大学, 2009.

[4] 范利锋, 王平仁, 兰培敏. 睡眠机制的研究概况 [J]. 临床内科杂志, 2005, 22 (10): 662-664.

[5] 失眠定义、诊断及药物治疗共识专家组. 失眠定义、诊断及药物治疗专家共识 (草案) [J]. 中华神经科杂志, 2006, 39 (2): 141-143.

[6] 谢永标, 刘破资. 原发性失眠的生活质量研究 [J]. 中国心理卫生杂志, 2004, 18 (5): 343-344.

[7] SCHWARTZ J R L, ROTH T. Neurophysiology of sleep and wakefulness : basic science and clinical implications[J]. Curr Neuropharmacol, 2008, 6 (4): 367-378.

[8] PRATHER A A, RABINOVITZ M, POLLOCK B G, et al. Cytokine-induced depression during IFN-alpha treatment: the role of IL-6 and sleep quality[J]. Brain Behav Immun, 2009, 23 (8): 1109-1116.

[9] KENTNER A C, MIGUELEZ M, JAMES J S, et al. Behavioral and physiological effects of a single injection of rat interferon-alpha on male Sprague-Dawley rats: a long-term evaluation[J]. Brain Res, 2006, 1095 (1): 96-106.

[10] 周伟东, 李荣姣, 黄国光. 失眠症药物治疗的进展 [J]. 华北煤炭医学院学报, 2008, 10 (2): 200-202.

[11] 陆峥. 失眠症的诊断和药物治疗现状 [J]. 世界临床药物, 2011, 32 (4): 193-199.

[12] 赵建军, 秦竹. 失眠症治疗方剂的历史回顾及现代研究进展 [J]. 云南中医中药杂志, 2010, 31 (3): 63-65.

[13] 何福龙, 李艳飞. 蒙医温针疗法治疗失眠 [J]. 中国民族民间医药, 2011 (1): 6.

第十二章

蒙医温针调节失眠大鼠 miR-101a 及 PAX8 蛋白治疗失眠症的机制研究

本项研究是笔者主持的 2016—2019 年国家自然科学基金项目：蒙医温针调节失眠大鼠 miRNAs 及 PAX8/APP 蛋白治疗失眠症的机制研究（编号 81560801）。

失眠症是入睡和 / 或睡眠维持困难所致的睡眠质量或数量达不到正常生理需求而影响社会功能的一种主观体验，是最常见的睡眠障碍性疾患，并且患病率很高。据世界卫生组织调查，在世界范围内约 1/3 的人有睡眠障碍，而在中国患有各类睡眠障碍的人的比例明显高于世界 27% 的水平。因此，失眠的有效防治仍为全球关注的热点 [1]。

在临床上，现代医学主要采用镇静、催眠药物，而此类药物有许多副作用，远期疗效较差，长期服用还会造成成瘾性、耐受性等，并非一种理想的治疗方法 [2]。蒙古医学治疗失眠具有独特的理论和良好的疗效，蒙医认为"三根失衡，赫依偏盛而位于心和白脉，其功能紊乱致赫依血相搏"是本病的基本病因病机，紧张、忧虑、恐惧、抑郁、焦虑等负面情绪及社会环境、饮食、起居、运动情况等均是外因，镇赫依、调节"三根"平衡为主要治疗原则。温针疗法是蒙医治疗失眠的常用方法之一，具有温通经脉、调和气血、调理体素、增强抵抗力以及防治疾病的作用 [3]。温针疗法对于失眠的治疗具有疗效显著、安全、简单、经济等优势。

本课题以蒙医温针对对氯苯丙氨酸（PCPA）致失眠大鼠模型的催眠作用为切入点，从基因水平对温针治疗前后相关 miRNAs 及靶基因进行探讨，同时对失眠相关细胞因子、神经递质含量进行观察，并结合临床试验探讨蒙医温针治疗失眠症的生物学基础，初步阐明蒙医温针疗法的多层面复杂机制。主要研究成果如下。

一、miR-101a 在蒙医温针治疗失眠大鼠前后脑组织中的表达差异

芯片数据分析发现，相对于正常大鼠，蒙医温针治疗后，有 141 个 miRNAs

表达存在差异；变化最为显著的为 miR-101a，相比模型组升高了 98 倍。我们接下来对 15 只温针治疗失眠大鼠的 miR-101a 的水平进行了荧光实时定量 PCR 研究，发现中位数由模型组的 2.9 倍上升到了 3.2 倍（$P<0.001$）（见图 12-1）。

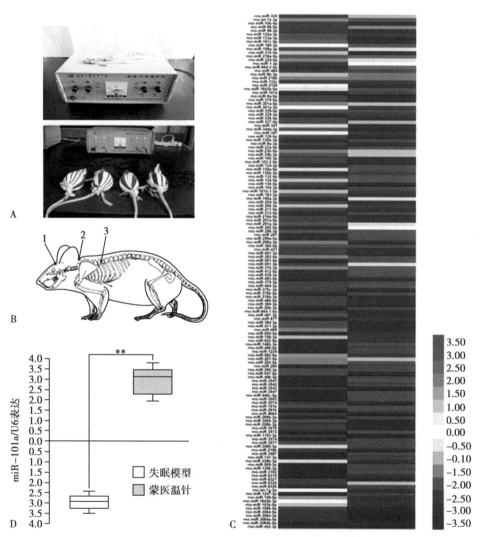

注：A. 蒙医电热温针器及大鼠针灸套袋；B. 针刺穴位选择，1 为顶会穴，2 为赫依穴，3 为心穴；C. 用数字化 miRNAs 表达谱的方法高通量分析了 15 对蒙医温针治疗失眠大鼠与未治疗失眠大鼠脑组织中 miRNA 的表达情况，在肝癌中表达显著改变的 miRNA 列出，红色表示上调，蓝色表示下调，其中 miR-101a 表达上调最高；D. 15 对温针治疗及未治疗失眠大鼠经过 qPCR 技术进行测定，治疗组中位值 2.9 倍，而未治疗组的中位值为 3.2 倍（$P<0.01$）。

图 12-1 蒙医 miR-101a 的数字化表达谱情况

二、miR-101a 在蒙医温针治疗失眠大鼠前后海马中的表达

为下一步研究 miR-101a 的生物学功能,我们用荧光实时定量 PCR 检测了 miR-101a 在蒙医温针治疗失眠大鼠前后海马中的表达情况。结果发现,相对于正常大鼠的脑组织细胞,失眠模型组大鼠脑组织 miR-101a 的表达水平明显下调($P < 0.05$);经过温针治疗后,miR-101a 的表达水平明显上升,恢复到接近正常值($P < 0.05$)(图 12-2A)。空白神经细胞中,相对于阴性对照组,转染 miR-101a mimics 的细胞中 72 小时后 miR-101a 的表达量明显升高($P < 0.05$),转染 miR-101a inhibitor 显著降低($P < 0.05$);在失眠模型组中,相对于阴性对照组,转染 miR-101a mimics 的细胞中 72 小时后 miR-101a 的表达量明显升高($P < 0.05$),转染 miR-101a inhibitor 无显著变化;蒙医温针治疗后,相对于阴性对照组,转染 miR-101a mimics 的细胞中 72 小时后 miR-101a 的表达量明显升高($P < 0.05$),转染 miR-101a inhibitor 显著降低($P < 0.05$)(图 12-2B)。

体外培养的模型组及蒙医温针组神经元细胞在最初 24 小时荧光素酶活性未存在差异,在 48 小时检测,蒙医温针组的细胞活力比模型组细胞强;在 72 小时,蒙医温针组的细胞活力比模型组细胞显著增强($P < 0.05$)(图 12-2C)。为了进一步证实 miR-101a 对于神经细胞活性的影响,在蒙医温针大鼠培养的神经元细胞中转染 miR-101a inhibitor 和 scramble,从图 12-2D 中我们可以看出,48 小时后与 scramble 相比,转染 miR-101a inhibitor 的细胞活性比较高。72 小时检测,转染 miR-101a inhibitor 的细胞活性显著升高($P < 0.05$)。

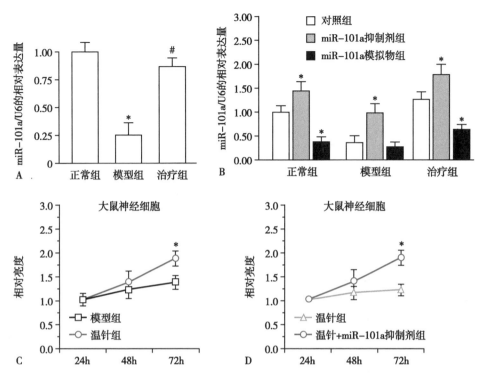

注：A. 应用荧光实时定量 PCR 检测空白对照组、失眠模型组及温针组大鼠体外培养的神经细胞中 miR-101a 的表达水平，失眠模型组显著下降（$P<0.01$），温针组显著上升（$P<0.01$）；B. 三组大鼠体外培养的神经细胞转染 miR-101a inhibitor 和 mimics，除失眠模型 mimics 组外，均呈正负相关表达；C. 对比失眠模型组，温针组大鼠体外培养的神经细胞 24 小时后呈现较强的生长活力，48 小时呈现显著性生长活力（$P<0.05$）；D. 温针组大鼠体外培养的神经细胞分别转染空白质粒和 miR-101a inhibitor 后，24 小时后与对照组相比，inhibitor 组出现抑制了细胞的生长活力，48 小时后显著抑制了神经细胞的生长活力（$P<0.05$）。

图 12-2 外源性 miR-101a 分子对大鼠神经细胞调控的实验验证

三、miR-101a 能够抑制 PAX8 蛋白的表达

蛋白印迹结果显示，体外培养失眠模型大鼠神经元细胞，对比加入 scramble 组加入 miR-101a mimics 72 小时后，PAX8 蛋白的表达出现抑制，呈显著的下调（$P<0.01$）（图 12-3A/B）。293T 细胞中荧光素酶报告结果显示，相对于空白质粒组 pGL3M，阴性对照组 pGL3M-MUT-PAX8-3'UTR 及 pGL3M-WT-PAX8-3'UTR 均没有显著性变化，加入 miR-101a mimics 后，MUT 组的活性没有出现显著性的变化，而 WT 组荧光强度显著下降，说明 miR-101a 能够与 WT-PAX8-

3'UTR 启动子中特异顺序结合，而改变了启动子的特异序列，则 miR-101a 不起作用（图 12-3C/D）。

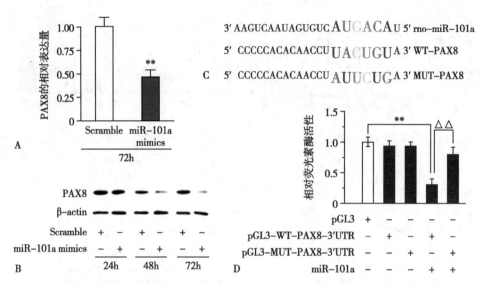

注：A/B. 温针组大鼠体外培养的神经细胞蛋白印迹结果显示，加入 miR-101a mimics 72 小时后 PAX8 蛋白出现了显著的下调（P<0.01）；C. WT-PAX8 和 MUT-PAX8 质粒设计；D. 293T 细胞中荧光素酶报告结果显示，相对于空白质粒组 pGL3M，阴性对照组 pGL3M-MUT-PAX8-3'UTR 及 pGL3M-WT-PAX8-3'UTR 均没有显著性变化，加入 miR-101a mimics 后，MUT 组的活性没有出现显著性的变化，而 WT 组荧光强度显著下降（P<0.01）。

图 12-3　miR-101a 抑制 PAX8 蛋白的表达

四、IL-1、IL-2、IL-6 和 TNF-α 水平检测结果

用酶联免疫吸附法检测白细胞介素 IL-1、IL-2、IL-6 和肿瘤坏死因子 -α（TNF-α）水平，结果如图 12-4 所示，失眠大鼠下丘脑、海马和大脑前额叶皮质组织中白细胞介素 IL-1、IL-2、IL-6 和 TNF-α 水平与空白对照组相比明显降低，有显著差异（P<0.05）。经过治疗，无论是温针治疗还是西药治疗，各部位白细胞介素 IL-1、IL-2、IL-6 和 TNF-α 水平与模型组相比均显著提升，有统计学差异（P<0.05）。说明温针对治疗大鼠失眠有显著效果，与药物治疗基本效果相当。

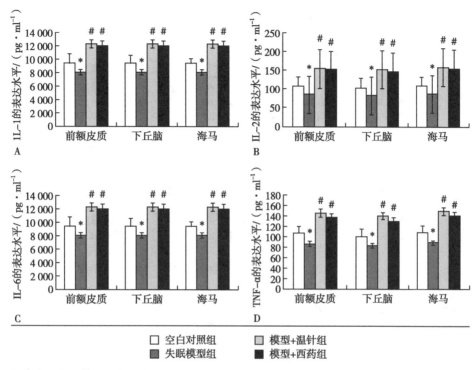

注：* 表示失眠模型组与空白对照组比较，有显著差异，$P < 0.05$；# 表示温针组和药物治疗组与失眠模型组比较，有显著差异，$P < 0.05$。

图 12-4　大鼠下丘脑、海马和大脑前额叶皮质组织 IL-1、IL-2、IL-6 和 TNF-α 水平

五、5-HT、NE、ACh、DA、Glu、GABA 水平检测结果

对大鼠下丘脑、海马和大脑前额叶皮质组织中 5-HT、NE、ACh、DA、Glu、GABA 水平检测结果如图 12-5 所示。失眠模型组大鼠 NE、DA、Glu 水平明显高于空白对照组，差异显著，具有统计学意义（$P < 0.05$），而经过温针或西药治疗，NE、DA、Glu 水平则与失眠模型组相比有了明显降低，差异显著，具有统计学意义（$P < 0.05$）；温针治疗效果和西药治疗效果差异不明显，说明两者治疗效果相近。失眠模型组大鼠 5-HT、GABA、ACh 水平明显低于空白对照组，具有统计学意义，差异显著（$P < 0.05$）；与失眠模型组比较，温针或西药治疗后失眠大鼠 5-HT、GABA、ACh 水平明显升高，差异显著，具有统计学意义（$P < 0.05$）；温针治疗与西药治疗比较差异不明显，证明蒙医温针治疗效果与西药效果相近 [4-5]。

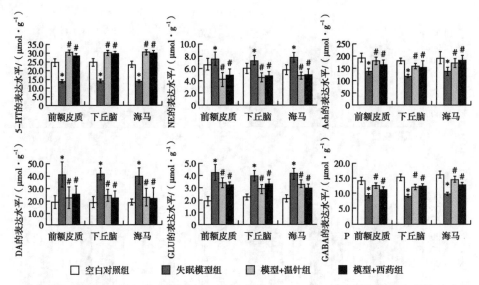

注：*表示失眠模型组与空白对照组比较，有显著差异，$P<0.05$；#表示温针组和药物治疗组与失眠模型组比较，有显著差异，$P<0.05$。

图12-5 大鼠下丘脑、海马和大脑前额叶皮质组织中5-HT、NE、Ach、DA、Glu、GABA水平

六、讨论

蒙医温针通过针刺效应、温热效应以及穴位特异性刺激的相互作用，对机体产生一些生物学效应，而达到治疗疾病的目的[6]。大量临床研究表明，蒙医温针治疗失眠具有简便、高效、安全等特点。

蒙医通过辨证论治"镇赫依、疏通赫依血、平衡三根"以达到改善睡眠、治疗失眠症的目的。蒙医学认为温针疗法有疏通经脉、调和气血、调理体素、增强抵抗力之功，现代研究证实针灸有调节神经体液、增强和激发调动机体抗病能力和提高机体免疫力等作用，是失眠患者较佳的选择。关于蒙医温针治疗失眠症的临床报道较多，这些临床报道中多数选择头顶会穴、赫依穴、前顶穴针刺治疗失眠症，得到满意的疗效。可见，蒙医温针对治疗失眠症的作用十分显著。

传统蒙医对针灸治疗指标的定量定性并无统一标准，只考察几个神经递质的指标不能完全代表整个机体的生理指数，不符合整体观的蒙医理论。针灸机制十分复杂，较难从某个生理指标去分析掌握，但机体内miRNAs的改变可以进行标准化、客观化的测定，所以以miRNAs为介质研究蒙医温针既能体现出宏观性和整体性，又符合现代分子生物技术的微观性和针对性[7-10]。

本实验中发现，相对于失眠大鼠模型组，蒙医温针治疗组中miR-101a的表

达水平相对升高，转染 miR-101a inhibitor 能成功降低细胞中内源性 miR-101a 的表达。我们通过 TargetScan、PicTar、miRanda 等软件，推测 miR-101a 的靶基因可能为配对盒基因 8（paired box gene 8，PAX8）。巧合的是，在 2014 年底的一项报道中，研究人员调查了超过 47 000 个欧洲血统的人及近 5 000 名非洲裔美国人，研究人员将他们的遗传信息与晚上睡觉时间作了对比，结果显示"睡眠模式受遗传差异影响"，某个基因区域可能会通过调节甲状腺激素水平影响睡眠模式，这个 DNA 区域靠近一个名为 PAX8 的基因，PAX8 与甲状腺发育和功能有关。甲状腺功能减退的患者容易过度嗜睡，而那些甲状腺功能亢进的患者可能会失眠[11-12]。我们本次试验验证了蒙医温针改善失眠的原理与 miR-101a 调节 PAX8 基因有直接关联。

现代医学对失眠的研究发现，睡眠 - 觉醒是一个涉及多系统、多中枢的协调整合的生理过程，具有复杂的调节机制，主要与位于脑干网状系统视前区的睡眠激活细胞、位于乳头结节区的组胺能神经元、大脑皮质等特殊神经结构，γ- 氨基丁酸、乙酰胆碱、5- 羟色胺、多巴胺、去甲肾上腺素、组胺和食欲素等与睡眠 - 觉醒密切相关的神经递质，IL-1 和 TNF 的睡眠调节作用，以及非肽类物质对睡眠的调节机制有关。我们同时证明了蒙医温针治疗失眠还与上述相关神经递质有关。

蒙医温针集针刺效应、温热效应以及穴位特异性刺激为一体，通过对血液循环、神经系统、免疫功能等多系统、多渠道、多途径的复杂作用机制，达到调节机体、治疗疾病的目的。本研究证明 miR-101a 在温针治疗大鼠中表达上调与 PAX8 调控有直接关联，对多种神经递质调节网络进行了验证，为今后蒙医温针的现代治疗提供了生物学的研究证明，为传统民族医药的现代化发展提供了科学支持。

参 考 文 献

[1] WANG Y M，CHEN H G，SONG M，et al. Prevalence of insomnia and its risk factors in older individuals: a community-based study in four cities of Hebei Province，China[J]. Sleep Med，2016，19：116-122.

[2] HAN K H，KIM S Y，CHUNG S Y. Effect of acupuncture on patients with insomnia: study protocol for a randomized controlled trial[J]. Trials，2014，15：403.

[3] KIM T H，JUNG S Y. Mongolian traditional-style blood-letting therapy[J]. J Altern Complement Med，2013，19：921-924.

[4] MURRAY N M，BUCHANAN G F，RICHERSON G B. Insomnia caused by serotonin depletion is due to hypothermia[J]. Sleep，2015，38：1985-1993.

[5] SI L G, WANG Y H, WUYUN G, et al. The effect of Mongolian medical acupuncture on cytokines and neurotransmitters in the brain tissue of insomniac rats[J]. Eup J Integr Med, 2015, 7: 492-498.

[6] YU E, AMRI H. China's other medical systems: Recognizing Uyghur, Tibetan, and Mongolian Traditional Medicines[J]. Glob Adv Health Med, 2016, 5 (1): 79-86.

[7] SUN X, LUO S, HE Y, et al. Screening of the miRNAs related to breast cancer and identification of its target genes[J]. EurJ Gynaecol Oncol, 2014, 35: 696-700.

[8] ZHU X, ZHAO H, LIN Z, et al. Functional studies of miR-130a on the inhibitory pathways of apoptosis in patients with chronic myeloid leukemia[J]. Cancer Gene Ther, 2015, 22: 573-580.

[9] MARRELLI M, PADUANO F, TATULLO M. Human periapical cyst-mesenchymal stem cells differentiate into neuronal cells[J]. J Dent Res, 2015, 94: 843-852.

[10] BURENBATU, BORJIGIN M, EERDUNDULENG, et al. Profiling of miRNA expression in immune thrombocytopenia patients before and after Qishunbaolier (QSBLE) treatment[J]. Biomed Pharmacother, 2015, 75: 196-204.

[11] RIESCO-EIZAGUIRRE G, WERT-LAMAS L, PERALES-PATON J, et al. The miR-146b-3p/PAX8/NIS regulatory circuit modulates the differentiation phenotype and function of thyroid cells during carcinogenesis[J]. Cancer Res, 2015, 75: 4119-4130.

[12] GOTTLIEB D J, HEK K, CHEN T H, et al. Novel loci associated with usual sleep duration: the CHARGE Consortium Genome-Wide Association Study[J]. Mol Psychiatry, 2015, 20: 1232-1239.

第十三章

蒙医温针对 PCPA 诱导失眠大鼠肠道菌群及代谢产物的影响

本项研究是笔者主持的 2021—2024 年国家自然科学基金项目：LncRNA CCAT1/miR-101a/GAT-1 介导蒙医温针治疗失眠的作用及机制研究（编号 82074577）。

本研究在 2021 年度主要以蒙医温针对氯苯丙氨酸（PCPA）致失眠模型大鼠的催眠作用为切入点，对大鼠肠道微生物以及代谢产物进行探讨，同时对相关蛋白进行定量分析，探讨蒙医温针治疗失眠症的生物学基础。

方法：取 6 周龄雄性 SD 大鼠（体重 160～180g），适应性饲养 7 天后，随机分为 3 组，空白对照组、失眠模型组和蒙医温针治疗组。使用 PCPA 诱导失眠大鼠模型，给模型大鼠腹腔注射 PCPA（300mg/kg），连续 3 天；空白对照组用等量生理盐水代替。治疗组于造模后开始在大鼠顶会穴、赫依穴和心穴给予蒙医温针刺激，每次 15min，加热温度为 40℃左右。进行旷场实验，记录大鼠 5min 内的运动距离、运动时间和站立次数；使用 2% 戊巴比妥钠麻醉大鼠后取腹主动脉血分离血清、新鲜粪便、大脑各区组织。使用 ELISA 试剂盒检测血清样本中的 5-羟色胺（5-HT）、去甲肾上腺素（NE）、乙酰胆碱（ACh）和 γ-氨基丁酸（GABA）水平；使用 PCR 技术对粪便样本中细菌 16s rRNA 基因进行扩增后，在 Illumina MiSeq 平台进行测序；非靶向代谢组学分析用于评估血清代谢组的变化与短链脂肪酸（丁酸）含量；并使用 Spearman 分析代谢产物与肠道菌群的相关性；Western-blot 检测脑组织中 γ-氨基丁酸转运体-1（GAT-1）的表达，并分析蒙医温针对丁酸产生和 GAT-1 表达的影响；采用 SPSS21.0 软件对数据进行统计分析。

一、蒙医温针治疗改善 PCPA 诱导的失眠大鼠睡眠

如图 13-1 所示，与对照组相比，失眠模型组食物摄入较少，体重增加较低

（$P<0.05$）。蒙医温针治疗能够显著增加大鼠体重（$P<0.05$）。旷场实验表明，失眠模型组大鼠的运动时间、运动距离和站立次数均较对照组增加（$P<0.05$）。这些自主活动测试指数在治疗组中呈下降趋势（$P<0.05$）。与对照组相比，模型组大鼠的 5-HT 和 GABA 水平较低，ACh 和 NE 含量较高（$P<0.05$）；相反，与失眠模型组相比，治疗组 5-HT 和 GABA 水平升高，ACh 和 NE 含量降低（$P<0.05$）。这些结果表明，蒙医温针对失眠有治疗作用。

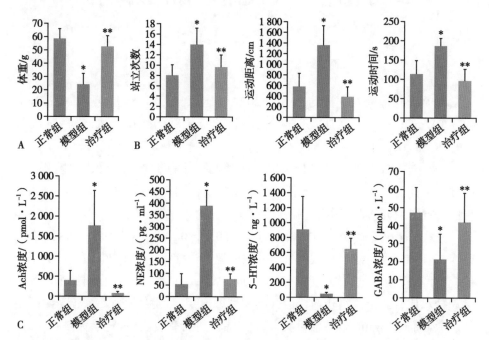

注：A. 3 组大鼠体重增加情况的比较；B. 3 组大鼠的站立次数、运动距离、运动时间的比较；C. 3 组大鼠血清中 ACh、NE、5-HT、GABA 神经递质的比较（值为 $\bar{x}\pm s$，每组 8 只大鼠）。

图 13-1 蒙医温针对失眠症大鼠的治疗作用

二、蒙医温针治疗改善 PCPA 诱导的失眠大鼠肠道微生物

通过细菌 16S rRNA 测序确定粪便微生物组成。共保留 16S rRNA 基因的 163 228 次读取，每个样本的总数在 68 192 和 70 198 之间。此外，从所有样本中总共鉴定出 1 513 个 OTU。图 13-2 通过 α 多样性指数显示了肠道微生物群的多样性。对照组、模型组和处理组中，反映物种丰富度和均匀度的香农指数分别为 1.29±0.30、1.07±0.21 和 1.10±0.28（图 13-2A）。同样，反映 3 组社区均匀性的辛普森指数分别为 0.35±0.12、0.47±0.11 和 0.42±0.13（图 13-2B）。在 3 组

中, 加权 unifrac 分析 ($P=0.008$) 和未加权 unifrac 分析 ($P=0.817$) 中观察到 β 多样性存在显著差异 (图 13-2C)。

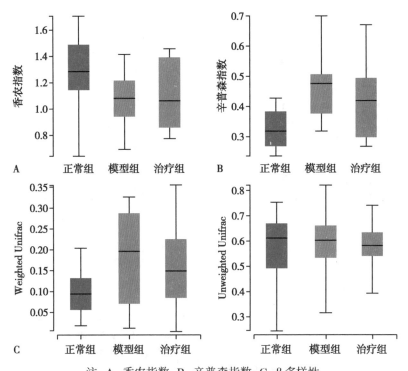

注: A. 香农指数; B. 辛普森指数; C. β 多样性。

图 13-2 蒙医温针对各组大鼠肠道菌群多样性的影响

门级的微生物组成如图 13-3A 所示, 厚壁菌是最丰富的细菌群, 在对照组、模型组和治疗组中分别平均占 98.1%、98.7% 和 99.7% 的序列。同时, 在这 3 组中, 变形菌是第二优势菌群, 分别占平均 1.1%、1.0% 和 0.2% 的序列。其他门的相对丰度较低 (小于 3%)。在属级, 微生物组成如图 13-3B 所示, 乳杆菌属 (lactobacillus)、罗姆布茨菌属 (romboutsia)、梭菌属 (clostridium_sensu_stricto)、绿脓杆菌属 (turicibacter) 在这三组中都很丰富。与对照组相比, 模型组粪便样本中的 romboutsia 计数显著增加, 乳杆菌属和梭菌属数量减少 ($P<0.05$)。相反, 蒙医温针处理逆转了这些菌属的丰度。

根据 LDA Effect Size 分析 (LEfSe 分析), 空白组和模型组之间有 13 个分类群存在显著差异: 空白组 9 个, 模型组 4 个 (图 13-4A)。对照组大鼠主要表现出较高的气球菌、棒状杆菌科、肉核杆菌科、棒状杆菌、微球菌科、罗斯氏菌、葡萄球菌和颗粒细胞, 而模型大鼠的变形菌门、梭菌属 XIVa、蓝藻和毛螺菌科的丰度较高。同样,模型组和治疗组之间的差异也被确定了(图 13-4B),模型组与治疗组只有 1 个分类群存在明显差异。模型组大鼠表现出较高的变形菌门富集,提示蒙医温针可能通过影响大鼠变形菌门的含量调节失眠症。

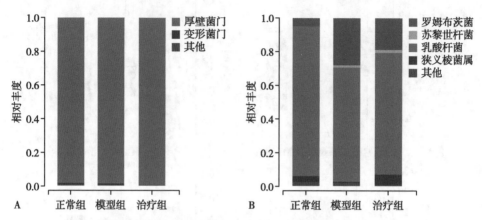

注:A. 在门水平上的分类学组成;B. 在属水平上的分类学组成。

图 13-3　蒙医温针对肠道菌群组成的影响

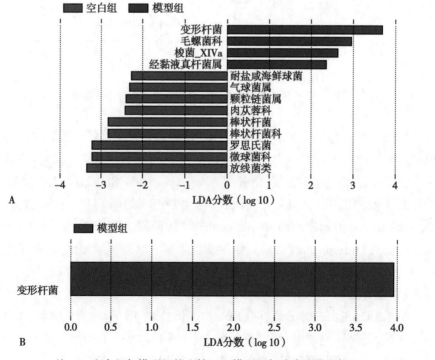

注:A. 空白组与模型组的比较;B. 模型组与治疗组的比较。

图 13-4　LEfSe 分析确定的不同组中显著富集的细菌类群

三、蒙医温针对 PCPA 诱导的失眠大鼠血清代谢物的调节

首先确定了正离子和负离子模式下的代谢物谱。由于在负离子模式下观察到高基线，因此在本研究中选择正离子模式进行进一步分析。在对照组和模型组之间共注释了 88 种代谢物（图 13-5A）。OPLS-DA 评分图和热图显示，模型大鼠可与对照大鼠分离（图 13-5B、图 13-5C）。在 88 种代谢物中，与对照组相比，模型组中 57 种代谢物的水平显著升高，而其他 31 种代谢物的水平显著降低。相比之下，在治疗组和模型组之间总共注释了 35 种代谢物（图 13-5D）。治疗组也可以从模型组中分离出来（图 13-5E、图 13-5F）。结果表明，经蒙医温针处理后，6 种代谢物的含量发生逆转，包括鹰嘴豆芽素 A、细辛脑、琥珀酸酐、西维因、油酰乙醇酰胺和磺基水杨酸。其中 3 种代谢物（鹰嘴豆芽素 A、细辛脑和琥珀酸酐）在模型组与对照组相比上调，但在治疗组与模型组相比下调。与对照组相比，模型组的其他 3 种（西维因、油酰乙醇酰胺和磺基水杨酸）表达下调，而治疗组与模型组相比表达上调。

KEGG 通路富集分析表明，失眠的发生与多种通路有关，其中代谢通路和信号通路被认为特别重要（图 13-6A）。相反，蒙医温针治疗可以改变 cAMP 信号通路，对失眠产生有益的影响（图 13-6B）。此外，如图 13-7 所示，与对照组相比，模型组的 cAMP 信号通路上调。然而，经蒙医温针治疗后，情况逆转。

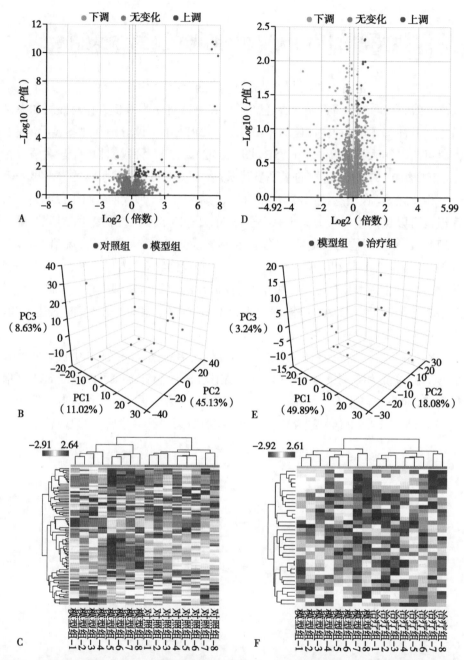

注：A. 对照组与模型组之间差异代谢物的火山图；B. 对照组和模型组阳离子模式血清样本的 OPLS-DA 评分图；C. 对照组与模型组间差异代谢物的热图分析；D. 模型组与治疗组之间差异代谢物的火山图；E. 阳离子模式下来自模型组和治疗组的血清样本的 OPLS-DA 评分图；F. 模型组与治疗组间差异代谢物的热图分析。

图 13-5　蒙医温针对失眠大鼠血清代谢物水平的影响

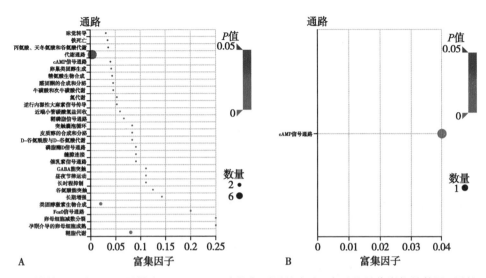

注：横轴表示富因子，纵轴表示 KEGG 通路的各项圆的大小，表示差异代谢物的数量，圆的颜色表示 P 值。

图 13-6　对照组与模型组（A）、模型组与治疗组（B）之间的差异代谢物的 KEGG 通路富集分析

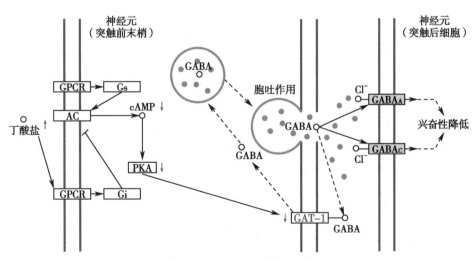

图 13-7　cAMP 信号通路图

四、血清代谢物与肠道微生物群的相关性

如表 13-1 所示，代谢产物，如酰胺 c18、N,N- 二甲基精氨酸、苯甲酰氯和胞嘧啶，在失眠症大鼠中明显增加，并与梭状芽孢杆菌和 Blautia 呈正相关。相反，酰胺 c18 的增加和 N- 乙酰血清素的减少分别与双歧杆菌和弯曲杆菌呈负相关。经蒙医温针处理后，代谢产物 1-（14- 甲基十六烷基）吡咯烷增加，并与类杆菌和弯曲杆菌呈正相关。同时，治疗组中 3-（{[（2s）-2,3- 二羟基丙氧基]（羟基）磷酰基}氧基）-2- 羟基丙基棕榈酸酯、4- 乙烯基环己烯、氨氧酸盐、卡米罗芬和环己酮的减少与梭状芽孢杆菌、对羟基丁酸杆菌、细脉菌、不动杆菌、棒状杆菌、伊丽莎白菌属、假单胞菌和红球菌呈正相关（表 13-2）。

表 13-1 模型组与对照组的代谢物水平与肠道代谢物丰度的相关性

名称	基因	相关性	P 值
酰胺 c18	双歧杆菌	−0.766 758	0.000 530
酰胺 c18	梭状芽孢杆菌 *XIVa*	0.668 651	0.004 627
N,N - 二甲基精氨酸	布劳特氏菌	0.765 262	0.000 551
N,N- 二甲基精氨酸	梭状芽孢杆菌 *XIVa*	0.695 278	0.002 788
苯甲酰氯	梭状芽孢杆菌 *XIVa*	0.721 906	0.001 591
胞嘧啶	布劳特氏菌	0.697 319	0.002 677
2- 氨基 -1,3,4- 植物鞘胺醇	*GpI*	−0.694 634	0.002 825
丁二酸酐	*GpI*	−0.693 140	0.002 910
N- 乙酰血清素	弯曲杆菌	−0.668 781	0.004 616

表 13-2 治疗组与模型组的代谢物水平与肠道代谢物丰度的相关性

名称	基因	相关性	P 值
3-（{[（2s）-2,3- 二羟基丙基]（羟基）磷酰}氧）-2- 羟丙基棕榈酸酯	梭状芽孢杆菌 *XIVa*	0.766 920	0.000 527
3-（{[（2s）-2,3- 二羟基丙基]（羟基）磷酰}氧）-2- 羟丙基棕榈酸酯	副拟杆菌	0.570 110	0.021 123
3-（{[（2s）-2,3- 二羟基丙基]（羟基）磷酰}氧）-2- 羟丙基棕榈酸酯	韦荣氏球菌属	0.578 145	0.018 984
4- 乙烯环己烯	不动杆菌	0.758 516	0.000 659

续表

名称	基因	相关性	P 值
氨基甲酸酯	棒状杆菌	0.651 492	0.006 255
氨基甲酸酯	伊丽莎白金菌	0.573 944	0.020 080
卡米罗芬	假单胞菌	0.634 234	0.008 323
环己酮	红球菌	0.573 944	0.020 080
1-(14-甲酯十六烷酰基)吡咯烷	类杆菌	0.625 954	0.009 490
1-(14-甲酯十六烷酰基)吡咯烷	弯曲杆菌	0.582 225	0.017 964

五、蒙医温针治疗对 PCPA 诱导的失眠大鼠丁酸盐水平及 GAT-1 表达影响

粪便丁酸盐的水平如图 13-8A 所示。模型组大鼠粪便丁酸盐含量较对照组有下降趋势（$P<0.05$）。然而，治疗组的粪便丁酸盐水平高于模型组（$P<0.05$）。

蒙医温针治疗降低 PCPA 诱导失眠大鼠 GAT-1 的表达：如图 13-8B 所示，与对照组相比，模型组大鼠的 GAT-1 水平更高（$P<0.05$），但治疗组 GAT-1 水平低于模型组（$P<0.05$）。

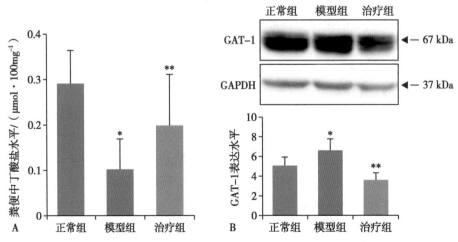

注：A. 粪便中丁酸盐水平；B. GAT-1 在脑组织中的表达水平

图 13-8　蒙医温针对丁酸盐水平和 GAT-1 表达的影响

六、讨论

虽然蒙医温针疗法历史上用于治疗失眠，但对其潜在机制的了解仍然有限。最近，多项研究结果表明，肠道微生物群及其相关代谢物在失眠症的发病机制中起着重要作用。本研究旨在从肠道菌群和代谢物的角度评价蒙医温针的治疗效果，阐明其抗失眠的作用机制。本研究建立了 PCPA 诱导的失眠大鼠模型，证明了蒙医温针的干预防止了体重的减轻，并对行为产生了有益的影响。本实验还表明，蒙医温针处理显著降低了 ACh 和 NE 水平，提高了 5-HT 和 GABA 水平。众所周知，神经递质的功能障碍与失眠有关，在失眠症患者的大脑中 5-HT 和 GABA 显著降低，而 ACh 和 NE 的水平增加。因此，我们的观察表明，蒙医温针的干预对失眠有令人满意的效果。

本实验基于 16S rRNA 基因扩增测序，进一步分析了肠道微生物区系的组成和多样性。厚壁菌门和变形菌门是最主要的细菌门，这与之前的报道[1]一致。在属水平上，与对照组相比，失眠症大鼠中乳酸菌属和梭菌属的相对丰度显著下降。乳酸菌作为益生菌被广泛应用，具有改善睡眠的作用[2]。此外，乳酸菌和梭菌属的丰度与丁酸盐[3]的浓度有关。有趣的是，研究表明这些细菌种类与昼夜节律有关，越来越多的证据表明丁酸盐调节宿主生物钟基因[4]的表达。根据文献记载，细菌倾向于通过丁酸盐[5]来影响宿主。综上所述，乳酸菌和梭状梭菌可能至少部分通过其代谢物丁酸调节宿主的昼夜节律。此外，该属的成员可能参与了肠道微生物群的生态失调[6]，这与我们的研究结果一致。有趣的是，蒙医温针的干预导致了罗姆布茨菌属的丰度的减少，显著增加了乳酸菌和梭菌的丰度，提示其可能在肠道微生物群平衡中发挥作用。先前的一项研究表明，针灸治疗在属水平上促进了乳酸菌属的产生。

采用 LEfSe 算法对类群间相对丰度差异显著的重要微生物类群进行鉴定。在门水平上，变形菌门在模型类群中起着重要的作用。在睡眠碎片[7]大鼠模型中观察到肠道菌群中促炎变形菌门的相对丰度增加。在家族水平上，XIVa 梭菌和 Blautia 是模型组的特征。在目水平上，毛螺菌科是模型群的特征。青光眼和毛螺菌科已被证明与人类的睡眠效率呈负相关[8]。据我们所知，XIVa 梭菌在失眠症中的作用尚未见报道。然而，值得注意的是，XIVa 梭状芽孢杆菌在自闭症谱系障碍[9]儿童中富集，提示其在神经病理生理学中的潜在作用。为了进一步验证蒙医温针治疗是否能使 PCPA 诱导的失眠大鼠模型的肠道菌群重新平衡，我们获得了对照组和治疗组之间基于 LEfSe 分析的 LDA 评分。令人惊讶的是，治疗组的大鼠主要特征是较高的丰度。肠道微生物群弹性的概念已经在文献中描述过，据报道[10]，有弹性的微生物群在受到扰动后，会恢复到原来的平衡状态，而非有弹性的微生物群将转移到另一种稳定状态[11]。因此，我们认为，Blautia 在模型组中含量丰富，这在某种程度上取决于某些宿主因素的影响，但采用蒙医温针干预后，该微生物则转移到另一种稳定状态。然而，微生物群恢复力的机制仍有待阐明[12]。

失眠大鼠肠道微生物群的改变伴随着血清代谢组的紊乱[13-15]。相关分析表明，失眠大鼠的代谢物升高，如酰胺 c18、苯甲酰氯、胞嘧啶、N,N- 二甲基精氨酸与失眠大鼠 XIVa 和 Blautia 的丰度呈正相关。经蒙医温针处理后，3-（{[(2s)-2,3- 二羟基丙氧基]（羟基）磷酸基}氧)-2- 羟基丙基棕榈酸酯降低，并与 XIVa 梭菌呈正相关。这些结果进一步证实了这些细菌可能在失眠症中起着重要的作用。

对血清样本的代谢组学分析显示，蒙医温针处理降低了 PCPA 诱导的大鼠模型中的 cAMP 信号通路。先前的一项研究报道，cAMP 参与调节睡眠 - 觉醒周期[16]。与清醒状态下[17] 相比，快速眼动（REM）睡眠时的 cAMP 水平最低，这与我们的研究结果一致。先前的研究也发现，丁酸盐可以通过 Gi 蛋白[18] 抑制 cAMP 信号通路。我们检测了蒙医温针干预对失眠症大鼠丁酸盐水平的影响。我们的结果显示，蒙医温针显著增加了丁酸盐的含量。我们进一步证实，丁酸盐减弱了 PCPA 诱导的 cAMP 水平的升高。这些结果表明，蒙医温针至少部分地通过上调丁酸盐来抑制 cAMP 信号通路。

最新的研究也表明，cAMP 信号通路在 GAT-1 功能[19] 的调控中发挥了重要作用。众所周知，γ- 氨基丁酸能突触有助于失眠症的发展。GAT-1 在调节 GABA 水平中发挥关键作用，并参与 GABA A 受体（GABAAR）介导的抑制[20]。在本研究中，我们证实了蒙医温针干预降低了 GAT-1 的表达，这与之前的报道一致[19]。

结论：本研究表明，蒙医温针干预可调节与失眠相关的多种微生物属和代谢产物，从而逆转丁酸介导的由失眠引起的 cAMP 信号通路异常和 GAT-1 表达异常。这些发现将有助于更好地理解蒙医温针有效治疗失眠症的分子机制。

参 考 文 献

[1] HE W Q, XIONG Y Q, GE J, et al. Composition of gut and oropharynx bacterial communities in Rattus norvegicus and Suncus murinus in China[J]. BMC Vet Res, 2020, 16（1）: 413.

[2] LIN A, SHIH C T, HUANG C L, et al. Hypnotic effects of Lactobacillus fermentum PS150TM

on pentobarbital-induced sleep in mice[J]. Nutrients, 2019, 11(10): 2409.

[3] APPERT O, GARCIA A R, FREI R, et al. Initial butyrate producers during infant gut microbiota development are endospore formers[J]. Environ Microbiol, 2020, 22(9): 3909-3921.

[4] PARKAR S G, KALSBEEK A, CHEESEMAN J F. Potential role for the gut microbiota in modulating host circadian rhythms and metabolic health[J]. Microorganisms, 2019, 7(2): 41.

[5] LEE S M, KIM N, NAM R H, et al. Gut microbiota and butyrate level changes associated with the long-term administration of proton pump inhibitors to old rats[J]. Sci Rep, 2019, 9(1): 6626.

[6] WEI D, XIE L, ZHUANG Z, et al. Gut microbiota: a new strategy to study the mechanism of electroacupuncture and moxibustion in treating ulcerative colitis[J]. Evid Based Complement Alternat Med, 2019, 2019: 9730176.

[7] MAKI K A, BURKE L A, CALIK M W, et al. Sleep fragmentation increases blood pressure and is associated with alterations in the gut microbiome and fecal metabolome in rats[J]. Physiol Genomics, 2020, 52(7): 280-292.

[8] SMITH R P, EASSON C, LYLE S M, et al. Gut microbiome diversity is associated with sleep physiology in humans[J]. PLoS One, 2019, 14(10): 0222394.

[9] ZOU R, XU F, WANG Y, et al. Changes in the gut microbiota of children with autism spectrum disorder[J]. Autism Res, 2020, 13(9): 1614-1625.

[10] DOWNING A S, VAN NES E H, MOOIJ W M, et al. The resilience and resistance of an ecosystem to a collapse of diversity[J]. PLoS One, 2012, 7(9): 46135.

[11] DOGRA S K, DORE J, DAMAK S. Gut microbiota resilience: definition, link to health and strategies for intervention[J]. Front Microbiol, 2020(11): 572921.

[12] FISHER C K, MEHTA P. Identifying keystone species in the human gut microbiome from metagenomic timeseries using sparse linear regression[J]. PLoS One, 2014, 9(7): 102451.

[13] SI Y, CHEN X, GUO T, et al. Comprehensive 16S rDNA sequencing and LC-MS/MS-based metabolomics to investigate intestinal flora and metabolic profiles of the serum, hypothalamus and hippocampus in p-chlorophenylalanine-induced insomnia rats treated with lilium brownie[J]. Neurochem Res, 2022, 47(3): 574-589.

[14] ZHOU J, WU X, LI Z, et al. Alterations in gut microbiota are correlated with serum metabolites in patients with insomnia disorder[J]. Front Cell Infect Microbiol, 2022(12): 722662.

[15] SI Y, WEI W, CHEN X, et al. A comprehensive study on the relieving effect of Lilium brownii on the intestinal flora and metabolic disorder in p-chlorophenylalanine-induced insomnia rats[J]. Pharm Biol, 2022, 60(1): 131-143.

[16] AMICI R，PEREZ E，ZAMBONI G，et al. Changes in cAMP concentration in the rat preoptic area during synchronized and desynchronized sleep[J]. Experientia，1990，46（1）：58-59.

[17] OGASAHARA S，TAGUCHI Y，WADA H. Changes in the levels of cyclic nucleotides in rat brain during the sleep-wakefulness cycle[J]. Brain Res，1981，213（1）：163-171.

[18] LU N，LI M，LEI H，et al. Butyric acid regulates progesterone and estradiol secretion via cAMP signaling pathway in porcine granulosa cells[J]. J Steroid Biochem Mol Biol，2017，172：89-97.

[19] BORGES-MARTINS V P P，FERREIRA D D P，SOUTO A C，et al. Caffeine regulates GABA transport via A1R blockade and cAMP signaling[J]. Neurochem Int，2019，131：104550.

[20] GHIRARDINI E，WADLE S L，AUGUSTIN V，et al. Expression of functional inhibitory neurotransmitter transporters GlyT$_1$, GAT-1, and GAT-3 by astrocytes of inferior colliculus and hippocampus[J]. Mol Brain，2018，11（1）：4.

第十四章

蒙医温针疗法治疗失眠症的临床试验研究

临床资料表明，长期失眠将导致心脏病、高血压、高脂血症、阿尔茨海默病、抑郁、焦虑多种疾病的患病风险上升[1]。失眠症是由于各种原因造成控制睡眠的解剖结构的破坏和递质传递功能障碍导致的睡眠障碍。近年来，在临床中运用各种治疗手段（包括药理和非药理性）改善睡眠的报道不胜枚举[2]，但是，除了临床疗效外，与其治疗作用机制有关的研究尚不够全面。目前，寻找安全、有效的防治失眠方法是临床和实验研究的重要课题之一。

蒙医将失眠症称为"无眠""不得眠""睡眠不安"等，是指"身、心、语"功能紊乱而引起人体"三根"平衡失调，导致经常性不能获得正常睡眠的一种病。温针疗法是蒙医治疗失眠的常用方法之一，本研究为首次针对蒙医温针治疗失眠所做的临床试验，通过考察蒙医证候病情、匹兹堡睡眠质量指数及多导睡眠监测指标对蒙医温针治疗失眠症作出评估。

一、试验方法

（一）诊断标准

根据《中医病证诊断疗效标准》及美国睡眠研究协会《睡眠障碍国际分类（ICSD-2）》标准进行诊断[3]；蒙医诊断标准参照全国高等医药院校蒙医药（本科）专业规划教材《蒙医内科学》中失眠症的诊断标准。

主要症状为赫依偏盛引起赫依血和赫依希拉相搏的症状，即入睡困难、不易入睡或容易醒、醒后不能再睡、彻夜不眠。次要症状包括头痛头昏、心悸、健忘多梦、烦躁易怒、神疲乏力等。

（二）纳入标准

1. 年龄在20～75岁。

2. 病程在 1 个月至 2 年之间。

3. 入睡困难,入睡时间超过 30 分钟。

4. 睡眠维持障碍,整夜觉醒次数≥2 次。

(三)排除标准

1. 孕妇,哺乳期女性。

2. 病情危笃或疾病晚期患者。

3. 重度抑郁症患者(参照《中国精神障碍分类与诊断标准(CCMD-3)》)。

4. 有严重慢性疾病的患者。判断标准为患者是否定期使用药物治疗。

5. 疼痛症状患者(如风湿、类风湿性疾病,坐骨神经痛,腰椎间盘突出症等患者)。

6. 夜班工作者。

(四)分组及患者一般资料

所有病例为 2015 年 9 月至 2015 年 12 月在内蒙古医科大学附属医院蒙医科确诊为失眠症的门诊以及住院患者。80 例病例使用统计学中分层随机的方法,分为针灸组和艾司唑仑组。每组中依病情之轻重各分为轻、中、重 3 层。

(五)干预方法

1. 温针组 使用加温灸的特制银针针刺治疗。取穴:顶会穴、赫依穴、心穴。针具:蒙医银针(银质,0.5mm×30mm)。

2. 针刺方法 患者取坐位,75% 酒精常规消毒皮肤后,于顶会穴斜刺,以患者头皮有紧捏感或重胀感为度;于赫依穴和心穴针向下平刺。用 MLY-Ⅰ型蒙医疗术温针仪加温,蒙医疗术温针仪温度控制在 38℃,每次 30 分钟,每天 1 次,9 天为 1 个疗程;治疗 6 个疗程,每个疗程之间间隔 3 天。

3. 药物组 艾司唑仑:常用剂量 1mg,睡前 15～30min 服用,治疗时间 56 天。

(六)观察指标

1. 蒙医学指标观察 参照《蒙医内科学》,根据蒙医证候积分判定蒙医证候病情。轻度:不大于 5 分;中度:6 分到 10 分;重度:11 分到 15 分。

2. 匹兹堡睡眠质量指数量表(PSQI) 匹兹堡睡眠质量指数量表用于评定被试者最近 1 个月的睡眠质量。本量表积分之满分为 21 分,疗效的判断标准为:治疗前积分减去治疗后积分,与治疗前积分的比值×100%,无效 <30%;有

效≥30%；显效≥70%；痊愈≥90%[4]。

3. 多导睡眠指标检测（PSG）　使用 Embletta 13（X100）导联便携式多导睡眠监测系统对睡眠结构分析，指标包括：睡眠总时间、醒起时间、醒觉时间、运动觉醒时间、醒觉次数、NREM、REM 睡眠时间、NREM S3/S4 期时间等，温针及药物干预前测量 1 次，温针及药物干预结束后间隔 7 天再测 1 次。

（七）统计分析方法

所有数据采用 SPSS18.0 统计软件分析。数据采用配对 t 检验分析每组患者治疗前后的变化情况，$P < 0.05$ 为显著性差异。实验数据用均数 ± 标准差（$\bar{x} \pm s$）表示；两组的组间差异用 Student's t 检验。组间计数资料的比较采用卡方检验或威尔科克森符号秩检验。$P < 0.05$ 认为差异有统计学意义，$P < 0.01$ 认为差异有显著性统计学意义。

二、结果

1. 患者一般资料　本试验纳入病例共 80 例，其中蒙医温针治疗组 40 例，艾司唑仑对照组 40 例，其中 1 组为蒙医温针组，男性患者 24 例，女性患者 16 例，21～65 岁之间，年龄范围：43.25 ± 9.56 岁，病程时间范围在 3.15 ± 1.24 年，轻度 4 例，中度 22 例，重度 14 例；2 组为艾司唑仑对照组，男性患者 22 例，女性患者 18 例，19～67 岁之间，平均年龄 47.21 ± 8.31 岁，平均病程在 4.10 ± 1.06 年，轻度 4 例，中度 19 例，重度 17 例（见表 14-1）。

表 14-1　患者一般资料

组别	病例数	性别		病程	年龄	病情		
		男	女			轻	中	重
温针组	40	24	16	3.15 ± 1.24 年	43.25 ± 9.56 岁	4	22	14
药物组	40	22	18	4.10 ± 1.06 年	47.21 ± 8.31 岁	4	19	17
		$\chi^2 = 0.292$		$t = 0.651$	$t = 0.717$	$z = -1.303$		
		$P = 0.587$		$P = 0.534$	$P = 0.536$	$P = 0.319$		

注：2 组性别比较采用卡方检验；病程、年龄比较采用 t 检验；病情比较采用秩和检验。两组病例经过统计分析，在年龄、病程、病情等统计学指标无具有统计学意义的差异，即具有可比性。病情评估，对秩和检验进行编秩，以轻为 1，中为 2，重为 3。温针组和药物组经过秩和检验，$z = -1.303$，$P = 0.319$，2 组病情差别无统计学意义（$P > 0.05$）。

2. 蒙医证候病情指标 治疗前经过 t 检验，2 组患者蒙医学证候积分未见明显差异（$P > 0.05$），说明 2 组具有可比性；治疗后 t 检验显示两组患者仍无显著差异（$P > 0.05$），具有可比性。温针组和药物组治疗前后比较，蒙医学证候积分 $P < 0.01$，具有极显著差异（见表 14-2）。

表 14-2 蒙医证候病情指标

分组	病例数	治疗前积分	治疗后积分	t	P
温针组	40	11.56 ± 3.64	3.64 ± 1.08	6.302	0.000
药物组	40	12.27 ± 4.25	4.25 ± 1.69	10.524	0.000
		t=0.647	t=0.631		
		P=0.421	P=0.596		

3. 临床疗效结果的分析 疗效结果的判定使用积分法。积分之满分为 21 分。疗效判定：治疗前积分减去治疗后积分的差值，与治疗前积分的比值 ×100%。结果：痊愈 $\geq 90\%$；明显有效 $\geq 70\%$；有效 $\geq 30\%$；无效 $< 30\%$（见表 14-3）。

表 14-3 临床疗效结果的分析

分组	病例数	痊愈	明显有效	有效	无效	有效率
温针组	40	2	18	14	6	85%
药物组	40	0	13	15	12	70%

4. 匹兹堡睡眠质量指数评价 治疗前 2 组 PSQI 总分相近，经 t 检验，$t=-0.314$，$P=0.847$，2 组匹兹堡睡眠质量指数未见明显差异，说明 2 组具有可比性；治疗后，2 组睡眠质量指数均呈显著下降（$P < 0.05$），可以认为治疗有效，蒙医温针组分数略低，但 2 组之间未见明显差异（$P > 0.05$）。治疗后，睡眠质量指标蒙医温针组显著好转（$P < 0.01$），优于艾司唑仑组（$P < 0.01$）；入睡时间显著缩短（$P < 0.05$），睡眠时间显著增加（$P < 0.01$），睡眠障碍评分显著降低（$P < 0.05$），但此 3 项指标显示治疗效果不如艾司唑仑组；治疗后，睡眠效率和日间功能蒙医温针组患者均显著提高（$P < 0.01$），对比艾司唑仑组同样具有显著提高的作用（$P < 0.01$）（见图 14-1）。

5. 多导睡眠指标检测（PSG） 治疗前所有多导睡眠检测指标 2 组患者均值经 t 检验，P 均 > 0.05，说明 2 组具有可比性；治疗后，2 组总睡眠时间均呈现显著上升趋势，其中蒙医温针组睡眠时间显著延长（$P < 0.01$）；治疗后只有蒙医温针组夜间觉醒显著减少，停药后艾司唑仑组仍然保持较多的觉醒次数，2 组存在

显著性差异（$P<0.01$）；与治疗前比较，或与治疗后艾司唑仑组比较，NREM 期睡眠时间蒙医温针组显著提高（$P<0.01$）；NREM 期睡眠时间百分率 2 组治疗前后无明显变化；REM 期睡眠时间均呈下降趋势，其中蒙医温针组呈显著性下降（$P<0.01$）；REM 期睡眠时间占总睡眠时间的百分率 2 组均呈下降趋势，其中艾司唑仑组呈显著下降（$P<0.05$）；NREM3＋4 期睡眠时间占总睡眠时间的百分率来看，治疗后 2 组均有所提高，其中蒙医温针组呈显著提高（$P<0.01$），与艾司唑仑组比较也呈显著提高（$P<0.01$），可以认为治疗有效（见图 14-2）。

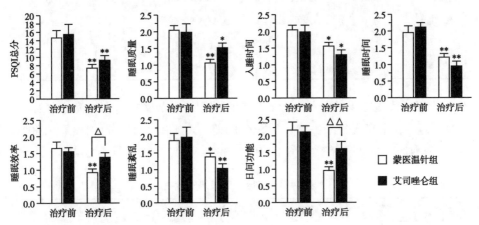

注：* 表示治疗后对比治疗前数值呈显著性差异，* 表示 $P<0.05$，** 表示 $P<0.01$；△ 表示蒙医温针组对比艾司唑仑组数值呈显著性差异，△ 表示 $P<0.05$，△△ 表示 $P<0.01$。

图 14-1 2 组间匹兹堡睡眠质量指数评价

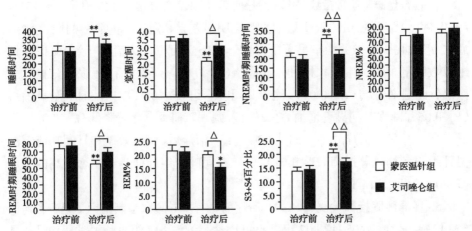

注：* 表示治疗后对比治疗前数值呈显著性差异，* 表示 $P<0.05$，** 表示 $P<0.01$；△ 表示蒙医温针组对比艾司唑仑组数值呈显著性差异，△ 表示 $P<0.05$，△△ 表示 $P<0.01$。

图 14-2 2 组间多导睡眠指标检测评价

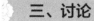
三、讨论

　　失眠是一种显著的公共健康问题,发病率高,如果失眠不加以治疗,最终会导致心理、生理和职业健康问题的发生。导致失眠的相关因素众多,生理 - 心理因素、遗传基因、机体素质、环境条件、社会人际关系、精神刺激、认知过程、躯体疾患、精神疾病、药物不良反应及睡眠习惯等都可引起。失眠症的发病机制复杂,至今仍有许多未完全明了。药物治疗仍是目前国内外治疗失眠的主要方法。当前治疗失眠的药物主要是针对 γ- 氨基丁酸(GABA)的受体,褪黑激素受体,组胺受体,食欲肽和血清素受体[5]。药物包括第一代巴比妥类、第二代苯二氮䓬类及第三代非苯二氮䓬类。

　　由于口服药物多数疗效持续时间短,长期服用会有药物依赖、停药反应,因而优先选择非药物治疗的患者不在少数。经过本次临床试验验证,蒙医温针组和艾司唑仑组比较而言,蒙医温针组能够更好地改善患者的睡眠时间和日间功能,并且提高睡眠时间方面也优于停药后的艾司唑仑组,能够比催眠药物更有效的帮助失眠患者。

　　失眠症与脑电图的关联已受到广泛重视,国外文献进一步认为,REM 潜伏期缩短是失眠症的特征性改变[6],另外,还有 S3、S4 期睡眠减少,REM 密度增加,睡眠效率降低及 REM 时间增多等异常。失眠症 PSG 的特征性改变是睡眠的连续性发生改变和结构上的异常,表现为夜间觉醒次数增多、实际睡眠时间减少、睡眠效率低;睡眠结构比例失衡,浅睡多即 S1、S2 期睡眠占整个睡眠期的比例增多,而深睡明显减少[7]。本次试验干预前数据证明了以上观点。

　　蒙医温针可以减少觉醒次数、缩短 REM 期睡眠时间、REM 睡眠百分比;增加 NREM 睡眠时间;同时睡眠质量、入睡时间、睡眠时间、睡眠效率、睡眠障碍、日间功能、总分评分与治疗前相比均有显著改善。在这些指标上均优于艾司唑仑组。

　　本实验首次针对蒙医温针治疗失眠症采用多导睡眠监测具有重要意义,对于失眠症睡眠生理指标改变明显的患者要长时间的温针治疗能够使部分睡眠指标趋于正常,如 REM 睡眠时间、睡眠效率、觉醒时间等;同时对于失眠症的特征性指标,如 NREM3 + 4 期也有好的改善作用,在某种程度上可以优于目前的安眠药物治疗。本试验为今后蒙医温针的现代治疗提供了临床的研究证明,为传统民族医药的现代化发展提供了科学支持。

参 考 文 献

[1] CHUNG K F, YEUNG W F, HO F Y, et al. Cross-cultural and comparative epidemiology of insomnia: the Diagnostic and statistical manual (DSM), International classification of diseases (ICD) and International classification of sleep disorders (ICSD) [J]. Sleep medicine, 2015, 16 (4): 477-482.

[2] VINIEGRA DOMINGUEZ M A, PARELLADA ESQUIUS N, MIRANDA DE MORAES RIBEIRO R, et al. An integral approach to insomnia in primary care: Non-pharmacological and phytotherapy measures compared to standard treatment[J]. Atencion primaria, 2015, 47 (6): 351-358.

[3] YEH Z T, CHIANG R P, KANG S C, et al. Development of the Insomnia Screening Scale based on ICSD-II[J]. International Journal of psychiatry in clinical practice, 2012, 16 (4): 259-267.

[4] ZHONG Q Y, GELAYE B, SANCHEZ S E, et al. Psychometric Properties of the Pittsburgh Sleep Quality Index (PSQI) in a Cohort of Peruvian pregnant women[J]. Journal of clinical sleep medicine, 2015, 11 (8): 869-877.

[5] SHI Y, DONG J W, ZHAO J H, et al. Herbal Insomnia Medications that Target GABAergic Systems: A Review of the Psychopharmacological Evidence[J]. Current neuropharmacology, 2014, 12 (3): 289-302.

[6] PERUSSE A D, PEDNEAULT-DROLET M, RANCOURT C, et al. REM sleep as a potential indicator of hyperarousal in psychophysiological and paradoxical insomnia sufferers[J]. International Journal of psychophysiology, 2015, 95 (3): 372-378.

[7] MAI E, BUYSSE D J. Insomnia: Prevalence, impact, pathogenesis, differential diagnosis, and evaluation[J]. Sleep medicine clinics, 2008, 3 (2): 167-174.

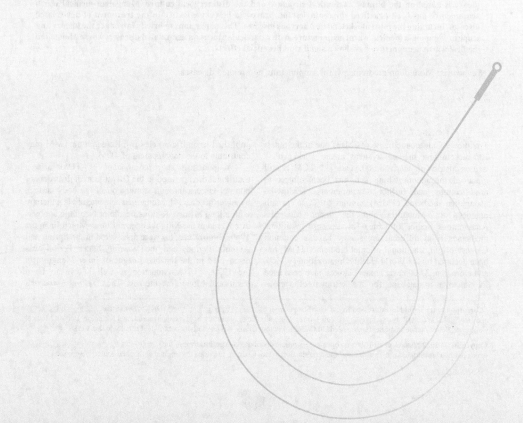

附录

Aging and Disease
www.aginganddisease.org

Volume 13, Number 4; 1030-1041, August 2022
http://dx.doi.org/10.14336/AD.2022.0115

Commentary

Overview of Traditional Mongolian Medical Warm Acupuncture

Guo Shao[1,2,3,#,*], Wei Xie[2,3,#], Xiaoe Jia[2,3], Rengui Bade[2,3], Yabing Xie[2,3], Ruifang Qi[2,3], Kerui Gong[4], Haihua Bai[5], Lengge Si[5], Yingsong Chen[5], Kai Sun[1*], Agula Bo[2*]

[1]Center for Translational Medicine and Department of Laboratory Medicine, the Third People's Hospital of Longgang District Shenzhen, Shenzhen, China. [2]Inner Mongolia Key Laboratory of Hypoxic Translational Medicine, Baotou Medical College of Neuroscience Institute, Baotou Medical College, Baotou, China. [3]Beijing Key Laboratory of Hypoxic Conditioning Translational Medicine, Xuanwu Hospital, Capital Medical University, Beijing, China. [4]Department of Oral and Maxillofacial Surgery, University of California San Francisco, San Francisco, USA. [5]Inner Mongolia Minzu University, Tongliao, China.

[Received December 2, 2021; Revised January 6, 2022; Accepted January 7, 2022]

ABSTRACT: Mongolian medical warm acupuncture is a traditional therapy of Mongolian medicine and was developed by people living on the Mongolian Plateau. This kind of traditional oriental medicine has a long history. The main characteristics of Mongolian medical warm acupuncture are the acupoints and the needles used. Its theory is based on the human anatomical structure and the distinct local culture. Mongolian medical warm acupuncture has been practiced for centuries and proved to be very effective in the treatment of age-related diseases, including the musculoskeletal and nervous diseases. This paper aims to briefly introduce the history and scope of Mongolian medical warm acupuncture, with a particular focus on age-related diseases, where Mongolian medical warm acupuncture has shown significant beneficial effects.

Key words: Mongolian medicine, warm acupuncture, age-related diseases

Traditional Chinese medicine (TCM) is one of the oldest and most unique medical systems in the world with a written history of nearly 3,000 years [1]. TCM is still practiced throughout China and has been subject to modifications and further developments. Traditional Mongolian medicine (TMM), similar to TCM, is still practiced in Mongolia and the Inner Mongolia Autonomous Region of China [2]. Because traditional medicines from different areas may have a common Chinese origin, traditional oriental medicine (TOM) has been declared by the World Health Organization (WHO), and more than 3,000 basic nomenclatures have been used to construct a database for the retrieval of various published scientific articles [3]. Research on TMM may contribute to the development of TOM.

Acupuncture is a component of TOM and a traditional therapy used in the Orient to treat disorders of internal viscera through stimulation of the body surface by silver needles [4]. Mongolian acupuncture is a therapy with a long history. A stone needle of Neolithic age was discovered in the Xiligol League of Inner Mongolia in the 1960s, bronze needles were discovered in the Spring and Autumn Period, and the Warring States Period was discovered in the Ikezhao League of Inner Mongolia in the 1970s [5]. Moxibustion is well known to be a traditional Mongolian therapy. The *"Yellow Emperor's*

Correspondence should be addressed to: Dr. Guo Shao (Email: shao.guo.china@gmail.com), Dr. Kai Sun (Email: Henrysk@163.com), and Dr. Agula Bo (Email: bagulaimmu@163.com), Inner Mongolia Key Laboratory of Hypoxic Translational Medicine, Baotou Medical College of Neuroscience Institute, Baotou Medical College, Baotou, China. #These authors contributed equally to this work.

ISSN: 2152-5250

1030

Classic of Internal Medicine" states that the origin of warm acupuncture is "North." We can infer that the "North" region refers to the Mongolian Plateau because of the descriptions of nomadic living and the cold climate. Mongolian moxibustion was recorded in *"Four Medical Tantras"* written by Yutuo Yundan-Kampot, a famous physician of the 8th century AD. Therefore, Mongolian warm acupuncture may have been employed by people living on the Mongolian Plateau for centuries [6].

The use of warm acupuncture to treat disease depends on the culture of Mongolian people. People living on the Mongolian Plateau have achieved an understanding of the human anatomical structure through celestial burials and hunting. They also adopted medical practices from TCM, most prominently implementing the Yin and Yang theory for their diagnoses and treatments. They combined their anatomic knowledge and Tibetan Buddhism with TCM theories to create a medical system that has unique cultural features [2]. The TMM theory is based on the idea that the "Black Meridian" and "White Meridian" systems connect the body with the surrounding environment; they control the exchange of matter and information between the inside and the outside. Currently, the "Black Meridian" and "White Meridian" systems are regarded as the circulation and neural systems, respectively, in the modified TMM theory [7]. In TMM, the "White Meridian" system comprises the brain and spinal cord, and includes the inner and outer "White Meridian"[8]. The inner "White Meridian" controls internal organs (heart, small intestine, lungs, colon, liver, gallbladder, spleen, stomach, kidneys, and bladder), thus its function is similar to that of the autonomic nervous system.

Acupuncture is a set of medical treatments and an ideology based on the principle of applying small needles or pressure to specific points, presenting a dermal projection of the body's internal viscera [9]. In the TMM system, there are certain special points (acupoints) to which warm needles may be applied to treat different diseases. Some models were set up for Mongolian physicians to practice the identification of acupoints [10]. There are more than 42 acupoints on the neck and more than 150 on the trunk, with most of these acupoints on the "White Meridian" (Fig. 1).

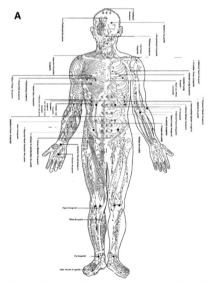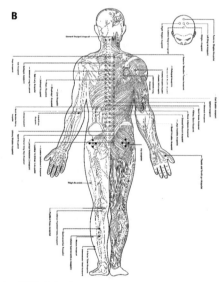

Figure 1. The map of Mongolian medicine acupoints. (A) Anterior view. **(B)** Posterior view.

Acupoints in TMM are those points that can balance the internal environment and regulate temperature when stimulated. The selection of acupoints is based on dialectical treatment, which uses the etiology and pathological changes for theoretical guidance. These factors, including the "Black Meridian" and "White Meridian," pain location, and diseased areas are to be considered in the choice of the acupoints. For example, the Dinghui acupoint mainly treats symptoms such as those of the Heyi fever, which causes dumbness, confusion, and memory loss, based on the records of the *"Encyclopedia of Mongolian Studies (Medical)."* Stimulation of the Heyi acupoint can be used to treat dizziness and headaches, including those caused by disease. The basic principle for acupoint choice is maximizing the effects with fewer points. The selection of the acupoints on behalf of the doctors is based on recorded documentation or their own experience.

During the past 3,000 years, many cases of various diseases have been treated by acupuncture in Asian countries. These diseases are often considered to be neurovegetative disorders. Mongolian warm acupuncture has diverse effects on the body: (1) it can reduce inflammation and promote the reabsorption of chronic inflammation; (2) it may have analgesic effects and raise the pain threshold; and (3) can have a regulatory effect on the immune system [11]. Mongolian warm acupuncture was effective in treating certain diseases related with aging, such as bone [12], neuronal [13], and metabolic diseases.

Basic principles of Mongolian medicine and its anti-aging effects

Mongolian medicine is a type of TOM. Its characteristics are based on the experience accumulated by the Mongolian ancestors in their long-term life practice, while absorbing the essence of other (Chinese medicine, Tibetan medicine) ethnic and ancient Indian medicines. TMM is guided by simple materialism and spontaneous dialectics. A unique ethnic medicine gradually formed and developed. The basic theories of Mongolian medicine are based on experience from clinical practice. These theories include those of Yin and Yang, the five Yuan (earth, water, fire, air, empty) and the five elements (gold, wood, water, fire, earth), the three roots (Heyi, Shila, Badagan) and seven Su (food, blood, muscle, fat, bone, bone marrow, energy), among others. The three roots and seven Su are the most important theories in Mongolian medicine. The three roots control different parts of the body (Heyi and Badagan each control the upper and lower body, respectively above the heart and under the navel, while Shila controls the trunk, between the heart and navel). The seven Su are the materials that build the body. The three roots and seven Su are the foundation of the Mongolian medicine theory. A disorder in these elements is considered the reason for disease in TMM [14].

The three methods of diagnosis generally adopted by TMM doctors are the basic methods for illness diagnosis: observation, inquiry, and palpation. These basic methods are very similar to the four methods of diagnosis used in TCM. There are four treatment methods used in TMM, namely oral medicine (such as herb), therapeutic techniques (such as acupuncture and bloodletting),

beverages and food (such as yogurt made with horse milk), and movement (such as Andai dancing). Mongolian warm acupuncture is part of the therapeutic techniques of the Mongolian medicine system. Traditional Chinese acupuncture has been shown to be useful in clinical therapy and to possess anti-aging properties [15]. The imbalance of the three roots was regarded as the reason for aging. It has been demonstrated that six Mongolian acupoints, including Heyi, Dinghui, and Huoshuai, have stable anti-aging effects in Mongolian warm acupuncture [16].

History of Mongolian acupuncture and warm acupuncture

Mongolian ancestors invented acupuncture therapy. Acupuncture therapy belongs to TMM, has a long history and unique curative effects. Mongolian acupuncture can conduct heat or cold and produce stimulation at fixed acupoints on the human body. Archaeology has proven, in recent years, that Mongolian ancestors made and used special tools for traditional medicine as early as 6,000 years ago, in the Neolithic age or even earlier [17]. Medical stone needles, bone needles, bronze flint needles and other cultural relics unearthed in Inner Mongolia all explain the origin of acupuncture and moxibustion [18], showing that the ancestors living in the Xiligol and the Ikezhao Leagues of Inner Mongolia had mastered these techniques [19]. From the 11th to the 3rd century B.C., people already knew how to treat certain diseases with acupuncture and bloodletting therapies. Between the 17th and 18th century, the famous Mongolian physician Yixibalajur wrote the first record of indications, contraindications, efficacy, and acupoints of Mongolian acupuncture, which laid the foundation for the widespread use of acupuncture in clinical practice. *"Four Medical Tantras · Blue Beryl"* quotes that *"acupuncture is to correct the five kinds of surgical treatment errors."* The *"Encyclopedia of Chinese Medicine · Mongolian Medicine"* reports the use of iron, bone, bronze, copper, silver, and gold needles in the process of development of Mongolian medicine acupuncture. Among these needles, the silver needles are mainly used [20]. The silver needle has a strong bactericidal effect, does not deteriorate over long periods of time, presents appropriate hardness and good elasticity, and is therefore widely used in the clinical practice.

Due to the late definition of Mongolian characters, there are only scattered fragments of records in literature regarding the ancient medical activities of Mongolians and the process of development of acupuncture therapy. Ancient books written in Chinese and Tibetan in the Zhanguo and Qin/Han Dynasties contained records of Mongolian medicine and medical treatment, but the content of such records was relatively fragmented and did not form a theoretical system. The prescriptions and treatments, such as Mongolian moxibustion and Xiongnu sleeping pills commonly used by northern people, are recorded in the *"Four Medical Tantras"* and *"Bei Ji Qian Jin Yao Fang: Essential Prescriptions worth a Thousand in Gold for Every Emergency."* In the 13th century, *"The Secret History of the Mongol"* reports that, before the Yuan Dynasty, Mongolians used kefir to treat injured patients with bleeding and fainting. Because of the Indian medical book *"Ashtanga Hridya Samhita"* and Tibetan medicine *"Four Medical Tantras,"* the theoretical system of Mongolian medicine improved and further developed. Many Mongolian medical scientists emerged, and medical works about Mongolian medicine written in Tibetan or Mongolian were published. The monograph *"Zhu Shi Chu Hei Ming Deng"* edited by Darimaomaremba Lobsang Asahiga reports content related to the acupuncture techniques of Mongolian medicine from different perspectives and has had a great influence on the development of Mongolian medicine acupuncture techniques in later generations. Mongolian acupuncture therapy, guided by the basic theories of Mongolian medicine and based on syndrome differentiation, uses special needles to penetrate specific parts of the human body to stimulate and regulate the three roots, and dredge the "White Meridian," achieving a traditional therapy for preventing and curing diseases.

Before the 1950s, warm acupuncture was only one of the TMM techniques in Mongolian medicine. The existence of warm acupuncture was based on the geographical environment and living habits of a nomadic people. Moxibustion and acupuncture in Mongolian medicine have a long history. The development of warm acupuncture in Mongolian medicine can be divided into an accumulation period (before the 1950s), a formation period (between the 1950s and the end of the 20th century), and a prosperity period (from the 21st century to the present). The name of "warm acupuncture" is not ancient but gradually became clear with the development of Mongolian medicine. The evolution of the name has gone through different phases: hot needling plus fire moxibustion, hot needle assisting heat, warm moxibustion needle, warm needle, warm needling, and finally warm acupuncture. Mongolian medicine warm acupuncture was listed on the national intangible cultural heritage list, which allowed it to have a formal identity. As an invented tradition, the Zanbula Dorje warm acupuncture aims to create the identity of "national medicine - traditional status."

Modern needles used in Mongolian warm acupuncture have been continuously modified with the advancement of science and technology. Modern Mongolian "warm acupuncture" is used safely and

effectively in hospitals. The needle is heated electronically (Fig. 2C) and the diameter of the silver needle has been reduced. The method for temperature control has been improved, and resistance heating is used to replace mugwort burning. The new heating technology can not only achieve the thermal efficiency of traditional silver needle heating, but is also easy to operate and smoke-free, overcoming the issue of moxa grass smoke [21]. These thin silver needles can reduce damage as effectively as those used in traditional warm acupuncture.

Types of Mongolian acupuncture and warm acupuncture

Warm acupuncture is a needle method where the tail of a filiform needle is wrapped with moxa, the combustion of which generates heat to cure diseases. Warm acupuncture combines the effects of acupuncture and moxibustion; the needles are passed through the body acupoints to warm the meridians and promote the circulation of Qi and blood. Warm acupuncture is used to treat cold stagnation in the meridians, Qi and blood blockage, and other diseases [22]. With the increase in acupuncture research, a variety of needles have emerged. In *"Modern Acupuncture Equipment and Special Therapy,"* nine ancient, nine new, and various modern needles are systematically classified according to the purpose, shape of the needle handle, material of the needle body, and specifications [23]. The needles used in Mongolian medicine acupuncture are generally silver or gold. In the development process, bone, iron, bronze, copper, silver, and gold needles were used (Fig. 2A). There were eight types of Mongolian acupuncture needles recorded in the *"Gan Lu Si Bu,"* and these types were divided into three types with holes and five without. Mongolian medicine silver needles are widely used clinically because they do not rust easily, are hard but present good elasticity, have strong thermal conductivity and are suitable for warm acupuncture [24–28]. In the research *"Origin of Acupuncture Technique,"* the opinions of various experts are also divided. TCM acupuncture techniques were first recorded in the *"Yellow Emperor's Classic of Internal Medicine."* The theory of acupuncture techniques, symptoms, acupunctures and moxibustion methods are also described in the *"Yellow Emperor's Classic of Internal Medicine."* Especially in *"Ling Shu,"* significant space is devoted to acupuncture techniques. In the Wei and Jin Dynasties, Huang Fu Mi (215–282)[29] systematically explained acupuncture and moxibustion and compiled the *"A-B Classic of Acupuncture and Moxibustion."* This valuable text is the earliest existing monograph on acupuncture and moxibustion integrating theory with practice. Known as the ancestor of TCM acupuncture, it provides specific guidance and a theoretical basis for clinical treatments performed by acupuncturists. Modern TCM acupuncture techniques employ ancient traditional acupuncture,

enriched, and perfected by the combination with modern science and technology.

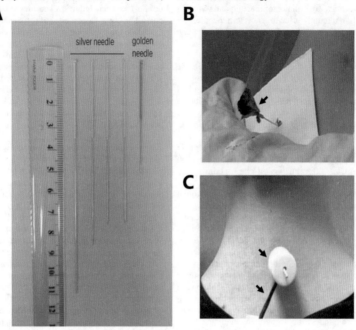

Figure 2. Illustration of Mongolian acupuncture needle and Mongolian warm acupuncture. (A) The acupuncture needles commonly used in Mongolian acupuncture. **(B)** The representative image showing Traditional Mongolian warm needles, which heated by burned moxa. The arrow indicated that the burned moxa was heating up the needle. **(C)** The representative image showing Modern Mongolian warm needle, which heated by electronically. Tthe arrows indicated that the electric heating unit was heating up the needle.

Mongolian medicine acupuncture is divided into hot and cold, with hot acupuncture comprehending fire needle, hot moxibustion combined with acupuncture, and hot moxibustion combined with fire needle, while cold acupuncture includes pure acupuncture, warm acupuncture, and cold acupuncture. Since the 16th century, Mongolian medicine scholars have paid increasing attention to the theory and operation of warm acupuncture. In the book *"Gan Lu Si Bu"* we find written that *"acupuncture has two kinds of cold needling amounts and hot acupuncture,"* explaining that "cold acupuncture" is acupuncture alone, while "hot acupuncture" is fire acupuncture deriving from a combination of acupuncture and combustion. Among these types of acupuncture, warm acupuncture has a long history. Warm acupuncture is based on the basic theory of Mongolian medicine and the treatment principle of TMM. It uses a special needle to heat the body surface through fixed acupoints so that

warm stimulation can be transmitted into the body through the needle to treat diseases, also known as "turimu" [30,31].

Developed in modern Mongolian medicine, the therapeutic use of acupuncture is recorded in detail in the *"Mongolian Medicine Clinic"* edited by Ce Su Rongzhabu. This book has a high theoretical and practical clinical value. Warm needling therapy is a type of acupuncture in both TCM and TMM, first seen in TCM in the *"Shang Han Lun Treatise on Febrile Diseases Caused by Cold"* by Zhang Zhongjing in the Eastern Han Dynasty. The method used fragrant *Angelica dahurica* as round cake and moxibustion on the trocar to obtain the effect on the acupoints. A moxa rod was placed at the end of the needle, and, after the rod was ignited, the heat was transmitted to the body through the needle to prevent diseases. Warm acupuncture was regarded as a method capable of gathering and regulating Qi. Therefore, this method is still widely applied to treat diseases related to Qi.

In addition to the different acupuncture methods in TCM, warm acupuncture therapy, the forms of moxa used, and the methods of application in TMM warm acupuncture are also different. It can be divided into moxa moxibustion and moxibustion moxibustion [22]. Moxibustion takes advantage of the mild heat of moxibustion fire and the pharmacological effects of mugwort leaves through the meridian conduction. This method can warm the blood, strengthen the body, and eliminate disease, achieving its curative purpose. The Mongolian warm acupuncture is an excellent treatment with national and regional characteristics that the Mongolian people have developed through thousands of years. In accordance with the living environment and lifestyle, the Mongolian people have created warm acupuncture to treat diseases related to the cold temperatures. Mongolian warm acupuncture therapy is a combination of acupuncture and warm moxibustion and maintains the functions of both techniques. Mongolian medicine moxibustion is a treatment consisting in a needle, made of gold or silver, pierced into the target acupoint, and the needle handle is heated by moxa combustion or candle fire.

Through the inheritance and development of Mongolian medicine over several generations, the warm needle of Mongolian medicine has become an important treatment in contemporary Mongolian rehabilitation medicine. *"Gan Lu Zhi Quan,"* part of the *"Gan Lu Si Bu,"* is the earliest record of the types of acupuncture techniques, correction of acupuncture errors, acupuncture methods, acupoints, contraindications, and efficacy, among others [32]. Mongolian warm acupuncture has also undergone continuous development and innovation through the improvement and transformation of traditional techniques. Consequently, the therapeutic effect of Mongolian warm acupuncture has been reinforced. The method has been progressively upgraded from the original Mongolian warm moxa acupuncture to the current 1st and 2nd generation methods. At present, modern Mongolian medicine warm acupuncture therapy devices can easily control acupuncture temperature according to the different patients and their condition [33-36]. However, both TCM warm acupuncture and Mongolian warm acupuncture are adapted to the requirements of current times and the standardization of scientific research. Both are based on the idea that "innovation is not separated from the source" and seek common ground while keeping their differences.

Effects of Mongolian warm acupuncture on age-related diseases

Bone diseases

Degenerative osteoarthrosis, which includes gonarthrosis, cervical spondylosis (CS), and lumbar disc herniation (LDH), is a degenerative disease characterized by degenerative injury of articular cartilage and reactive hyperplasia of the articular margin and subchondral bone [37]. Clinical manifestations are mainly joint pain, tenderness, stiffness, joint swelling, limited movement derived from aging, obesity, strain, and trauma [38]. This disease often causes great pain and seriously affects the quality of life of patients. However, to date, there is still no effective drug to prevent disease progression, but only for alleviating pain [39]. However, Mongolian medicine has unique advantages and rich experience in the treatment of degenerative osteoarthrosis [40]. In particular, Mongolian warm acupuncture, as a safe and noninvasive therapy, has been widely used in the clinical treatment of degenerative osteoarthrosis and has achieved significant therapeutic effects [41].

According to TCM, LDH is caused by liver and kidney deficiencies, Qi stagnation, blood stasis, and external pathogenic factors [42]. Warm needle moxibustion, as one of the treatment methods in TCM, has been reported to have a better therapeutic effect in relieving lumbago and lumbar dysfunction, and can upregulate blood β-EP levels [43]. However, LDH is considered to depend on the imbalance between Heyi, Xila, and Badagan at the TMM acupoint. The Qi and Xieriwu factors are concentrated in the lumbar joint, surrounding tissue, muscle, and fascia, resulting in the obstruction of the White Meridian function. Because of this, LDH is regarded as a "White Meridian" disease [44]. At present, some studies have found that Mongolian warm acupuncture can effectively treat LDH. In a clinical experiment, warm acupuncture was used to treat 73 cases of LDH by puncturing three spinal and Badagan acupoints. After 20 days of treatment (once daily), the overall effectiveness rate was 94.59% in all patients. The VAS score and IL-1β and TNF-α levels in the serum of patients were significantly lower than before treatment [45]. In addition, other studies also showed that Mongolian warm acupuncture might improve the curative effect on LDH in a short period of time and reduce the degree of pain in patients [46].

Knee osteoarthritis (KOA) has been included in the category of "GuBi" in TCM. Due to aging or working for extended periods of time, KOA often stems from liver and kidney deficiencies, Yang deficiency, and blood stasis [47]. Four interventions of TCM, acupuncture, moxibustion, herbs, and massage may alleviate symptoms such as pain, swelling, and dysfunction in KOA [48]. Furthermore, TMM has also been studied in KOA for many years and is believed to be a Xieriwu factor disease.

On one hand, the obstruction of Qi and blood circulation, the siltation of diseased blood, and Xieriwu factors may induce joint swelling or articular effusion. On the other, a reduction in joint lubricating fluid and joint cavity stenosis may occur due to the decrease in blood supply and Badagan [49]. Recent studies have shown that Mongolian warm acupuncture might be an effective method to treat KOA by puncturing the Xiyan acupoints (EX-LE5), Jingneice acupoints, and Qiangshen acupoints. For example, in a clinical experiment involving 1,500 KOA patients, the overall effective can reach 98.6% after one month of continuous treatment with Mongolian medicine warm acupuncture, and the VAS score of patients was significantly decreased compared with before treatment [50]. Moreover, compared with certain physical therapies, Mongolian warm acupuncture might quickly relieve pain and improve joint discomfort caused by KOA [51].

CS often results in neck pain. Nevertheless, four weeks of optimized acupuncture treatment, which is an important part of TCM, can alleviate CS-related neck pain [52]. There are two types of CS in TMM: cervical spondylotic radiculopathy and CS of the vertebral artery type. Between these, cervical spondylotic radiculopathy has the highest incidence. CS is caused by damage to the "White Meridian" of the head and neck resulting from the disorder of the three roots (Heyi, Xila and Badagan), which eventually leads to the loss of physiological functions. Therefore, CS belongs to the head and neck "White Meridian" disease group [53]. Mongolian medicine warm acupuncture can conduct heat stimulation to the diseased area and dredge the "White Meridian," playing a therapeutic role in the treatment of cervical spondylotic radiculopathy [54]. A series of clinical experimental results also supports these effects, where 170 cases of CS were treated with Mongolian medicine warm acupuncture by puncturing the Dazhui, Fengfu, Tianzhu, Fengmen, Fengchi, and Jianjing points. Following up to seven treatments (one time every two days), Mongolian warm acupuncture might effectively relieve neck spasms, exert analgesic effects, and improve microcirculation functions [55].

Although Mongolian warm acupuncture is an effective method to treat degenerative osteoarthrosis, the detailed mechanism remains to be investigated. Some studies have speculated that the temperature of the tip of the needle in Mongolian warm acupuncture is 39–41 °C. This heat may penetrate through the muscle and be transmitted to the pathological tissue around the bone and joint, causing edema and atrophic degeneration of skeletal muscle cells to disappear [56]. In addition, Mongolian warm acupuncture may also destroy the collagen protruding outside the vertebral nucleus pulposus, thus alleviating the pressure of induced by the LDH

protrusions on the nerve root and dural sac [57]. Self-repair of articular cartilage and reduction of joint friction may be activated by Mongolian warm acupuncture to protect the knee joint cartilage and articular surface in KOA patients [50]. Studies have indicated that Mongolian warm acupuncture may also suppress ischemia and inflammatory stimulation by promoting local blood circulation and down-regulating the expression of inflammatory factors (such as IL-1β, IL-6,TNF-α, IFN-γ) and iNOS [58], relieving pain by inhibiting the apoptosis of nucleus pulposus cells, or accelerating the release of analgesic substances such as the morphine peptide [59,60]. In particular, Mongolian warm acupuncture needles are generally made of silver, which plays an anti-inflammatory and bacteriostatic role [61]. In brief, more research on the mechanisms underlying the effects of Mongolian medicine warm acupuncture should be performed to advance its clinical application.

Nervous system diseases

Effects on insomnia

Insomnia is a common disease caused by various factors, such as difficulty falling asleep, short sleep depth or frequency, early awakening, insufficient sleep time, or poor quality sleep [62]. Insomnia has become one of the most common diseases in neurological clinics, according to recent studies. Mongolian warm acupuncture may improve sleep quality and has few toxic side effects compared to hypnotic medications.

In one clinical trial study on insomnia conducted by Gula et al., Mongolian warm acupuncture significantly improved the quality of sleep by decreasing the awakening times and the sleep hours in the rapid eye movement (REM) period. The Pittsburgh sleep quality index (PSQI) and polysomnography indexes (PSGs) have been measured in Mongolian warm acupuncture clinical trials. The index of sleep quality, time for falling asleep, sleep hours, sleep efficiency, sleep disorders, and daytime functions in the Mongolian warm acupuncture group all improved significantly compared with those in the estazolam tranquilizer group [13].

Mongolian warm acupuncture may improve insomnia symptoms by upregulating the expression of certain genes in the hypothalamus. In the *p*-chlorophenylalanine (PCPA)-induced rat model of insomnia, the transcription levels of *Egr1*, *Btg2*, and *BDNF* were upregulated in the Mongolian warm acupuncture-treated group [63].

As proteins are executors of biological functions, it is necessary to identify the protein expression levels, modifications, and interactions in the Mongolian warm acupuncture-treated insomnia group. As reported by Gula A et al., in the hypothalamus of a rat insomnia model, 36 proteins showed increased levels and 45 proteins showed decreased levels in the insomnia model group compared with the healthy control. Twenty-eight proteins showed increased levels, while 17 proteins showed decreased levels in the Mongolian warm acupuncture-treated insomnia group compared with the insomnia model. The Mongolian warm acupuncture-treated insomnia group showed obvious recovery in protein expression levels and insomnia symptoms. Mongolian warm acupuncture may upregulate neuroactive ligand-receptor expression and oxytocin signaling to recover insomnia [64]. Another group also confirmed that warm acupuncture could improve sleep quality of patients with insomnia by promoting the expression of brain neurotransmitters (5-HT and GABA/Glu) and reducing that of norepinephrine (NE) [65].

Gula and colleagues showed that 141 miRNAs were changed when treated with Mongolian warm acupuncture in a rat insomnia model. The upregulation of miR-101a expression has been demonstrated to be directly associated with PAX8 regulation in rats treated with Mongolian warm acupuncture. Additionally, the levels of noradrenaline, dopamine, and glutamic acid and the interleukins IL-1, IL-2, and TNFα were decreased significantly in rats treated with Mongolian warm acupuncture [66].

Effects on neuropathic pain

Neuropathic pain is complex and chronic and is caused by damaged nerves. Acupuncture can relieve pain with few side effects and improve the quality of life of patients with neuropathic pain. In a double-blinded clinical trial, acupuncture relieved the pain of idiopathic trigeminal neuralgia. The mechanical thresholds were decreased, and the deep pain thresholds were increased in the acupuncture group. There was a reduction in secondary myofascial pain and mandibular limitations in the acupuncture group, and the changes could be maintained for more than six months [67]. In a clinical trial of angioneurotic headache patients, the efficacy index in headaches of the Mongolian warm acupuncture treatment group was superior to the efficacy index in the control groups. The total effectiveness rate was 90% in the research of Xiuping Bao [68]. As Li et al. reported Mongolian warm acupuncture could induce the recovery of idiopathic trigeminal neuralgia in the clinical observation of 80 patients, and the total effectiveness rate was 92.5% [69].

Effects on stroke sequelae

Stroke is emerging as a worldwide health issue threatening human health. Spastic paralysis after stroke

(SPAS) is a common sequela of stroke and has received wide attention. The common treatment methods for SPAS are medications, surgical interventions, and physical therapy. However, these methods present disadvantages, such as the side effects of drugs, the invasive nature of the surgery, and the high cost of treatment.

According to two clinical studies by Zhang et al., acupuncture can significantly improve cerebral palsy motor and comprehensive functions in children, and the effect of acupuncture combined with rehabilitation is evidently superior to the effect of simple rehabilitation training therapy alone [70,71]. Mongolian warm acupuncture can increase recovery by enhancing immunity, regulating blood circulation, relieving pain, and relaxing muscles. In a clinical study, 70 patients with hemiplegic sequelae of stroke were treated with Mongolian acupuncture. After treatment, the Fugl-Meyer and Barthel assessment scores were significantly higher than the comparable scores of the control group.

Mongolian warm acupuncture can significantly improve the clinical conditions of patients with hemiplegia stroke sequelae and has positive significance in ensuring patient quality of life along with physical and mental health [72]. In another study, 60 patients with sequelae of cerebral infarction were subjected to Mongolian warm acupuncture. After a course of treatment, of the 60 patients, 3 were cured, accounting for 5.00% of cases, in 15 the treatment was markedly effective, accounting for 25.00% of cases, in 40 it was effective, accounting for 66.67% of cases, and in two cases it was ineffective, accounting for 3.33% of cases [73]. In Wang et al.'s clinical observations of 120 patients with sequelae of cerebral infarction, the total effectiveness rate of treatment in the Mongolian warm acupuncture group was significantly higher than the total effectiveness rate of treatment in the control group. After treatment, the ADL and FMA scores of the experimental group were higher than those of the control group, while the NIHSS score was lower than that of the control group [74].

Other diseases

The main physiological characteristics of the elderly are the decline of the internal organs, the gradual depletion of essence and blood, the gradual loss of spirit, and the imbalance in Yin and Yang. However, multiple organ damage and multiple diseases often appear together and are the main pathological features in the elderly [75].

Mongolian warm acupuncture showed good therapeutic effects on lung function in elderly patients with stable chronic obstructive pulmonary disease. Through acupuncture and moxibustion, the main acupoints such as Beishu, Fengmen, Tanzhong, Dingchuan, Shenshu, and Zusanli were selected as matching acupoints for Xuehai, Fenglong, Chize, and Lieque. Mongolian warm acupuncture can regulate lung function, replenish lung Qi, remove wind pathogens, enhance Qi intake, and replenish vitality [76,77].

Diabetic peripheral neuropathy is a common chronic complication of diabetes, and its cause is mainly related to long-term high blood sugar levels, which lead to circulatory disturbances in nerve tissue metabolism, which in turn lead to peripheral neuropathy. At present, its pathogenesis is still in the research stage, and there is no clinical treatment for this disease. Studies have shown that Mongolian medicine warm acupuncture at the Zusanli, Sanyinjiao, Taixi, Waiguan, Shenshu, Pishu, Huantiao, Quchi, and Hegu acupoints can promote the smooth flow of the meridians and collaterals of the patient and increase the benign stimulation of the patient's body and limb blood circulation. The warm Yang medicinal power of wormwood can dredge collaterals and disperse silt, promote local tissue nutrition and the improvement of symptoms in patients [78].

Prostatitis is a common high-incidence disease that mainly affects the population under 50 years of age. The reason the patient has related diseases is mainly because the pathogen invades the patient's prostate through urine, causing the patient to develop an infection. Under normal circumstances, the treatment of prostatitis patients is performed with Western medicine. However, the effects of using antibiotics for treatment are not obvious, and at the same time, the use of antibiotics can cause complications that may have a certain impact on the patient's quality of life. Studies have shown that Mongolian warm acupuncture has a good effect on prostatitis, using mainly the Jingfuqian, Bladder, Wrist Acupoints, or 23 Zhui, Shen, and Elbow Neiwen acupoints for treatment [79].

Ischemic cerebrovascular disease has a high incidence and seriously threatens human health, being one of the three major causes of death. The mechanisms by which ischemia damages and causes the death of brain nerve cells are diverse and complex. Prevention and treatment of ischemic cerebrovascular disease is an urgent problem that needs to be solved. Mongolian warm acupuncture dealing with Dinghui and Heyi acupoints was found to significantly counteract the generation of free radicals in rats after ischemia, improve the body's ability to scavenge free radicals, and enhance SOD activity, which will help improve neurological deficits after stroke occurrence [80].

Conclusions

Mongolian warm acupuncture is a kind of acupuncture that is still popular in the Inner Mongolia Autonomous Region of China and Mongolia. The tail of the needle used

in Mongolian warm acupuncture is wrapped with moxa and burned (Fig. 2B) or, in nowadays, heated by electronics (Fig. 2C). Whether the needle tip temperature influences the therapeutic effect of acupuncture on disease is still unclear and needs to be further studied. At the same time, certain acupoints in TMM co-localize with those in TCM. Most acupoints in TMM include the brain and spinal cord, which are part of the "White Meridian" system. It has been proved that stimulating these acupoints can treat certain diseases in TMM, but the mechanisms still need to be further elucidated. With the development of technology and the standardization of scientific research, the physiological basis for the effect of Mongolian warm acupuncture will be better understood, contributing to the promotion of the therapy.

Acknowledgments

This study was supported by the National Natural Science Foundation of China (Nos.81660307, 81660204, 8190 1918, 81971114,82060337), Inner Mongolia Science Foundation (Nos.2018LH03029, 2019MS08052, 2019 MS03093, 2020MS08172, 2020MS08006, 2020MS08 010), Inner Mongolia Educational Research Foundation (Nos. NJZZ19189, NJZZ17243, NJZY17250, NJZY1 7251, NJZY18191, NJZY18192) and Baotou Medical College Foundation (BSJJ-201804, BSJJ-201706, BYJJ-QM-2018004, BYJJ-QM-2018026, BYJJ-YF-201719, BYJJ-QWB-201805).

Conflicts of interest

All the authors state that there is no potential conflict of interest.

References

[1] Sivin N (1989). A cornucopia of reference works for the history of Chinese medicine. Chin Sci, 9:29-52.

[2] Yu E, Amri H (2016). China's other medical systems: Recognizing Uyghur, Tibetan, and Mongolian traditional medicines. Glob Adv Health Med, 5:79-86.

[3] Choi SH, Chang IM (2010). A milestone in codifying the wisdom of traditional oriental medicine: TCM, Kampo, TKM, TVM-WHO International Standard Terminologies on Traditional Medicine in the Western Pacific Region. Evid Based Complement Alternat Med, 7:303-305.

[4] Toyama PM, Nishizawa M (1973). The traditional oriental medicine and acupuncture therapy. J Miss State Med Assoc, 14:488-495.

[5] Zhang H (1979). Investigation on several issues in medical history of Inner Mongolia. J Shaanxi Univ Chin Med, 3:45-59.

[6] Wu L, Guo L (2018). Modern application of Mongolian acupuncture therapy. Chin J Tradit Chin

Med, 33:223-225.

[7]   Bao Z, Su R, Hang S, Daina R (2017). A brief talk on the research status of "white meridian" disease in Mongolian medicine. World Lat Med Inform, 17:34-35.

[8]   Su R (2006). Discussion on regulating viscera function of white meridian system in Mongolian medicine. Chin Arch Tradit Chin Med, 24:127-128.

[9]   Sha T, Gao LL, Zhang CH, Zheng JG, Meng ZH (2016). An update on acupuncture point injection. QJM, 109:639-641.

[10] Bo A, Sa Q (2016). Acupuncture and moxibustion acupuncture on bronze man's upper arm acupoint location and safety evaluation of acupuncture. J Chin Natl Med, 3:74-75.

[11] Huo B (2006). The effects of Mongolian warm acupuncture on body. J Chin Natl Med, 5:76-77.

[12] Zhao S (2019). The clinical effect of Mongolian warm acupuncture therapy on cold-damp shoulder periarthritis. Electron J Clin Med Lit, 6:47.

[13] Bo A, Si L, Wang Y, Xiu L, Wu R, Li Y, et al. (2016). Clinical trial research on Mongolian medical warm acupuncture in treating insomnia. Evid Based Complement Alternat Med, 2016:6190285.

[14] Bao MJ, Bo A (2018). The basic theory characteristic of Mongolia medicine. J Med Pharm Chin Minor, 24:58-60.

[15] Yu J, Yu T, Han J (2005). Aging-related changes in the transcriptional profile of cerebrum in senescence-accelerated mouse (SAMP10) is remarkably retarded by acupuncture. Acupunct Electrother Res, 30:27-42.

[16] Wen M, Si QT (2009). Anti-aging thoughts and advantages of Mongolian medicine moxibustion therapy. Chin J Tradit Chin Med, 3:76-77.

[17] Bo A (2007). Overview of traditional therapy of Mongolian medicine. J Med Pharm Chin Minor, 1:23-26.

[18] Yao H, Bao L (2007). The similarities and differences between acupuncture and moxibustion in Mongolian medicine and traditional Chinese medicine. J Med Pharm Chin Minor, 5:24-26.

[19] Zhang HY (1979). Investigation on several issues in medical history of Inner Mongolia. J Shaanxi Univ Chin Med, 3:45-59.

[20] Saiyin C, Bao QL, Hou YM (2015). A brief talk on the differences and origins of acupuncture in traditional Chinese medicine and Mongolian medicine. J Med Pharm Chin Minor, 21:7-8.

[21] Hasi Q, Si Q (2013). Mechanism of Mongolian medicine warming needle therapy and ideas for improvement of apparatus. J Inner Mong Univ Natl (Nat Sci), 28:83-85.

[22] Gao XZ, Hu L (2010), editors. Chinese dictionary of acupuncture. Nanjing: Phoenix Science Press; 2010.

[23] Gan D, Yang HY, Cao Y, editors. Modern acupuncture equipment and special therapies. Beijing: Traditional Chinese Medicine Classics Press; 2004.

[24] Gao W (2018). Clinical observation on 60 cases of frozen shoulder treated by warm needle of Mongolian medicine. World Lat Med Inform, 18:227.

[25] Bai XF (2018). Clinical observation on 89 cases of insomnia treated by silver needle warm needle therapy combined with Mongolian medicine. J Med Pharm Chin Minor, 24:4-5.

[26] Su L (2017). Observation on the effect of warm needling of Mongolian medicine on lumbar disc herniation. Electron J Clin Med Lit, 4:2225.

[27] Ao T, Da G, Bo A, Meng H (2002). Clinical observation on 100 cases of osteoarthritis treated by Mongolian medicine silver needle warm moxibustion. J Med Pharm Chin Minor, 8:53.

[28] Qing G, Xin J, Zhang H (2019). Analysis of clinical application effect of Mongolian medicine Turi Muzha Sale (gold needle, silver needle). Electron J Clin Med Lit, 6:21-22.

[29] Huangfu M, Jia CW, editors. A-B classic of acupuncture and moxibustion. Guiyang: Guizhou Education Press; 2010.

[30] Bo A, editor. Mongolian medicine warm accupuncture therapy. Huhhot: Inner Mongolia Science and Technology Press; 2018.

[31] Chen YS, Bo A, Wu L (2008). New development of Mongolian medical technology research. Mod Tradit Chin Med Mater Med World Sci Technol, 1:117-121.

[32] Yeshes Palbyor, editor. Gan lu si bu (The four tantras of nectar) Mongolian version. Huhhot: Inner Mongolia People's Publishing House; 1998.

[33] Shui L, Wu Y, LU J, Wu QZ, Chen YS, Sa R, et al. (2020). Effect of Mongolian warm acupuncture on expression of caspase-3 and serum death receptor DR and fas in chroinic fatigue syndrome model rats. Liaoning J Tradit Chin Med, 48:192-195.

[34] Jin Q, Bo A (2020). Efficacy and mechanism of Mongolian medicine warm needling for sciatica caused by lumbar disc herniation. J Med Pharm Chin Minor, 26:13-15.

[35] Jin Q, Si L, Bo A (2020). Randomized controlled trial of warming acupuncture in the treatment of heyi partial insomnia patient by Mongolian medicine. Yunnan J Tradit Chin Med Mater Med, 41:77-81.

[36] Hasi G (2010). A comparative study of traditional Mongolian medicine warming needle and Mongolian medicine warming needle apparatus in treating rheumatic knee joint pain. J Med Pharm Chin Minor, 16:17-18.

[37] Pap T, Korb-Pap A (2015). Cartilage damage in osteoarthritis and rheumatoid arthritis--two unequal siblings. Nat Rev Rheumatol, 11:606-615.

[38] Hunter DJ, Bierma-Zeinstra S (2019). Osteoarthritis. Lancet, 393:1745-1759.

[39] Tryfonidou MA, de Vries G, Hennink WE, Creemers LB (2020). "Old Drugs, New Tricks"-Local controlled drug release systems for treatment of degenerative joint disease. Adv Drug Deliv Rev, 160:170-185.

[40] Bo A (2007). Overview about the traditaonal therapy of Monggolian medicine. J Med Pharm Chin Minor, 13:23-26.

[41] Kim TH, Kim DH, Lee SG (2018). Moxibustion therapy in traditional Mongolian medicine. Chin J Integr Med, 24:707-712.

Shao G., et al.   *Traditional Mongolian Warm Acupuncture*

[42]   Cai C, Gong Y, Dong D, Xue J, Zheng X, Zhong Z, et al. (2018). Combined therapies of modified Taiyi miraculous moxa roll and cupping for patients with lumbar intervertebral disc herniation. Evid Based Complement Alternat Med, 2018:6754730.

[43]   Zai FL, Wu RL, Zheng MF, Guo LY (2018). Warming needle moxibustion relieves symptoms of lumbar disc herniation patients and upregulates plasma beta-endorphin. Zhenci Yanjiu, 43:512-515.

[44]   Meng G (2017). Clinical study on Mongolian medicine acupuncture assisted treatment for the lumbar disc herniation. China Health Stand Manage, 8:78-80.

[45]   Jin Q, Bo A (2020). Therapeutic effect and mechanism of Mongolian medicine warm acupuncture on sciatica caused by lumbar disc herniation. J Med Pharm Chin Minor, 26:13-15.

[46]   Tu Y, Wu J, Du G (2019). Clinical observation of Mongolian medicine warm acupuncture and nursing in the treatment of lumbar disc herniation. J Med Pharm Chin Minor, 25:7-8.

[47]   Yang M, Jiang L, Wang Q, Chen H, Xu G (2017). Traditional Chinese medicine for knee osteoarthritis: An overview of systematic review. PLoS One, 12:e0189884.

[48]   Wang M, Liu L, Zhang CS, Liao Z, Jing X, Fishers M, et al. (2020). Mechanism of traditional Chinese medicine in treating knee osteoarthritis. J Pain Res, 13:1421-1429.

[49]   Chaoke B (2015). Clinical study on the treatment of knee osteoarthritis with Mongolian medicine warm acupuncture and Mongolian drug. J Med Pharm Chin Minor, 21:28-29.

[50]   Yao H, Hong G (2015). Clinical observation of Mongolian medicine warm acupuncture in the treatment of knee osteoarthritis. J Med Pharm Chin Minor, 21:7-9.

[51]   Chen G (2017). Effect of Mongolian medicine warm acupuncture on knee osteoarthritis. Cardiovasc Dis Electron J Integr Tradit Chin West Med, 5:75.

[52]   Chen L, Li M, Fan L, Zhu X, Liu J, Li H, et al. (2021). Optimized acupuncture treatment (acupuncture and intradermal needling) for cervical spondylosis-related neck pain: a multicenter randomized controlled trial. Pain, 162:728-739.

[53]   Ji R (2018). Clinical observation of Mongolian medicine warm acupuncture in the treatment of cervical spondylotic radiculopathy. Electron J Clin Med Lit, 5:82.

[54]   Tala, Wen D (2017). Clinical observation on the treatment of cervical spondylotic radiculopathy with Mongolian medicine warm acupuncture. J Med Pharm Chin Minor, 23:3-4.

[55]   Ye R (2020). Observation on therapeutic effect of Mongolian medicine combined with warm acupuncture on cervical spondylotic radiculopathy. J Med Pharm Chin Minor, 26:18-19.

[56]   Wulan, Yao H, Gerile (2015). Study the curative effect of Mongolian medicine warm needle in the treatment of lumbar disc prolapse. J Med Pharm Chin Minor,

21:1-4.

[57]   Dabu X, Hong G, Gerile, Wu L, Yao H (2019). Analysis of the application of Mongolian medicine warm acupuncture in the treatment of lumbar disc herniation. J Med Pharm Chin Minor, 25:21-23.

[58]   Shui L, Yi RN, Wu YJ, Bai SM, Si Q, Bo A, et al. (2019). Effects of Mongolian warm acupuncture on iNOS/NO and inflammatory cytokines in the hippocampus of chronic fatigue rats. Front Integr Neurosci, 13:78.

[59]   Huo B (2006). Study on the mechanism of Mongolian medicine warm acupuncture. J Med Pharm Chin Minor, 12:76-77.

[60]   Li S, Bao L, Si L, Wang X, Bo A (2018). Research on roles of Mongolian medical warm acupuncture in inhibiting p38 MAPK activation and apoptosis of nucleus pulposus cells. Evid Based Complement Alternat Med, 2018:6571320.

[61]   Wu H (2018). The observation of effect of Mongolian medicine warm acupuncture on the lumbar disc herniation. J Med Pharm Chin Minor, 24:13-14.

[62]   Buysse DJ (2013). Insomnia. JAMA, 309:706-716.

[63]   Bo A, Li X, Su B, Lian H, Bao M, Liang Y, et al. (2019). Effect of Mongolian warm acupuncture on the gene expression profile of rats with insomnia. Acupunct Med, 37:301-311.

[64]   Xu Y, Li X, Man D, Su X, Bo A (2020). iTRAQ-based proteomics analysis on insomnia rats treated with Mongolian medical warm acupuncture. Biosci Rep, 40:BSR20191517.

[65]   Yang JL, Zhang R, Du L, Yang YS, Liu XC (2014). Clinical observation on the neurotransmitters regulation in patients of insomnia differentiated as yang deficiency pattern treated with warm acupuncture and auricular point sticking therapy. Zhongguo Zhenjiu, 34:1165-1168.

[66]   Bo A, Si L, Wang Y, Bao L, Yuan H (2017). Mechanism of Mongolian medical warm acupuncture in treating insomnia by regulating miR-101a in rats with insomnia. Exp Ther Med, 14:289-297.

[67]   Ichida MC, Zemuner M, Hosomi J, Pai HJ, Teixeira MJ, de Siqueira JTT, et al. (2017). Acupuncture treatment for idiopathic trigeminal neuralgia: A longitudinal case-control double blinded study. Chin J Integr Med, 23:829-836.

[68]   Bao XP (2015). Observation on the clinical curative effect of Mongolian medicine on vascular headache. J Med Pharm Chin Minor, 21:7-8.

[69]   Li YM, Bao B (2010). Observation on the efficacy of Mongolian medicine in treating trigeminal neuralgia. J Med Pharm Chin Minor, 16:15-16.

[70]   Zhang NX, Liu GZ, Sun KX, Hao JD (2007). Clinical study of the treatment of infant cerebral palsy with warm-reinforcing needling combined with rehabilitation training. Zhenci Yanjiu, 32:260-263.

[71]   Zhang NX, Wang XY, Liu GZ, Li YB, Zhang HY (2014). Randomized controlled clinical trials of individualized treatment of cerebral palsy children by warm-reinforcing needling combined with Bobath rehabilitation training. Zhenci Yanjiu, 39:318-323.

Shao G., et al.　　　　　　　　　　　　　　　　　　　　　Traditional Mongolian Warm Acupuncture

[72]　Meng B (2017). Analysis of the curative effect of Mongolian medicine acupuncture on patients with hemiplegia (stroke) sequelae of Sar disease. Bip Health, 26:181+183.

[73]　Bai Y (2017). Clinical study on 60 cases of cerebral infarction sequelae treated by Mongolian medicine acupuncture. World Lat Med Inform, 17:203.

[74]　Wang CY, Su LD (2019). The clinical effect of Mongolian medicine combined with acupuncture rehabilitation training on the sequelae of ischemic Sa disease. J Med Pharm Chin Minor, 25:25-27.

[75]　Tian DZ (1985). Gerontology and acupuncture. Chin Acupunct, 1:31-33.

[76]　Yu Z (2014). Effect of warm acupuncture on lung function in elderly patients with stable chronic obstructive pulmonary disease. China J Chin med, 29:485-486.

[77]　Zhu JP (2017). Effect of warm acupuncture on lung function in elderly patients with stable chronic obstructive pulmonary disease. Shenzhen J Integr Chin West Med, 27:49-51.

[78]　Liu M (2020). Clinical observation of warm needle therapy for diabetic peripheral neuropathy. Diabetes New World, 23:8-10.

[79]　Tu Y (2017). Clinical nursing analysis of Mongolian medicine warming needle therapy combined with Mongolian medicine for treating prostatitis. World Lat Med Inform, 17:279-280.

[80]　Su D, Mo R, Li YT (2018). Mongolian medicine hot needle on focal cerebral ischemia-reperfusion injury in rats of protection. J Med Pharm Chin Minor, 24:56-58.

PLOS ONE

RESEARCH ARTICLE

Influence of warm acupuncture on gut microbiota and metabolites in rats with insomnia induced by PCPA

Hong Yu[1,2], Hui Yu[3], Lengge Si[4], Husileng Meng[4], Wensheng Chen[4], Zhanli Wang[3]*, A. Gula[1,3]*

1 College of Traditional Chinese Medicine, Beijing University of Chinese Medicine, Beijing, China, 2 School of Nursing, Baotou Medical College, Baotou, China, 3 Inner Mongolia Key Laboratory of Disease-Related Biomarkers, Baotou Medical College, Baotou, China, 4 Mongolian Medicine School, Inner Mongolia Medical University, Hohhot, Inner Mongolia, China

* wang.zhanli@hotmail.com (ZW); agula372000@126.com (GA)

Citation: Yu H, Yu H, Si L, Meng H, Chen W, Wang Z, et al. (2022) Influence of warm acupuncture on gut microbiota and metabolites in rats with insomnia induced by PCPA. PLoS ONE 17(4): e0267843. https://doi.org/10.1371/journal.pone.0267843

Editor: Chun Wie Chong, Monash University Malaysia, MALAYSIA

Received: December 16, 2021

Accepted: April 14, 2022

Published: April 28, 2022

Data Availability Statement: The data that support the findings of this study have been deposited into CNGB Sequence Archive (CNSA) of China National GeneBank DataBase (CNGBdb) with accession number CNP0002294.

Funding: This study was supported by the National Natural Science Foundation of China (no. 82074577). The funders had no role in study design, data collection and analysis, decision to publish, or preparation of the manuscript.

Abstract

Background

Insomnia is the most common of the sleep disorders. Current pharmacotherapy treatment options are usually associated with adverse effects and withdrawal phenomena. Therapeutic alternatives with a more favorable safety profile for patients are needed. Mongolian medical warm acupuncture (MMWA) is an emerging therapeutic option for treating insomnia. However, the underlying mechanisms responsible for the anti-insomnia efficacy of the MMWA remain unclear. This study aims to investigate the effect of the MMWA on the alterations of the gut microbiota and serum metabolome in rats with insomnia.

Results

We found that the relative abundances of gut bacteria and the concentrations of several serum metabolites were obviously altered in PCPA-induced insomnia rats. The MMWA treatment exerted an anti-insomnia effect. In addition, the dysbiosis of the gut microbiota and the serum metabolites were ameliorated by the MMWA. Correlation analysis between the gut microbiota and metabolites suggested that the levels of Amide c18, Benzoyl chloride, Cytosine, and N, n-dimethylarginine were positively correlated with the relative abundance of *Clostridium XIVa* and *Blautia*, which characterized the insomnia rats. KEGG enrichment analysis identified the cAMP signaling pathway involving anti-insomnia effect of the MMWA. Moreover, the MMWA intervention significantly increased contents of butyrate in feces, while effectively inhibited the expression level of GAT-1 in brain tissues.

Conclusion

This study reveals that the MMWA intervention might have a major impact on the modulation of host gut microbiota and metabolites, which in turn have a crucial role in the regulation of the host's signaling pathways associated with insomnia. The present study could provide useful ideas for the study of the intervention mechanisms of the MMWA in insomnia rat models.

Competing interests: The authors have declared that no competing interests exist.

Abbreviations: Ach, acetylcholine; ELISA, Enzyme-linked immunosorbent assay; FLASH, Fast Length Adjustment of SHort reads; GABA, Gamma-aminobutyric acid; GABAAR, GABA A receptor; GAT-1, Gamma-aminobutyric acid transporter-1; KEGG, Kyoto Encyclopedia of Genes and Genomes; LDA, Linear discriminant analysis; LEfSe, LDA effect size; MMWA, Mongolian medical warm acupuncture; NE, norepinephrine; OTUs, Operational units; PCPA, p-chlorophenylalanine; PICRSt, Phylogenetic Investigation of Communities by Reconstruction of Unobserved States; QC, Quality control; RDP, Ribosomal Database Project; REM, Rapid eye movement; SCFA, Short-chain fatty acid; SD, Sprague-Dawley; 5-HT, Serotonin.

Introduction

Insomnia is the most prevalent sleep disorder, which affects 6–10% of the general population worldwide [1]. It is characterized by difficulty with sleep initiation, maintenance, or early morning awakening, and accompanied by daytime impairment. Accumulating evidence indicated that insomnia was associated with a wide range of negative health consequences, such as mental disorder, cardiovascular dysfunction, type 2 diabetes, and obesity [2–4]. Many studies have suggested that multifactorial causes are involved in the etiology of insomnia, and the detailed pathological aspects of insomnia remain unclear [5].

The gut microbiota and its metabolites have long been recognized as a key component involved in various diseases [6]. Dysbiosis of the gut microbiota perturbs the host metabolism and immune balance, leading to the occurrence of diseases [7]. Several studies have also provided preliminary support for an association between gut microbiota and sleep disorder. It was reported that the structure, composition, and function of the gut microbiota, as well as the bacterial interaction network were significantly changed in insomnia patients [8]. In another study with acute and chronic insomnia patients between 26–55 years, the microbial richness and diversity were lower with the depletion of short-chain fatty acid (SCFA)-producing bacteria [9]. These studies provide a theoretical basis for the application and development of novel strategies for insomnia therapy.

Mongolian medicine, one of the traditional medicines, showed a favorable safety profile and beneficial therapeutic effects on insomnia [10]. In Mongolian medicine, warm acupuncture is one of the main treatment methods for insomnia. It prevents and treats diseases by stimulating specific anatomic sites (acupoints) using warm silver needles [11]. It has been widely accepted by insomnia patients due to its advantages, such as efficiency, safety, and no drug dependence [12]. In a recent study, acupuncture inhibited the neuroinflammation in a mouse model of Parkinson's disease by modulating gut microbial dysbiosis [13]. Another study reported that acupuncture might be beneficial for insomnia through modulating the gut microbiota to regulate the host inflammatory response [14]. However, the role of the gut microbiota and its metabolites on the effects of the Mongolian medicine warm acupuncture (MMWA) in insomnia is still unknown.

Our study aims to investigate the effects of the MMWA on the gut microbiota and metabolites in p-chlorophenylalanine (PCPA)-induced insomnia rats, which may help to elucidate the biological mechanisms of the gut microbiota-mediated sleep regulation.

Methods

Ethics

Ethical approval was obtained from Baotou Medical College Research and Ethical Review Committee (no. 2021039). At the end of the experiment, the animals were euthanized using 2% pentobarbital sodium (prepared in normal saline, 40 mg/kg, intraperitoneal injection.

Animals and PCPA-pretreated rat model

Six-week-old male Sprague-Dawley (SD) rats (body weight, 160 to 180 g) were obtained from Vital River Laboratory Animal Technology Co., Ltd. (Beijing, China). Animals were housed individually in a temperature-controlled room ($24 \pm 2°C$) under a 12/12-h light-dark cycle. The rats were allowed free access to food and water throughout the experiment. After one week of acclimatization, animals were randomly allocated into three groups: the control group (n = 8), the model group (n = 8), and the treatment group (n = 8). For the PCPA-induced insomnia model, rats received PCPA (300 mg/kg, dissolved in saline) via intraperitoneal injection in the morning of each day for 3 consecutive days [15]. The vehicle control group received an injection of the same volume of normal saline.

Acupuncture treatment

In the treatment group, rats were treated with the MMWA on the acupoints of Dinghui, Heyi, and Xin acupoints once daily for seven consecutive days. Detailed acupoint locations were shown in S1 Fig. Acupoint Dinghui has been used to alleviate daftness, dizziness, and headache. Acupoint Heyi is often used to treat palpitation, agitation, and insomnia. Acupoint Xin is stimulated to alleviate delirium, anorexia, and insomnia in traditional Mongolian medicine [16]. Recent studies have verified that stimulating these three acupoints improves the sleep quality of rats with PCPA-induced insomnia [11, 12]. The acupoints were stimulated with the MMWA for 15 min each time at ~40°C with the instrument of Mongolian Model MY-I electric heating needle warmers (Shanghai, China). The needle was evenly inserted 5 mm depth for each acupoint as described previously [15]. In the other groups, these three acupoints without acupuncture treatment were slightly lifted and twisted under the same conditions. Rats were weighed before the establishment of the insomnia model and at the end of the experiment.

Open field test

The rats were acclimated to the environment for 10 min before being subjected to an open-field test. Then, rats were placed in the center of a wooden open field box. The video tracking analysis system was used to record rat activity within the 5 min for calculating exercise distance, exercise time, and number of arm lifting.

Sample collection

At the end of the experiment, the animals were euthanized using 2% pentobarbital sodium (prepared in normal saline, 40 mg/kg, intraperitoneal injection). Fresh feces of rats were collected directly into the sterilization centrifuge tube and were immediately stored in liquid nitrogen, then transferred to –80°C refrigerator for determination of intestinal flora. Blood was collected from the abdominal aorta. Serum was collected in a refrigerator at –80°C for serum metabolomics analysis or neurotransmitters determination. The whole brain was quickly removed on ice, and then the brain stem was separated by precision forceps. The isolated brain stem segment was quickly frozen in liquid nitrogen and stored at -80°C for later use.

Enzyme-linked immunosorbent assay (ELISA) analysis

The neurotransmitter array kits (Absci, MD, USA) were used to detect serotonin (5-HT), norepinephrine (NE), acetylcholine (ACh), and gamma-aminobutyric acid (GABA) in serum samples according to the manufacturer's instructions. Moreover, the concentration of cAMP was determined using an ELISA kit according to the manufacturer's protocol [17]. The 5-HT, NE, Ach, GABA, and cAMP contents were measured at 450 nm on a microplate reader.

Gut microbiota analysis

The total microbial DNA was extracted from fecal samples using the MagPure Stool DNA KF kit B (Magen, China). The extracted DNA was quantified with a Qubit Fluorometer by using Qubit dsDNA BR Assay kit (Invitrogen, USA), and DNA quality was examined by 1% agarose gel electrophoresis (Solarbio, Beijing, China). The V3–V4 hypervariable regions of the bacterial 16S rRNA gene were amplified by PCR with the primers 341F (5'-ACT CCT ACG GGA GGC AGC AG-3') and 806R (5'-GGA CTA CHV GGG TWT CTA AT-3'). PCR reactions were performed using the following program: 3 min of denaturation at 94˚C, 30 cycles of 30 sec at 94˚C, 45 sec for annealing at 56˚C, 45 sec for elongation at 72˚C, and final extension at 72˚C for 10 min. PCR products were purified using the AmpureXP beads (Beckman Coulter, Fullerton, CA, USA) according to the manufacturer's instructions and quantified by the Agilent 2100 bioanalyzer (Agilent, USA). Then, the validated libraries were used for sequencing on the Illumina MiSeq platform (BGI, Shenzhen, China) according to the standard protocols.

Raw fastq files were quality-filtered to remove adaptors and low-quality and ambiguous bases and then merged by the Fast Length Adjustment of SHort reads program (FLASH, version 1.2.11) [18]. Operational units (OTUs) were clustered with a cutoff value of 97% using UPARSE (version 7.0.1090) [19]. The taxonomy of each 16S rRNA gene sequence was classified using Ribosomal Database Project (RDP) Classifier algorithm (version 2.2) using a confidence threshold of 60%. Alpha and beta diversity were calculated by MOTHUR (version 1.31.2) and QIIME (version 1.8.0) at the OTU level, respectively. The linear discriminant analysis (LDA) or LEfSe cluster was performed by LEfSe software. Phylogenetic Investigation of Communities by Reconstruction of Unobserved States (PICRUSt) based on Kyoto Encyclopedia of Genes and Genomes (KEGG) database was used to predict the microbiota functions [20].

Metabolomics analysis

After being fully thawed at room temperature, 100 μL serum samples were extracted three times by directly adding 300 μL of precooled methanol and acetonitrile (2:1, v/v). The mixture was vortexed for 1 min and incubated at -20˚C for 2 h. The samples were then centrifuged at 4000 rpm for 20 min at 4˚C and the supernatant was transferred for dryness by vacuum centrifugation. The metabolites were redissolved in 150 μL of 50% cold methanol and centrifuged at 4000 rpm for 30 min. The supernatant was transferred into autosampler vials for metabolism analysis. A quality control (QC) sample was prepared by pooling the same volume of each sample to monitor the stability of the instrument.

This experiment used the ultra-performance liquid chromatography (Waters 2D UPLC, Waters, USA) tandem high-resolution mass spectrometer (Q Exactive, Thermo Fisher Scientific, USA) for separation and detection of metabolites. The separation was performed on a Waters ACQUITY UPLC BEH C18 column (100 mm × 2.1 mm, 1.7 μm, Waters, USA), which was maintained at 45˚C. The mobile phase was composed of 0.1% formic acid (A) and acetonitrile (B) in the positive mode and was composed of 10 mM ammonium formate (A) and acetonitrile (B) in the negative mode. The gradient elution conditions were as follows: 0–1 min, 2% B; 1–9 min, 2%-98% B; 9–12 min, 98% B; 12–12.1 min, 98% B to 2% B; and 12.1–15 min, 2% B. The flow rate was 0.35 mL/min and the injection volume was 5 μL. The mass spectra conditions were as follows: spray voltage, 3.8/-3.2 kV; aux gas heater temperature, 350˚C; capillary temperature, 320˚C; sheath gas flow rate, 40 arbitrary units; aux gas flow rate, 10 arbitrary units. The full scan range was 70–1050 m/z with a resolution of 70000.

The original chromatographic peak data were processed using the Compound Discoverer 3.1 (Thermo Fisher Scientific, USA) software, which mainly included over-lapping peak resolution, peak alignment, and compound identification. Data pre-processing, statistical analysis, metabolite classification annotations, and functional annotations were performed using the metabolomics R package metaX [21] and the metabolome bioinformatic analysis pipeline [22].

Correlation analysis between metabolites and gut microbiota

Spearman correlation analysis was performed to reveal the correlation between two variables (such as metabolite level and microbial abundance). Sparse generalized canonical correlation analysis was used to calculate the overall correlation between metabolites and microorganisms.

附　录

Butyrate determination

Approximately 100 mg of fresh fecal contents was weighed and then mashed in acidic water (pH = 2.4). The sample was centrifuged at 12,000 g for 20 min at 4°C. The supernatants were then taken for analysis as previously described [23].

Administration of butyrate

The insomnia model was induced by PCPA as described previously. Sodium butyrate (Sigma Aldrich, Carlsbad, CA, USA) was dissolved in physiological saline and was intraperitoneally administrated to rats at a dose of 0.6 g/kg for seven consecutive days. Animal groups included the following: PCPA-treated rats with vehicle administration (Vehicle) (n = 8) and PCPA-treated rats with sodium butyrate administration (Butyrate) (n = 8). At the end of the experiment, the animals were euthanized using 2% pentobarbital sodium and the concentration of cAMP in the brain was determined using the ELISA method [17].

Western blot analysis

Western blot was used to examine the expression of gamma-aminobutyric acid transporter-1 (GAT-1) in the brain tissues. Frozen tissues were homogenized and total protein was extracted. Protein concentrations were measured using the BCA method. The supernatant samples containing 20 μg of protein were electrophoresed in 10% SDS polyacrylamide gels, transferred to polyvinylidene difluoride membrane (Millipore, Bedford, MA), blocked with 5% milk, and incubated overnight at 4°C with anti-GAT-1 primary antibody (1:1000, Cell Signaling Technology, MA, USA). Then the membranes were washed and incubated with the HRP-conjugated secondary antibody (1:5000; Santa Cruz Biotechnology, CA, USA), and visualized by enhanced chemiluminescence.

Statistical analysis

SPSS 21.0 software was used to analyze the data. The significant differences between multiple groups were analyzed using one-way ANOVA, and two groups were calculated using Student's unpaired t-test. Results are expressed as means ± SD, and a value of $P < 0.05$ is considered as statistically significant.

Results

MMWA treatment ameliorates insomnia induced by PCPA in rats

As shown in Fig 1A, the insomnia models exhibited less food intake and lower weight gain when compared with the control group ($P < 0.05$). Treatment with the MMWA was able to substantially increase weight gain ($P < 0.05$) (Fig 1A). The open field test demonstrated that the rats in the model group showed an increase in the movement distance, movement time, and the number of arm lifting compared with the controls ($P < 0.05$). These autonomous activity test indexes trended to decrease in the treatment group ($P < 0.05$) (Fig 1B). As shown in Fig 1C, the rats in the model group showed lower levels of 5-HT and GABA, and higher contents of ACh and NE compared with the controls ($P < 0.05$). Conversely, the treatment group showed higher levels of 5-HT and GABA, and lower contents of ACh and NE than the model group ($P < 0.05$). These results indicated that the MMWA had a therapeutic effect on insomnia.

PLOS ONE

Influence of warm acupuncture on gut microbiota and metabolites in insomnia rats

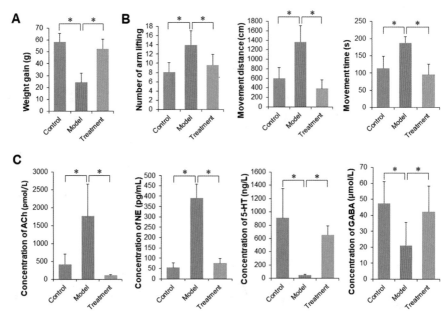

Fig 1. The therapeutic effect of the MMWA on insomnia rats. (A) Comparison of body weight gain of rats among three groups. (B) Comparison of the movement distance, movement time, and the number of arm lifting of rats among three groups. (C) Comparison of neurotransmitters in the serum of rats among three groups. Values are expressed as the means ± SD, n = 8 rats in each group (*P < 0.05).

https://doi.org/10.1371/journal.pone.0267843.g001

MMWA treatment improves gut microbiota in PCPA-induced insomnia rats

The fecal microbial composition was determined by bacterial 16S rRNA sequencing. A total of 1,632,128 reads of 16S rRNA gene were retained and each sample totaled between 68,192 and 70198 (S1 Table). In addition, a total of 1513 OTUs were identified from all samples (S2 Table). Species accumulation curve based on the OTUs reached saturation, indicating that the sequencing data were sufficient to cover the majority of microbe species (S2A Fig). The rank abundance curve representing species abundance and distribution evenness was shown in S2B Fig. Fig 2 showed the diversity of gut microbiota by the alpha diversity indices. The Shannon index reflecting the species richness and evenness was 1.29 ± 0.30, 1.07 ± 0.21, and 1.10 ± 0.28 in the control, model, and treatment groups, respectively (Fig 2A). Similarly, the Simpson index reflecting community evenness in the three groups was 0.35 ± 0.12, 0.47 ± 0.11, and 0.42 ± 0.13, respectively (Fig 2B). A significant difference was observed in beta diversity based on the weighted_unifrac (P = 0.008) but not unweighted_unifrac (P = 0.817) among the three groups (Fig 2C).

The microbial compositions at the phylum level were shown in Fig 3A. *Firmicutes* were the most abundant bacterial group, accounting for an average of 98.1%, 98.7%, and 99.7% sequences in the control, model, and treatment groups, respectively. Meanwhile, *Proteobacteria* represented the second dominant bacterial community in the three groups, accounting

附　　录

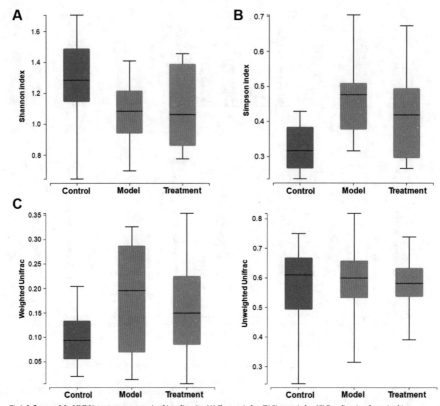

Fig 2. Influence of the MMWA treatment on gut microbiota diversity. (A) Shannon index. (B) Simpson index. (C) Beta diversity of gut microbiota.

https://doi.org/10.1371/journal.pone.0267843.g002

for an average of 1.1%, 1.0%, and 0.2% sequences, respectively. Other phyla were detected at low relative abundances (less than 3%). At the genus level, the microbial compositions were shown in Fig 3B. *Romboutsia*, *Lactobacillus*, *Clostridium sensu stricto* and *Turicibacter* were abundant in the three groups. Compared with the control group, a significant increase in the *Romboutsia* counts and reduction in *Lactobacillus* and *Clostridium sensu stricto* were observed in the fecal samples from the model group (P < 0.05). In contrast, the abundances of these genera were reversed by the MMWA intervention.

According to the LDA effect size (LEfSe) analysis, 13 taxa were significant different between the model group and the control group: 9 for the control group and 4 for the model group (Fig 4A). The control rats primarily showed higher enrichment of *Aerococcus*, *Corynebacteriaceae*, *Carnobacteriaceae*, *Corynebacterium*, *Micrococcaceae*, *Rothia*, *Jeotgalicoccus*, *Granulicatella*,

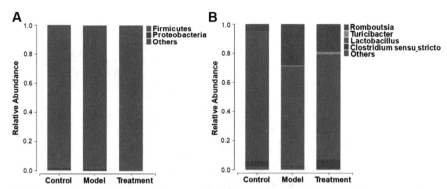

Fig 3. Influence of the MMWA treatment on gut microbiota composition. (A) Taxonomic composition at the phylum level. (B) Taxonomic composition at the genus level.

https://doi.org/10.1371/journal.pone.0267843.g003

and *Granulicatella*, whereas the model rats were mainly characterized by higher abundance of *Proteobacteria*, *Clostridium XlVa*, *Blautia*, and *Lachnospiraceae*. Similarly, the differences between the model group and the treatment group were also identified (Fig 4B). We observed that the *Proteobacteria* was significantly affected by the MMWA treatment. However, the proportion of *Blautia* in the MMWA-treated rats was closer to that in the model group (S3 Fig), indicating that the warm acupuncture intervention did not regulate the structure of intestinal flora to reach a healthy state.

MMWA treatment regulates serum metabolites in PCPA-induced insomnia rats

The metabolite profiles in both positive and negative ion modes were identified. Because a high baseline in the negative ion mode was observed (S4 Fig), the positive ion mode was selected for further analysis in this study. A total of 88 metabolites were annotated between the control group and the model group (Fig 5A). Score plots of OPLS-DA and Heatmap showed that the model rats could be separated from the control rats (Fig 5B and 5C). Among the 88 metabolites, the levels of 57 metabolites significantly increased in the model group compared to the control group, whereas the other 31 metabolite levels dramatically decreased (S3 Table). In contrast, a total of 35 metabolites were annotated between the treatment group and the model group (Fig 5D). The treatment group could also be separated from the model group (Fig 5E and 5F). The results showed that the contents of 6 metabolites were reversed after treatment of the MMWA, including Biochanin a, Asarone, Succinic anhydride, Carbaryl, Oleoylethanolamide, and Sulfosalicylic acid (S4 Table).

KEGG pathway enrichment analysis showed that the occurrence of insomnia was associated with multiple pathways, among which the metabolic pathways and signaling pathways were considered to be especially important (Fig 6A). In contrast, the MMWA treatment could modify the cAMP signaling pathway to exert beneficial effects on insomnia (Fig 6B). Moreover, as shown in S5 Fig, the cAMP signaling pathway was upregulated in the model group compared with the control group. However, it was reversed after the treatment with the MMWA. To verify the effects of MMWA on cAMP levels in PCPA-induced insomnia rats, the

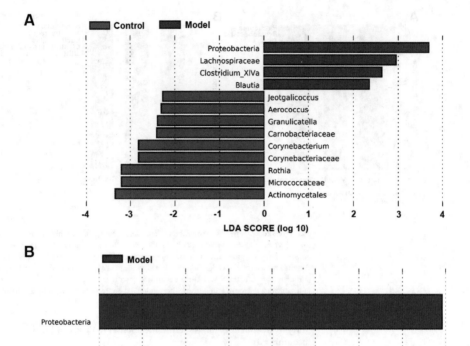

Fig 4. The significantly enriched bacterial taxa in different groups as determined by LEfSe analysis. (A) Pairwise taxonomic LEfSe analysis of the control and the model groups. (B) Pairwise taxonomic LEfSe analysis of the model and the treatment groups. (LDA score > 2.0, P < 0.05).

https://doi.org/10.1371/journal.pone.0267843.g004

concentrations of cAMP were evaluated using ELISA. Compared with the control group, the levels of cAMP were significantly increased in PCPA-induced insomnia rats (P < 0.05). However, the level of cAMP was significantly decreased in the treatment group (P < 0.05) (S6 Fig).

It is noteworthy that, after receiving MMWA treatment, there were significant differences in the metabolite profiles and enrichment KEGG pathways between the control group and the treatment group (P < 0.05) (S6 Fig), indicating that the serum levels of metabolites did not return to a normal state after treatment with the MMWA. This is consistent with our observations of intestinal flora.

Association of serum metabolites and gut microbiota

As shown in Table 1, the metabolites, such as Amide c18, Benzoyl chloride, Cytosine, and N, n-dimethylarginine were obviously increased in insomnia rats and showed a positive

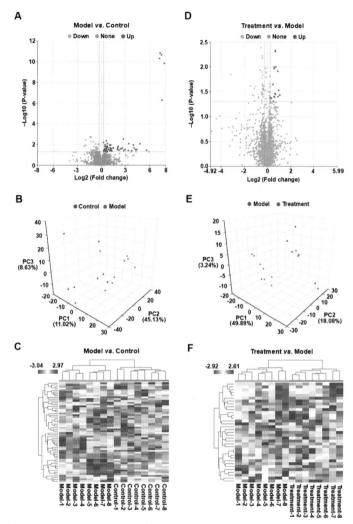

Fig 5. **Influence of the MMWA treatment on the levels of serum metabolites.** (A) Volcano plot of differential metabolites between the control group and the model group. (B) OPLS-DA score plots of serum samples from the control group and the model group in positive ion mode. (C) Heatmap analysis of differential metabolites between the control group and the model group. (D) Volcano plot of differential metabolites between the model group and the treatment group. (E) OPLS-DA score plots of serum samples from the model group and the treatment group in positive ion mode. (F) Heatmap analysis of differential metabolites between the model group and the treatment group.

https://doi.org/10.1371/journal.pone.0267843.g005

附　　录

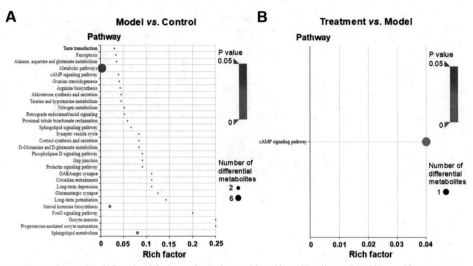

Fig 6. KEGG enrichment analysis of differential metabolites between the control group and the model group (A), and between the model group and the treatment group (B). The X-axis indicates rich factor and the Y-axis represents the terms of the KEGG pathways. The size of circle indicates the number of differential metabolites and the color of circle represents P-value.

https://doi.org/10.1371/journal.pone.0267843.g006

correlation with *Clostridium XIVa* and *Blautia*. Meanwhile, decreased 3-({[((2s)-2,3-dihydroxy-propoxy] (hydroxy) phosphoryl}oxy)-2-hydroxypropyl palmitate in the treatment group showed a positive correlation with *Clostridium XIVa* (Table 2).

MMWA treatment elevates the butyrate level in PCPA-Induced insomnia rats

The level of fecal butyrate was shown in Fig 7A. The contents of fecal butyrate in the model group tended to decrease compared with the control group (P < 0.05). However, there was higher fecal butyrate in the treatment group than in the model group (P < 0.05). To verify the

Table 1. Correlation of the metabolite levels with the abundance of gut microbiota in the control and model groups.

Description	Genus	Correlation
Amide c18	*Bifidobacterium*	-0.766758
Amide c18	*Clostridium_XIVa*	0.668651
N, n-dimethylarginine	*Blautia*	0.765262
N, n-dimethylarginine	*Clostridium_XIVa*	0.695278
Benzoyl chloride	*Clostridium_XIVa*	0.721906
Cytosine	*Blautia*	0.697319
2-amino-1,3,4-octadecanetriol	*GpI*	-0.694634
Succinic anhydride	*GpI*	-0.693140
N-acetylserotonin	*Campylobacter*	-0.668781

https://doi.org/10.1371/journal.pone.0267843.t001

202

PLOS ONE Influence of warm acupuncture on gut microbiota and metabolites in insomnia rats

Table 2. Correlation of the metabolite levels with the abundance of gut microbiota in the model and treatment groups.

Description	Genus	Correlation
3-({[[(2s)-2,3-dihydroxypropoxy](hydroxy)phosphoryl}oxy)-2-hydroxypropyl palmitate	Clostridium_XIVa	0.766920
3-({[[(2s)-2,3-dihydroxypropoxy](hydroxy)phosphoryl}oxy)-2-hydroxypropyl palmitate	Veillonella	0.578145
4-vinylcyclohexene	Acinetobacter	0.758516
Amiloxate	Elizabethkingia	0.573944

https://doi.org/10.1371/journal.pone.0267843.t002

effects of butyrate on cAMP levels in PCPA-induced insomnia rats, sodium butyrate was administered to the insomnia rats. As shown in S7 Fig, the production of cAMP was increased after PCPA treatment, which was dramatically attenuated by sodium butyrate, suggesting sodium butyrate suppressed PCPA -induced production of cAMP.

MMWA treatment reduces the GABA transporter 1 (GAT-1) expression in PCPA-induced insomnia rats

As shown in Fig 7B, the rats in the model group showed higher GAT-1 levels compared with the controls (P < 0.05). In contrast, the treatment group showed a lower GAT-1 level than the model group (P < 0.05).

Discussion

Although the MMWA therapy has been historically used for the treatment of insomnia, the understanding of the underlying mechanisms is still limited [11]. More recently, the results of multiple studies have demonstrated that the gut microbiota and its related metabolites played

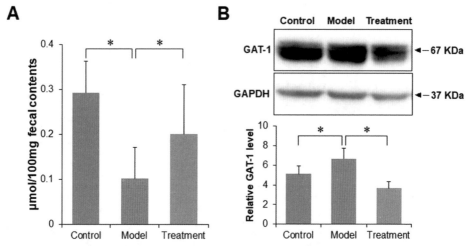

Fig 7. Influence of the MMWA treatment on the level of butyrate and the expression of GAT-1. (A) The level of butyrate in feces. (B) The expression levels of GAT-1 in brain tissues. Values are expressed as the means ± SD, n = 8 rats in each group (*P < 0.05).

https://doi.org/10.1371/journal.pone.0267843.g007

203

important roles in the pathogenesis of insomnia [24]. The aim of this study is to evaluate the therapeutic effect of the MMWA and to elucidate its anti-insomnia mechanism from the perspective of intestinal flora and metabolomics.

In our study, the insomnia rat models induced by PCPA were established. We demonstrated that the intervention of the MMWA prevented the loss of body weight and produced a beneficial impact on behavior. The present experiment also showed that the MMWA treatment significantly decreased ACh and NE levels and enhanced 5-HT and GABA levels. It is well known that dysfunction of neurotransmitters is nearly concerned with insomnia. 5-HT and GABA have been found to decrease significantly in brains of insomnia, whereas the levels of ACh and NE increased [25]. Therefore, our observations suggested that the intervention of the MMWA had a satisfactory effect on insomnia.

The present experiment further analyzed gut microbiota composition and diversity based on 16S rRNA gene amplicon sequencing. *Firmicutes* and *Proteobacteria* were the most dominant bacterial phylum, which is consistent with the previous reports [26]. At the genus level, a drastic decrease in the relative abundance of the genera *Lactobacillus* and *Clostridium sensu stricto* were detected in insomnia rats when compared with the controls. *Lactobacillus* species have been widely used as probiotics, which exhibit sleep-improving effects [27]. Additionally, the abundance of *Lactobacillus* and *Clostridium sensu stricto* were associated with the concentration of butyrate [28]. Interestingly, studies have shown that these bacterial species are associated with circadian rhythms [24], and more and more evidence has indicated that butyrate regulates the expression of host circadian clock genes [29]. According to the literature, bacteria tend to affect the host through butyrate [30]. Taken together, these findings suggested that *Lactobacillus* and *Clostridium sensu stricto* might modulate host circadian rhythm at least in part via their metabolite butyrate. Moreover, the abundance of *Romboutsia* was observed to increase in insomnia rats. Members of the genus *Romboutsia* may be involved in dysbiosis of gut microbiota [30], which is consistent with our results. However, the association between *Romboutsia* and insomnia in rats has yet to be elucidated. Interestingly, the intervention of the MMWA caused a reduction in the abundance of *Romboutsia* as well as a significant increase in the abundance of *Lactobacillus* and *Clostridium sensu stricto*, suggesting its potential role in the balance of gut microbiota. Consistently, a previous study showed that acupuncture treatment facilitated *Lactobacillus* on genus level [31].

LEfSe algorithm was used to identify important microbial taxa whose relative abundances differ significantly between groups. At the phylum level, *Proteobacteria* played an essential role in the model group. An increase in the relative abundance of pro-inflammatory *Proteobacteria* in the intestinal microbiota has been observed in rat models of sleep fragmentation [32]. At the family level, *Clostridium XlVa* and *Blautia* characterized the model group. At the order level, *Lachnospiraceae* characterized the model group. *Blautia* and *Lachnospiraceae* have been shown to be negatively correlated with sleep efficiency in humans [33]. To the best of our knowledge, the roles of *Clostridium XlVa* in insomnia have not been reported yet. However, it is interesting to note that *Clostridium XlVa* was enriched in children with autism spectrum disorder [34], suggesting its potential role in neurological pathophysiology. To further verify whether the MMWA treatment rebalances the intestinal flora in the insomnia rat models induced by PCPA, the LDA scores based on LEfSe analysis were obtained between the control and the treatment groups. Surprisingly, the rats in the treatment group were mainly characterized by a higher abundance of *Blautia*. The concept of gut microbiota resilience has been described in the literature [35]. It has been reported that a resilient microbiota will return to its original state of equilibrium after being subjected to a perturbation, whereas a non-resilient microbiota will shift to an alternative stable state [36]. Therefore, we supposed that *Blautia* was quite abundant in the model group, depending on certain host factors, and shifted to an altered

PLOS ONE

state after the MMWA intervention. However, the mechanism of microbiota resilience remains to be elucidated [37].

The alteration of the gut microbiota in insomnia rats was accompanied by the disorders of serum metabolome, as described in other studies [38–40]. Correlation analysis demonstrated that the metabolites elevating in insomnia rats, such as Amide c18, Benzoyl chloride, Cytosine, and N, n-dimethylarginine were positively associated with the abundance of *Clostridium XIVa* and *Blautia*, which characterized the insomnia rats. After treatment with the MMWA, 3-({[(2s)-2,3-dihydroxypropoxy] (hydroxy) phosphoryl}oxy)-2-hydroxypropyl palmitate decreased and showed a positive correlation with *Clostridium XIVa*. These results further confirmed that these bacteria might play an essential role in insomnia.

Metabolomics analysis of serum samples revealed that the MMWA treatment reduced the cAMP signaling pathway in PCPA-induced rat models. A previous study has reported that cAMP is involved in regulating the sleep-wake cycle [41]. The cAMP levels were lowest during rapid eye movement (REM) sleep compared with wakefulness [42], which is consistent with our results. A previous study also found that butyrate could inhibit the cAMP signaling pathway via Gi proteins [43]. We then examined the effect of the MMWA intervention on the butyrate level in insomnia rats. Our results showed that the MMWA significantly increased the

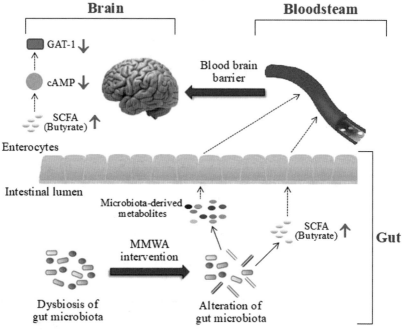

Fig 8. Schematic illustration of potential signaling pathways regulated by the MMWA.

https://doi.org/10.1371/journal.pone.0267843.g008

PLOS ONE   Influence of warm acupuncture on gut microbiota and metabolites in insomnia rats

content of butyrate. We further confirmed that butyrate treatment attenuated the PCPA-induced increase of the cAMP levels. These results implied that the MMWA inhibited the cAMP signaling pathway at least in part by upregulation of butyrate.

The latest research also indicated that the cAMP signaling pathway played an important role in the regulation of GAT-1 function [44]. It is well known that GABAergic synapse contributed to the development of insomnia. GAT-1 play a key role in regulating GABA levels and is responsible for GABA A receptor (GABAAR)-mediated inhibition [45]. In the present study, we confirmed that the MMWA intervention decreased the expression of GAT-1, which is in agreement with a previous report [44].

Conclusion

The present study suggested that the MMWA intervention could regulate a variety of microbial genera and metabolites related to insomnia, resulting in the reversal of butyrate-mediated abnormalities of the cAMP signaling pathway and GAT-1 expression (Fig 8). These findings would provide a better understanding of the molecular mechanism underlying the intervention of MMWA as an effective therapy for insomnia.

Supporting information

S1 Table. The number of reads of 16S rRNA gene retained from all samples.
(XLSX)

S2 Table. The number of OTUs identified from all samples.
(XLSX)

S3 Table. Number of up- or down-regulated metabolites in the control and model groups.
(XLSX)

S4 Table. Number of up- or down-regulated metabolites in the model and treatment groups.
(XLSX)

S1 Fig. Detailed acupoint locations.
(TIF)

S2 Fig. Species accumulation curve (A) and OTU rank-abundance distribution curve (B) of the intestinal microbiota in rats from the various groups.
(TIF)

S3 Fig. Pairwise taxonomic LEfSe analysis of the control and the treatment groups.
(TIF)

S4 Fig. Analysis of metabolites in the negative ion mode.
(TIF)

S5 Fig. Number of up- or down-regulated pathways in the control and model groups (A) or in the model and treatment groups (B).
(TIF)

S6 Fig. Influence of the MMWA treatment on the levels of cAMP and serum metabolites.
(A) Comparison of cAMP levels among three groups. Values are expressed as the means ± SD, n = 8 rats in each group (*P < 0.05). (B) Volcano plot of differential metabolites between the control group and the treatment group. (C) OPLS-DA score plots of serum samples from the control group and the treatment group in positive ion mode. (D) Heatmap analysis of

differential metabolites between the control group and the treatment group. (E) KEGG enrichment analysis of differential metabolites between the control group and the treatment group. (TIF)

S7 Fig. Influence of the butyrate on the levels of cAMP in PCPA-induced insomnia rats. (TIF)

S1 Raw image. (TIF)

Acknowledgments

We thank the staff at Beijing Genomics institution for their support during the performance of metabolome analysis.

Author Contributions

Conceptualization: Zhanli Wang, A. Gula.

Data curation: Hong Yu.

Formal analysis: Hong Yu, Hui Yu.

Investigation: Hong Yu, Hui Yu, Lengge Si, Husileng Meng, Wensheng Chen, Zhanli Wang, A. Gula.

Methodology: Hong Yu, Hui Yu, Husileng Meng, Wensheng Chen.

Project administration: Lengge Si, Zhanli Wang, A. Gula.

Resources: Zhanli Wang, A. Gula.

Software: Hong Yu, Hui Yu.

Supervision: Lengge Si, Zhanli Wang, A. Gula.

Visualization: Hong Yu, Hui Yu.

Writing – original draft: Hong Yu, Hui Yu.

Writing – review & editing: Zhanli Wang, A. Gula.

References

1. Ohayon MM. Epidemiology of insomnia: what we know and what we still need to learn. Sleep Med Rev. 2002; 6(2): 97–111. https://doi.org/10.1053/smrv.2002.0186 PMID: 12531146

2. Cappuccio FP, D'Elia L, Strazzullo P, Miller MA. Quantity and quality of sleep and incidence of type 2 diabetes: a systematic review and meta-analysis. Diabetes Care. 2010; 33(2): 414–20. https://doi.org/10.2337/dc09-1124 PMID: 19910503

3. Kamphuis J, Karsten J, de Weerd A, Lancel M. Sleep disturbances in a clinical forensic psychiatric population. Sleep Med. 2013; 14(11): 1164–9. https://doi.org/10.1016/j.sleep.2013.03.008 PMID: 24045060

4. Clark A, Lange T, Hallqvist J, Jennum P, Rod NH. Sleep impairment and prognosis of acute myocardial infarction: a prospective cohort study. Sleep. 2014; 37(5): 851–8. https://doi.org/10.5665/sleep.3646 PMID: 24790263

5. Bollu PC, Kaur H. Sleep medicine: insomnia and sleep. Mo Med. 2019; 116(1): 68–75. PMID: 30862990

6. Tilg H, Cani PD, Mayer EA. Gut microbiome and liver diseases. Gut. 2016; 65(12): 2035–44. https://doi.org/10.1136/gutjnl-2016-312729 PMID: 27802157

7. Thaiss CA, Zmora N, Levy M, Elinav E. The microbiome and innate immunity. Nature. 2016; 535 (7610): 65–74. https://doi.org/10.1038/nature18847 PMID: 27383981

8. Liu B, Lin W, Chen S, Xiang T, Yang Y, Yin Y, et al. Gut microbiota as an objective measurement for auxiliary diagnosis of insomnia disorder. Front Microbiol. 2019; 10: 1770. https://doi.org/10.3389/fmicb.2019.01770 PMID: 31456757

9. Li Y, Zhang B, Zhou Y, Wang D, Liu X, Li L, et al. Gut microbiota changes and their relationship with inflammation in patients with acute and chronic insomnia. Nat Sci Sleep. 2020; 12: 895–905. https://doi.org/10.2147/NSS.S271927 PMID: 33177907

10. Bo A, Si L, Wang Y, Xiu L, Wu R, Li Y, et al. Clinical trial research on Mongolian medical warm acupuncture in treating insomnia. Evid Based Complement Alternat Med. 2016; 2016: 6190285. https://doi.org/10.1155/2016/6190285 PMID: 28050194

11. A G, Li X, Su B, Lian H, Bao M, Liang Y, et al. Effect of Mongolian warm acupuncture on the gene expression profile of rats with insomnia. Acupunct Med. 2019; 37(5): 301–11. https://doi.org/10.1136/acupmed-2016-011243 PMID: 31225736

12. Xu Y, Li X, Man D, Su X, A G. iTRAQ-based proteomics analysis on insomnia rats treated with Mongolian medical warm acupuncture. Biosci Rep. 2020; 40(5): BSR20191517. https://doi.org/10.1042/BSR20191517 PMID: 32249904

13. Jang JH, Yeom MJ, Ahn S, Oh JY, Ji S, Kim TH, et al. Acupuncture inhibits neuroinflammation and gut microbial dysbiosis in a mouse model of Parkinson's disease. Brain Behav Immun. 2020; 89: 641–55. https://doi.org/10.1016/j.bbi.2020.08.015 PMID: 32827699

14. Hong J, Chen J, Kan J, Liu M, Yang D. Effects of acupuncture treatment in reducing sleep disorder and gut microbiota alterations in PCPA-induced insomnia mice. Evid Based Complement Alternat Med. 2020; 2020: 3626120. https://doi.org/10.1155/2020/3626120 PMID: 33178314

15. Bo A, Si L, Wang Y, Bao L, Yuan H. Mechanism of Mongolian medical warm acupuncture in treating insomnia by regulating miR-101a in rats with insomnia. Exp Ther Med. 2017; 14(1): 289–97. https://doi.org/10.3892/etm.2017.4452 PMID: 28672928

16. Si L, Wang Y, Wuyun G, Bao L, Bo A. The effect of Mongolian medical acupuncture on cytokines and neurotransmitters in the brain tissue of insomniac rats. Eur J Integr Med. 2015; 7: 492–8. https://doi.org/10.1016/j.eujim.2015.05.008

17. Wang Q, Qin F, Wang H, Yang H, Liu Q, Li Z, et al. Effect of electro-acupuncture at ST36 and SP6 on the cAMP-CREB pathway and mRNA expression profile in the brainstem of morphine tolerant mice. Front Neurosci. 2021; 15: 698967. https://doi.org/10.3389/fnins.2021.698967 PMID: 34512242

18. Magoč T, Salzberg SL. FLASH: fast length adjustment of short reads to improve genome assemblies. Bioinformatics. 2011; 27(21): 2957–63. https://doi.org/10.1093/bioinformatics/btr507 PMID: 21903629

19. Edgar RC. UPARSE: highly accurate OTU sequences from microbial amplicon reads. Nat Methods. 2013; 10(10): 996–8. https://doi.org/10.1038/nmeth.2604 PMID: 23955772

20. Wilkinson TJ, Huws SA, Edwards JE, Kingston-Smith AH, Siu-Ting K, Hughes M, et al. CowPI: A rumen microbiome focussed version of the PICRUSt functional inference software. Front Microbiol. 2018; 9: 1095. https://doi.org/10.3389/fmicb.2018.01095 PMID: 29887853

21. Wen B, Mei Z, Zeng C, Liu S. metaX: a flexible and comprehensive software for processing metabolomics data. BMC Bioinformatics. 2017; 18(1): 183. https://doi.org/10.1186/s12859-017-1579-y PMID: 28327092

22. Di Guida R, Engel J, Allwood JW, Weber RJ, Jones MR, Sommer U, et al. Non-targeted UHPLC-MS metabolomic data processing methods: a comparative investigation of normalisation, missing value imputation, transformation and scaling. Metabolomics. 2016; 12: 93. https://doi.org/10.1007/s11306-016-1030-9 PMID: 27123000

23. Bier A, Braun T, Khasbab R, Di Segni A, Grossman E, Haberman Y, et al. A high salt diet modulates the gut microbiota and short chain fatty acids production in a salt-sensitive hypertension rat model. Nutrients. 2018; 10(9): 1154. https://doi.org/10.3390/nu10091154 PMID: 30142973

24. Li Y, Hao Y, Fan F, Zhang B. The role of microbiome in insomnia, circadian disturbance and depression. Front Psychiatry. 2018; 9: 669. https://doi.org/10.3389/fpsyt.2018.00669 PMID: 30568608

25. Xu H, Wang Z, Zhu L, Sui Z, Bi W, Liu R, et al. Targeted neurotransmitters profiling identifies metabolic signatures in rat brain by LC-MS/MS: application in insomnia, depression and Alzheimer's disease. Molecules. 2018; 23(9): 2375. https://doi.org/10.3390/molecules23092375 PMID: 30227663

26. He WQ, Xiong YQ, Ge J, Chen YX, Chen XJ, Zhong XS, et al. Composition of gut and oropharynx bacterial communities in *Rattus norvegicus* and *Suncus murinus* in China. BMC Vet Res. 2020; 16(1): 413. https://doi.org/10.1186/s12917-020-02619-6 PMID: 33129337

27. Lin A, Shih CT, Huang CL, Wu CC, Lin CT, Tsai YC. Hypnotic effects of Lactobacillus fermentum PS150TM on pentobarbital-induced sleep in mice. Nutrients. 2019; 11(10): 2409. https://doi.org/10.3390/nu11102409 PMID: 31600934

28. Appert O, Garcia AR, Frei R, Roduit C, Constancias F, Neuzil-Bunesova V, et al. Initial butyrate produc- ers during infant gut microbiota development are endospore formers. Environ Microbiol. 2020; 22(9): 3909–21. https://doi.org/10.1111/1462-2920.15167 PMID: 32686173

29. Parkar SG, Kalsbeek A, Cheeseman JF. Potential role for the gut microbiota in modulating host circa- dian rhythms and metabolic health. Microorganisms. 2019; 7(2): 41. https://doi.org/10.3390/ microorganisms7020041 PMID: 30709031

30. Lee SM, Kim N, Nam RH, Park JH, Choi SI, Park YT, et al. Gut microbiota and butyrate level changes associated with the long-term administration of proton pump inhibitors to old rats. Sci Rep. 2019; 9(1): 6626. https://doi.org/10.1038/s41598-019-43112-x PMID: 31036935

31. Wei D, Xie L, Zhuang Z, Zhao N, Huang B, Tang Y, et al. Gut microbiota: a new strategy to study the mechanism of electroacupuncture and moxibustion in treating ulcerative colitis. Evid Based Comple- ment Alternat Med. 2019; 2019: 9730176. https://doi.org/10.1155/2019/9730176 PMID: 31354859

32. Maki KA, Burke LA, Calik MW, Watanabe-Chailland M, Sweeney D, Romick-Rosendale LE, et al. Sleep fragmentation increases blood pressure and is associated with alterations in the gut microbiome and fecal metabolome in rats. Physiol Genomics. 2020; 52(7): 280–92. https://doi.org/10.1152/ physiolgenomics.00039.2020 PMID: 32567509

33. Smith RP, Easson C, Lyle SM, Kapoor R, Donnelly CP, Davidson EJ, et al. Gut microbiome diversity is associated with sleep physiology in humans. PLoS One. 2019; 14(10): e0222394. https://doi.org/10. 1371/journal.pone.0222394 PMID: 31589627

34. Zou R, Xu F, Wang Y, Duan M, Guo M, Zhang Q, et al. Changes in the gut microbiota of children with autism spectrum disorder. Autism Res. 2020; 13(9): 1614–25. https://doi.org/10.1002/aur.2358 PMID: 32830918

35. Downing AS, van Nes EH, Mooij WM, Scheffer M. The resilience and resistance of an ecosystem to a collapse of diversity. PLoS One. 2012; 7(9): e46135. https://doi.org/10.1371/journal.pone.0046135 PMID: 23029410

36. Dogra SK, Doré J, Damak S. Gut microbiota resilience: definition, link to health and strategies for inter- vention. Front Microbiol. 2020; 11: 572921. https://doi.org/10.3389/fmicb.2020.572921 PMID: 33042082

37. Fisher CK, Mehta P. Identifying keystone species in the human gut microbiome from metagenomic timeseries using sparse linear regression. PLoS One. 2014; 9(7): e102451. https://doi.org/10.1371/ journal.pone.0102451 PMID: 25054627

38. Si Y, Chen X, Guo T, Wei W, Wang L, Zhang F, et al. Comprehensive 16S rDNA sequencing and LC- MS/MS-based metabolomics to investigate intestinal flora and metabolic profiles of the serum, hypo- thalamus and hippocampus in p-chlorophenylalanine-induced insomnia rats treated with *lilium brownie*. Neurochem Res. 2022; 47(3): 574–89. https://doi.org/10.1007/s11064-021-03466-z PMID: 34661797

39. Zhou J, Wu X, Li Z, Zou Z, Dou S, Li G, et al. Alterations in gut microbiota are correlated with serum metabolites in patients with insomnia disorder. Front Cell Infect Microbiol. 2022; 12: 722662. https://doi. org/10.3389/fcimb.2022.722662 PMID: 35252021

40. Si Y, Wei W, Chen X, Xie X, Guo T, Sasaki Y, et al. A comprehensive study on the relieving effect of Lilium brownii on the intestinal flora and metabolic disorder in p-chlorphenylalanine induced insomnia rats. Pharm Biol. 2022; 60(1): 131–43. https://doi.org/10.1080/13880209.2021.2019283 PMID: 34978949

41. Amici R, Perez E, Zamboni G, Parmeggiani PL. Changes in cAMP concentration in the rat preoptic area during synchronized and desynchronized sleep. Experientia. 1990; 46(1): 58–9. https://doi.org/10. 1007/BF01955415 PMID: 2153571

42. Ogasahara S, Taguchi Y, Wada H. Changes in the levels of cyclic nucleotides in rat brain during the sleep-wakefulness cycle. Brain Res. 1981; 213(1): 163–71. https://doi.org/10.1016/0006-8993(81) 91256-7 PMID: 6263409

43. Lu N, Li M, Lei H, Jiang X, Tu W, Lu Y, et al. Butyric acid regulates progesterone and estradiol secretion via cAMP signaling pathway in porcine granulosa cells. J Steroid Biochem Mol Biol. 2017; 172: 89–97. https://doi.org/10.1016/j.jsbmb.2017.06.004 PMID: 28602959

44. Borges-Martins VPP, Ferreira DDP, Souto AC, Oliveira Neto JG, Pereira-Figueiredo D, da Costa Calaza K, et al. Caffeine regulates GABA transport via A1R blockade and cAMP signaling. Neurochem Int. 2019; 131: 104550. https://doi.org/10.1016/j.neuint.2019.104550 PMID: 31563462

45. Ghirardini E, Wadle SL, Augustin V, Becker J, Brill S, Hammerich J, et al. Expression of functional inhib- itory neurotransmitter transporters GlyT1, GAT-1, and GAT-3 by astrocytes of inferior colliculus and hip- pocampus. Mol Brain. 2018; 11(1): 4. https://doi.org/10.1186/s13041-018-0346-y PMID: 29370841

Original paper

Effect of Mongolian warm acupuncture on the gene expression profile of rats with insomnia

Acupuncture in Medicine
1–11
DOI: 10.1136/acupmed-2016-011243
© The Author(s) 2019
Article reuse guidelines:
sagepub.com/journals-permissions
journals.sagepub.com/home/aim
⑤SAGE

Gula A[1], Xian Li[2], Budao Su[1], Hua Lian[1], Manjie Bao[1], Yabin Liang[2], Yingsong Chen[1], Yongfeng Jia[1], Lidao Bao[1] and Xiulan Su[2]

Abstract

Background: The mechanism of Mongolian warm acupuncture (MWA) for the treatment of insomnia has not been previously reported.

Objective: To investigate the effect of MWA on gene expression profile in the p-chlorophenylalanine (PCPA)-induced rat model of insomnia.

Methods: A rat model of insomnia was established and the animals were divided into five groups: control, PCPA (untreated), PCPA + estazolam, PCPA + MA (manual acupuncture), and PCPA + MWA. The rats were euthanased at 7 days after treatment, and hypothalamic tissue was harvested to extract total RNA for the analysis of gene expression profile. Micro-array and Partek Genomics Suite analysis system were used to analyse differential expression of genes between groups. Furthermore, ingenuity pathways analysis was used to analyse the main regulators.

Results: After treatment, in rats with improved sleep, micro-array data from the follow-up phase compared with baseline showed that MWA down-regulated 11 genes compared with the control group and 16 genes compared with the PCPA group. Six genes were selected following the micro-array detection to perform quantitative polymerase chain reaction (qPCR) verification, and the results showed that the coincidence rate was up to 90%, which verified the reliability of the microarray results. Compared with the PCPA group, transcription levels of Egr 1, Btg2 and BDNF in the PCPA + MWA group were up-regulated (P<0.05).

Conclusion: In combination, the findings of this study suggests that MWA is efficacious at improving sleep in an experimental rat model of insomnia.

Keywords

Mongolian warm acupuncture, cell biology, p-chlorophenylalanine, micro-array, insomnia

Accepted 2 December 2017

Introduction

Insomnia, characterised by a state of dissatisfaction with sleep quality, is a symptom that is frequently encountered by clinicians and has been attributed to increased stressors associated with modern lifestyles. The exact mechanism of insomnia has not yet been clarified although various hypotheses have been offered. Recently, the number of Chinese people suffering from insomnia has increased substantially; the incidence was 22% in 2014 and rose to 31.2% in 2015. In the USA, the incidence of insomnia is about 10–20%. Insomnia is not only a factor in many accidents, but it also has a role in the high incidence of lifestyle associated diseases such as diabetes, hypertension and malignant tumours. Insomnia is also an early clinical

[1]Inner Mongolia Medical University, Hohhot, China
[2]Clinical Medicine Research Center of Affiliated Hospital, Inner Mongolia Medical University, Hohhot, China

Corresponding author:
Xiulan Su, Clinical Medicine Research Center of Affiliated Hospital, Inner Mongolia Medical University, Hohhot, Inner Mongolia 010050, China.
Email: xlsu@hotmail.com

Acupuncture in Medicine, 00(0)

indicator of mental disorders such as anxiety, depression, schizophrenia and suicide.[1-4] The treatment for sleep disorders is diverse; although Western medicine is effective, it has many drawbacks. Previous studies have endorsed beneficial effects of acupuncture in insomnia. Traditional Chinese medicine (TCM), including acupuncture and moxibustion, has been used historically to treat insomnia. Chinese randomised controlled trials and clinical observations have suggested that moxibustion has the potential to be an effective and safe therapy for insomnia.[5] Estazolam is a triazolobenzodiazepine drug that acts on the central nervous system, and is mainly prescribed as a sedative and hypnotic agent.[6]

Similarly, Mongolian warm acupuncture (MWA) may improve sleep quality as it appears to have an equivalent therapeutic effect on insomnia when compared with TCM acupuncture, and may help spare patients the various drawbacks of hypnotic medications. Hypnotic drug therapy may induce a sense of 'hangover' the next morning, and can be complicated by drug dependence, resistance, or rebound withdrawal. The Mongolian medical literature and modern clinical experiments have demonstrated that Mongolian medical acupuncture has a significant therapeutic effect on insomnia while being non-toxic, safe, reliable and convenient.[7] However, Mongolian medical acupuncture differs from MWA, which heats the Mongolian acupuncture needle to 40°C for the treatment of insomnia.

The aim of this study was to explore the effect of MWA on genome-wide gene expression in the p-chlorophenylalanine (PCPA) rat model of insomnia. We hypothesised that MWA would improve sleep quality without side effects, and that its therapeutic mechanism may be related to the regulation of gene networks. The influence of MWA on gene profile was also addressed in this study. Some genes (Btg2, Egr1 and BNDF) may be important for the regulation of targets that affect insomnia, and may be potential markers of efficacy of MWA for insomnia. An additional aim of this work was to uncover potential therapeutic targets and provide a foundation for further study of the mechanism of action underlying the putative effects of MWA.

Methods

Ethics

All animal experiments were approved by the Institutional Animal Care and Use Committee of the Affiliated Hospital of Inner Mongolia Medical University (reference no. YKD2017289), performed in accordance with guidelines for animal welfare commensurate with the National Institutes for Health 'Guide for Care and Use of Experimental Animals' (National Academies Press, Washington DC, USA) and

reported according to the ARRIVE (Animal Research: Reporting In Vivo Experiments) guidelines.

Experimental animals and groups

A total of 70 healthy Wistar rats (male:female ratio 1:1), specific pathogen-free grade, weighing 200–280 g, and aged 8 weeks, were supplied by Beijing Vital River Laboratory Animal Technology Co, Ltd (licence no. SCXK-(Beijing)–2012–0001). The rats were randomly divided into five groups (n=14 each), stratified by weight and gender (to maintain a 1:1 male:female ratio), comprising one healthy control group and four PCPA-exposed groups that remained untreated (PCPA group), or received estazolam (PCPA + estazolam group), manual acupuncture (PCPA + MA group), or MWA (PCPA + MWA group).[8,9] Rats in each group were maintained in two cages and were regularly fed. Drinking water was freely provided. The untreated PCPA group and the PCPA + estazolam group were included as negative and positive (pharmacological) controls, respectively.

Modelling

Rats in the four PCPA groups received intraperitoneal injections of 450 mg/kg PCPA (Sigma No: C6506, CA, USA) suspended in weakly alkaline saline (pH 7~8) once daily for 2 consecutive days. Rats in the control group underwent intraperitoneal injections of the same volume of a weakly alkaline saline solution only. Around 28-30 hours after the first intraperitoneal injection of PCPA suspension, the rats' activity was monitored for evidence of successful modelling of insomnia, which included loss of circadian rhythm, increased excitability, enhanced aggression, increased urine and stool production, development of dishevelled and dull hair, and grey stools. Rats were weighed using an electronic balance (BS124S, Sartorius) before and after modelling.

Interventions

In the control group, the normal rats were intraperitoneally injected with weak alkaline saline on the second day, and were serially injected for 7 days.

In the PCPA group, the rats were intraperitoneally injected with weak alkaline saline on the second day after observing the successful modelling, and were serially injected for 7 days.

In the PCPA + estazolam group, the rats underwent intraperitoneal injection of 92 mg/kg estazolam (provided by Changzhou Second Pharmaceutical Factory, Jiangsu, China) dissolved in distilled water as a 9.2% aqueous solution, starting on the second day after successful modelling and continuing once daily (at 08:00 every morning) for a total of 7 days.

Rats in the PCPA+MA group received acupuncture treatment starting 1 day after successful modelling and lasting for 7 days. Based on TCM theory and clinical practice, the following acupuncture points were chosen: GV20 (*Baihui*); bilateral SP6 (*Sanyinjiao*); and bilateral ear *Shenmen*. GV20 was needled daily, and ipsilateral SP6 and *Shenmen* were alternately needled. Acupuncture treatment was performed at 08:00 every morning. Stainless steel acupuncture needles (0.35 mm × 20 mm, supplied by Inner Mongolia Yuanyang Traditional Chinese and Mongolian Science and Technology Development LLC) were used. Depth of needling at each point was 5 mm, and the needle was retained for 15 min. The treatment was performed at 08:00 every morning, and lasted for 7 days.

In the PCPA+MWA group, MWA was performed starting on the second day after successful modelling. According to classical Mongolian medical theory and clinical practice, and in keeping with previous research,[7] acupuncture points *Dinghui*, *Heyi*, and *Xin* (Supplementary Figure S1)[7] were selected. *Heyi* and *Xin* are located in the centre of the superior fovea of the first and seventh thoracic vertebrae (upward and downward concavities, respectively). *Dinghui* is located on the top of the head at the intersection of an imaginary line connecting the two earlobes and the midline of the two eyebrows, in the centre of the parietal bone (see Supplementary Figure S1). The rats were fixed in black bags in the PCPA+MWA group (Supplementary Figure S2), then a special Mongolian acupuncture needle (0.5 mm × 30 mm, stainless steel, supplied by Inner Mongolia Yuanyang Traditional Chinese and Mongolian Science and Technology Development LLC) was obliquely inserted and connected to the MWA needle device (MLY-I, developed by the College of Traditional Mongolia Medicine and Pharmacy of Inner Mongolia Medical University, patent no. ZL201120058078.0) set at a current intensity of 100 mA, temperature of 40°C. The needle was retained for 15 min. The treatment was performed at 08:00 every morning, and lasted for 7 days. Outcomes were measured 60 min after the last treatment.

Behavioural testing post-modelling and post-treatment

Open field test. An open field test was conducted as previously described,[4] under quiet and dark light conditions on the second day of insomnia (2 days after the first intraperitoneal injection of PCPA). Measurements comprised: (1) residence time at the central grid (s), defined as the time from when the rat was put into the middle grid until it crossed the grid within 3 feet; (2) standing time, defined as the total time the rat spent with its two forelegs lifted off the bottom of the box or climbing up on the side walls, using its hind legs to support its body in the upright posture; (3) horizontal activity time (exercise time, s), defined as the time the rat spent exercising on the horizontal plane.

Forced swimming test. Each rat was placed in a separate plastic vertical tube (40 cm in height and 18 cm in diameter) filled with water (25°C temperature) to a height of 30 cm, then the time from the beginning of the swim until the nose of the rat became submerged under the water was recorded.

Tail suspension test. The rat was suspended in a home-made barrel 50 cm in height; one third of the tail of the rat was suspended inside the barrel, and the immobility time(s) was recorded within 3 min.

Impact of pentobarbital sodium on sleep latency and total sleep time. Thirty-six hours after the first intraperitoneal injection of the PCPA model drugs, the control group and the modelling groups were all intraperitoneally injected with 35 mg/kg pentobarbital sodium (Sigma). Each rat was picked up by its tail and placed on a pad with its belly up, followed which the sleep latency and sleep duration were recorded; the disappearance and recovery of the righting reflex were taken to represent 'sleep' and 'awake' states, respectively. If the timing of restoration of the righting reflex was suspicious, then the rat was immediately replaced on its back. If it turned over automatically within 1 min, then the previous time was taken as the recovery time, otherwise the more accurate recovery time was considered to be the moment of the second turnover.

Sleep latency (the time after injection of pentobarbital sodium to the time of the disappearance of the righting reflex) and the duration of sleep (the time from the disappearance of the righting reflex to the time when the rat awakened) were calculated.

Microarray detection

After the last treatment, the rats were euthanased by cervical dislocation, and then the hypothalamus was removed and immediately placed into liquid nitrogen for later use. One third formalin was used to fix. RNA was extracted from the hypothalamic samples preserved in liquid nitrogen, and sent to CapitalBio to perform microarray detection and analysis of mRNA expression profile.

Detection of indices

Expression of Egr1, pc3 and BDNF in the hypothalamic tissues was evaluated with quantitative polymerase chain reaction (qPCR). Total RNA was isolated from the hypothalamus using TRIzol reagent (Invitrogen Life Technologies). According to the manufacturer's instructions, 2 μg of total RNA was used for reverse transcription using a cDNA synthesis kit (RevertAid First Strand cDNA Synthesis kit; Fermentas, Vilnius, Lithuania). The samples were quantified by qPCR in a 7500 Sequence Detection system (Applied Biosystems, Foster City, CA, USA) using a SYBR-Green PCR kit (Applied Biosystems). Primers were designed and synthesised by Sangon Biotech Co, Ltd (Shanghai, China). Primer sequences and amplification fragments of Btg2, Egr1, BDNF and GAPDH were as follows: Btg2 (forward GCGTGAGCGAGCAGAGAC, reverse TTGATGCGGATA CAGCGATAGC); Egr1 (forward GACCACCTTACCACCC ACATC, reverse TGCCTCTTGCGTTCATCACT); BDNF (forward AGGCACTGGAACTCGCAATG, reverse AAGG GCCCGAACATACGATT) and GAPDH (forward AAGTT CAACGGCACAGTCAAGG, reverse CATACTCAGCAC CAGCATCACC). The relative expression level was calculated using the comparative CT method.

Statistical analysis

All data were subjected to statistical analysis using SAS 8.0 software. Data were expressed as mean $\pm$ SD. Within group comparisons were performed using the two related sample test. Inter-group comparisons were performed with the test of least significance difference test (LSD). Differences were considered statistically significant at $P < 0.05$.

Results

Body weight

Comparison of body weights before and after modelling for rats in the PCPA, PCPA + estazolam, PCPA + MA and PCPA + MWA groups are shown in Figure 1A. Comparisons within each group pre- and post- modelling showed that the weights significantly decreased after modelling, and the difference was statistically significant ($P < 0.01$). The comparison of pre-treatment and post-treatment weights for rats in the PCPA + estazolam group, the PCPA + MA group and the PCPA + MWA group are shown in Figure 1B. Weights in each group increased after the treatment ($P < 0.01$). Figure 1C shows that, compared with the control group, body weight in the PCPA group was significantly decreased after modelling at 3 and 5 days ($P < 0.05$). After treatment at 5 days, body weight in the control, PCPA + estazolam, PCPA + MA and PCPA + MWA groups were significantly increased ($P < 0.05$) compared with the untreated PCPA group.

Open field test

Comparisons of exercise time, residence time at the central grid, and standing time in the open field test are shown in Figure 2A–C. After treatment, compared with the PCPA group, the horizontal activity time (exercise time) of rats in the treatment groups tended to decrease. When the PCPA + estazolam group was compared with the PCPA group, a statistically significant difference ($P < 0.05$) in horizontal activity was noted (Figure 2A). Compared with the control group, residence times at the central grid in the PCPA, PCPA + MWA and PCPA + estazolam groups were significantly increased ($P < 0.01$; Figure 2B). Compared

with the PCPA group, standing times of the PCPA + MWA group and the PCPA + estazolam group were significantly decreased ($P < 0.01$; Figure 2C).

Forced swimming test

Compared with the control group, the results showed that after treatment, the intensity of exercise in each group was enhanced (Figure 2D). Compared with the PCPA group, all treatment groups exhibited significantly longer swimming times, with the greatest increases observed in the PCPA + MWA group and the PCPA + estazolam group ($P < 0.01$).

Tail suspension test

After modelling and treatment, compared with the control group, there was a significant increase in the immobility time during tail suspension in the PCPA group, which was statistically significant ($P < 0.05$; Figure 2E). Compared with the PCPA group after treatment, immobility time in the treatment group significantly shortened ($P < 0.05$).

After treatment, sleep latency and total sleep time decreased and increased, respectively, in all groups, with the largest effects observed in the PCPA + MWA group (Figure 2F). Compared with the untreated PCPA group, the mental state of the rats during the open field test, forced swimming test and tail suspension test was highly reactive in the PCPA + estazolam, PCPA + MA and PCPA + MWA groups.

Quality control of microarray experiment

Microarray analysis of Affymetrix 3'IVT was performed to evaluate the impact of insomnia and MWA on gene expression profiles. The RNA degradation plot (Figure 3A) showed a smooth increase, indicating that the microarray experiment was normal. A box plot graph of the microarray before and after normalisation, is shown in Figure 3B,C, confirming there was no abnormal microarray. Quality control of hybridisation of the microarray experiment showed the curves were relatively parallel, and no crossing occurred, suggesting that the microarray experiment was normal (Figure 3D,E).

Differential genes in PCPA + MWA group vs. control groups

Statistical analysis was performed according to the fold difference (≥ 1.5 times) and the q value was $< 5\%$. Comparing the PCPA + MWA group with the control group, there were 11 differential screened genes (corresponding to the 13 probe clusters). There were no up-regulated genes, while there were 11 differential down-regulated genes > 1.5 times. Ignoring the q value, only the fold difference ≥ 1.5 times was used for statistical analysis. Comparing the

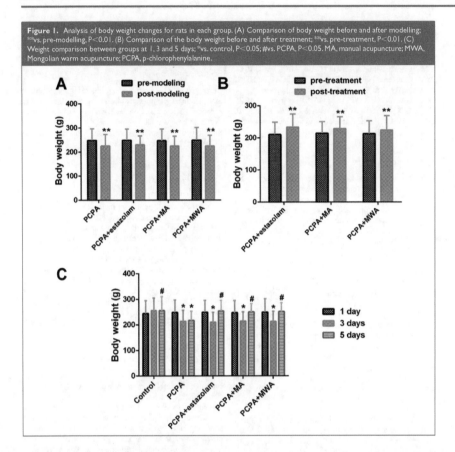

Figure 1. Analysis of body weight changes for rats in each group. (A) Comparison of body weight before and after modelling; **vs. pre-modelling, P<0.01. (B) Comparison of the body weight before and after treatment; **vs. pre-treatment, P<0.01. (C) Weight comparison between groups at 1, 3 and 5 days; *vs. control, P<0.05; #vs. PCPA, P<0.05. MA, manual acupuncture; MWA, Mongolian warm acupuncture; PCPA, p-chlorophenylalanine.

PCPA+MWA group with the control group, there were a total of 203 differential genes, of which 100 were up-regulated more than 1.5 times, and 103 were down-regulated more than 1.5 times.

Differential genes in PCPA+MWA vs. PCPA group

Statistical analysis was performed on the basis that the fold difference was ≥1.5 times, and q value was <5%. Comparing the PCPA+MWA group with the PCPA group, there were a total of 16 differential screened genes (corresponding to the 22 probe clusters). There were no up-regulated genes, while there were 16 differential genes that

were down-regulated more than 1.5 times. Without considering the q value, the statistic was carried out only for the fold difference ≥1.5 times. Comparing the PCPA+MWA group with the PCPA group, there were a total of 279 differential genes, of which 81 were up-regulated more than 1.5 times and 198 were down-regulated more than 1.5 times.

Comprehensive analysis of the affected differential genes in the PCPA+MWA group

Differential expression genes in PCPA+MWA vs. control groups included the following probes/genes: 1368321_at (Egr1), 1372389_at (Ier2), 1385240_at (Wdr33),

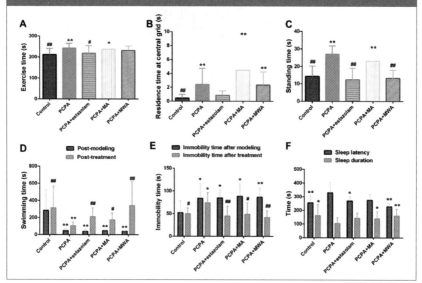

Figure 2. Exercise time (A), residence time at the central grid (B), and standing time during the open field test (C). (D) Swimming time post-modelling and post-treatment. (E) Immobility time during tail suspension after modelling and treatment. *vs. control group, P<0.05; **vs. control group, P<0.01; #vs. PCPA group, P<0.05; ##vs. PCPA group, P<0.01). (F) Sleep latency and duration in each group after treatment. *vs. PCPA group, P< 0.05; **vs. PCPA group, P<0.01. Comparing PCPA + estazolam with PCPA + MWA group, P=0.014 for sleep latency after treatment, and P=0.008 comparing PCPA + MA with PCPA + MWA group). MA, manual acupuncture; MWA, Mongolian warm acupuncture; PCPA, p-chlorophenylalanine.

1386935_at (Nr4a1), 1386994_at (Btg2), 1386995_at (Btg2), 1387260_at (Klf4), 1387870_at (Zfp36), 1389441_at (Bodl11), 1393324_at (Jam2), 1394814_at (Tpr), 1394964_at (Prrc2c). Differential expression genes in PCPA+MWA vs. PCPA groups included the following probes/genes: 1368321_ at (Egr1), 1373759_at (Fosb), 1381445_at (Esrrg), 1385240_ at (Wdr33), 1385825_at (Secisbp2l), 1386994_at (Btg2), 1386995_at (Btg2), 1387260_at (Klf4), 1389441_at (Bodl11), 1390706_at (Sptbn1), 1394814_at (Tpr), 1394964_at (Prrc2c), 1395154_at (Zc3h13), 1395557_at (Klf6).

In summary, the statistical analysis was performed on the basis that the fold difference was ⩾1.5 times, and q value was <5%. Compared with the control group, there were 11 down-regulated genes in the PCPA + MWA group, and there were 16 down-regulated genes compared with the PCPA group. Comparing the PCPA + MWA group with the control group and the PCPA + MWA group with the PCPA group, there were eight genes that were jointly down-regulated, including Egr1, Wdr33, Btg2, Klf4, Bodl11, Jam2, Tpr, and Prrc2c (Supplementary Figure S3).

qPCR verification

The following six genes were selected for qPCR verification following the results of the microarray test: Klf12, RGD1308706, Btg2, Dusp1, and LOC102548146. It can be seen that the specificity of the real-time PCR reaction was good from the amplification curve, melting curve and electrophoresis (Figure 4A–C). The coincidence rate of the result was >90%, reflecting the reliability of the microarray results (Figure 4D–G).

Changes in Btg2, Egr1 and BDNF mRNA expression in the hypothalamus

Figure 5 shows that the transcription levels of Egr 1, Btg2 and BDNF in the PCPA, PCPA+MA and PCPA+ estazolam groups were not significant, compared with the control group, while in the PCPA + MWA group they were up-regulated (P<0.05). Compared with the PCPA group, the transcription levels of Egr 1, Btg2 and BDNF in the PCPA + MWA group were up-regulated (P<0.05).

Figure 3. (A) RNA degradation plot. (B) Box plot graph of microarray experiment. (C) Box plot graph before and after normalisation. (D) Quality control of hybridisation of microarray experiment. (E) Quality control of Poly-A of microarray experiment.

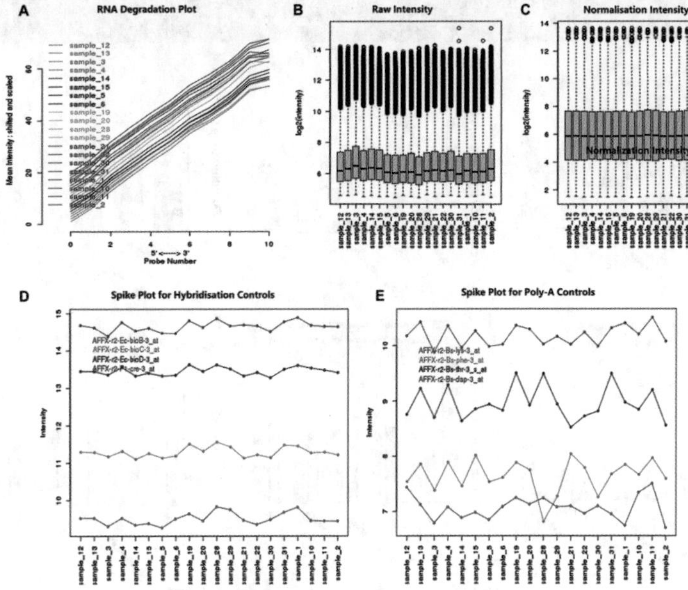

Enrichment analysis of the function of the differential genes

As described above, without the consideration of the q value, the statistical analysis was performed for the fold difference that was ≥1.5 times. There were differences in 203 genes in the PCPA+MWA group compared with the control group, and 279 genes compared with the untreated PCPA group. Enrichment analysis was conducted for these differential genes; the results are shown in supplemental Tables S1 and S2. Compared with the control group and the PCPA group, the genes with differential expression relative to the PCPA+MWA group were significantly gathered in pathways such as neuropeptide signals, interactions of nerve ligands and receptors, and dopamine receptor signalling pathways, indicating that PCPA+MWA may improve sleep by influencing nerve related pathways (Supplementary Figures S4 and S5).

Discussion

MWA has over 3000 years of history and has been anecdotally used to clinically treat insomnia effectively without side effects. MWA is a therapeutic option that differs from Western medicine and TCM acupuncture treatment. Clinical studies have confirmed that MWA can shorten the time taken to fall asleep in insomnia patients, and prolong sleep time, without the development of tolerance and side effects. It appears to have better efficacy for insomnia patients with co-morbid cardiovascular disease and tumours.[7] Mongolian medical acupuncture significantly decreases the cerebral excitability of rats with insomnia and promotes sleep, probably by regulating the contents of cytokines and neurotransmitters in brain tissues.[7] It is speculated that the MWA has a different mechanism from Western medicine and TCM acupuncture treatment, which may be related to certain biomarkers that can improve the quality of sleep, especially in insomnia patients who reject

Figure 4. The NM_001107281 genes for the amplification curve (A), melting curve (B), and electrophoresis (C) by real-time PCR reaction. Coincidence rate of PCPA + MWA vs. control group (D), PCPA + MWA vs. PCPA group (E), PCPA + MWA vs. PCPA + estazolam group (F), and PCPA + MA vs. control group (G). MA, manual acupuncture; MWA, Mongolian warm acupuncture; PCPA, p-chlorophenylalanine.

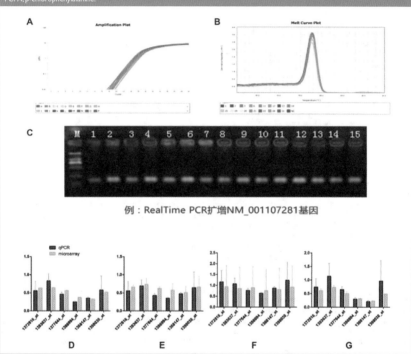

例：RealTime PCR扩增NM_001107281基因

other traditional treatments for insomnia. However, the precise mechanism of MWA for the treatment of insomnia has not been elucidated.

He and Li[10] treated 100 cases of insomnia using MWA, and reported that the overall efficiency of MWA reached 97%. Zhao and Sun[11] treated insomnia using MWA plus laser and *Tianwangbuxin*, and reported a clinical cure rate of 31% and overall efficiency of 100%, suggesting MWA had no side effects when combined with other treatments for insomnia, and was readily accepted by the patients who had satisfactory results. Wang et al.[12] observed the efficacy of dorsal and auricular MWA for insomnia and found that the cure rate of the experimental group was significantly higher than the control group. Jian[13] retrospectively analysed the clinical efficacy of MWA combined with the Mongolian drug Sugmel-3 for the treatment of insomnia,

demonstrating 94% improvement in the treatment group compared with 72% in the blank control group (P<0.05).

The choice of hypothalamic tissue for gene expression profiling was based on the study of Xiao et al.[14] Heinrich et al.[15] reported that the hypothalamic network, including the arcuate nucleus, ventromedial and lateral hypothalamus, and paraventricular nucleus (PVN), is crucial for regulating feeding behaviour and thermogenesis. Meanwhile, precise evaluation of the ascending reticular activating system (ARAS) is important for diagnosis, prediction of prognosis, and management of patients with disorders of impaired consciousness.[16] Acupressure seems to have a positive effect on sleep quality in haemodialysis patients.[17] Therefore, in this study, an animal model, microarray, and bioinformatics were used to study the relationship between the changes in genome-wide

Figure 5. Changes in Btg2, Egr1 and BDNF mRNA expression in the hypothalamus of each group. (A) Relative expression of Btg2 and Egr1. (B) Relative expression of BDNF.* P<0.05. MA, manual acupuncture; MWA, Mongolian warm acupuncture; PCPA, p-chlorophenylalanine.

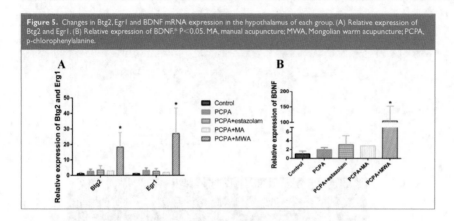

expression in the hypothalamic tissue and insomnia for the first time, and these changes in gene expression profile were compared with traditional western medicine and acupuncture treatment, in order to provide a foundation for further study to clarify the molecular mechanism of MWA for the treatment of insomnia.

In this study, rats underwent modelling of insomnia before being treated with MWA and the findings revealed a variety of ways by which MWA affected sleep. Neuropeptide signals, the interaction of nerve ligands and receptors, and the signalling pathway of dopamine receptors were implicated, suggesting that MWA can improve the quality of sleep by influencing nerve related pathways, as well as involving some inflammatory factors. The treatment of insomnia using MWA may be completed through the combined actions of the central nervous system, the endocrine system and the immune system, and some genes may become key genes for regulation. Therefore, it is particularly important to further the study of its mechanism.

Whitney et al.[18] measured changes in the gene expression profile of 68 soldiers diagnosed with insomnia using a gene microarray technique, showing that, after treatment, depression and the expression of altered genes were significantly reduced for the subjects whose sleep had been improved, and the most obvious result was a reduction in inflammatory cytokines. The study reported that there were 68 soldiers whose sleep was improved after decreasing activity of the genes, and compared with the group not experiencing sleep improvement, the expression of encoding genes in the sleep improvement group changed—suggesting that recovery of sleep may reduce the expression of inflammatory genes associated with ubiquitin. Although there are many other mechanisms that promote the

regulation and effectiveness of the production of protein, including epigenetic modification, altered gene expression is arguably the first step toward explaining the molecular mechanisms associated with the change in the activity of proteins, which may provide new insights into the complex relationships between the mechanisms of gene regulation.[19]

Among the most significant differentially expressed genes identified by microarray analysis after MWA were proliferation-related genes, Egr1, as well as an anti-proliferation gene, Btg2, which were found to be increased by qRT-PCR. These genes are regulated by BDNF, and Egr1 can also regulate the expression of BDNF. Our study shows that MWA therapy was able to reverse insomniac behaviours while concurrently increasing BDNF levels. mRNA levels of Egr1 and BDNF in our study were both up-regulated after MWA treatment of insomniac rats. Previous reports suggest that mRNA expression of Egr1 is induced by BDNF, since the Egr-1 gene promoter contains several splicing regulatory elements (SREs), the SRE-dependent transcription is activated by BDNF, and the ERK/MAP kinase pathway is involved in BDNF-induced Egr1 mRNA expression.[20] Levels of expression of Egr-1 in the normal brain is relatively low, but increased expression can be induced by a variety of stresses such as ischaemic stroke.[21] Previous studies also observed that Egr1 could suppress BDNF expression by binding to its promoter after ischaemic stroke.[22] We speculate that increased BDNF expression induced by MWA outweighs the inhibited effect of Egr1 on BDNF. Meanwhile, estazolam and MA appeared to have no effect on the expression of BDNF and Egr1. The Pc3/Tis21/Btg2 gene is expressed in many different tissues and cells in different ways. For example, Pc3/TIS21/BTG2 promotes neuronal differentiation.[25]

Acupuncture in Medicine, 00(0)

Levels of BDNF, Egr1 and Pc3 increased significantly after MWA, compared with the untreated PCPA group, and it is possible that MWA treatment could activate the transcript of genes such as Pc3 and Egr1 to protect the brain from the damage associated with insomnia. Up-regulation of BDNF may also play a role in protecting the brain and nervous system.

It has been shown that sleep disorders, post-traumatic stress disorder (PTSD) and depression are all related to high concentrations of inflammatory biomarkers, which confer an increased risk of inflammatory diseases, including metabolic syndrome, cardiovascular disease, obesity and type 2 diabetes.[23–25] Furthermore, it has been shown in healthy people that short-term reduction of sleep time also increases the production of inflammatory cytokines, including interleukin-6 (IL-6).[26–29] In this study, it was found that expressions of inflammatory factors was increased in insomniac rats in the PCPA group, while expression was decreased after MWA, as reported elsewhere in the literature. Moreover, this study showed differential effects on four specific regulatory genes (Wdr33, Bod1l1, Tpr, and Prrc2c) in the PCPA+MWA group. Although the results of our study support the relationship between the treatment of insomnia using MWA and the regulation of gene expression, the potential molecular mechanism underlying the changes in gene expression associated with the mitigation of insomnia after MWA was not fully elucidated. Our study of the gene expression profile of an animal model of insomnia has, for the first time, provided scientific data related to the stress exposure associated with insomnia and the change in gene activities associated with symptoms. This study confirmed that MWA improved sleep quality, associated with the regulation of gene expression. The function of the expected target genes in insomnia require further examination through subsequent in-depth studies.

Acknowledgements

We are grateful to all participants in this study.

Contributors

GA proposed the research plan and organised the implementation. XL wrote the text. XS wrote the outline, and organised the implementation and review. BS, HL, MB and YL participated in animal care and treatment. YC, YJ and LB conducted the animal behavioural observations and assessment. All authors approved the final version of the manuscript accepted for publication.

Funding

The authors disclosed receipt of the following financial support for the research, authorship, and/or publication of this article: This work was supported by a grant from the National Natural Science Foundation of China (ref. 81260571) and the Inner Mongolia Autonomous Region Mongolian medicine collaborative innovation special fund (ref. MYYXT201501).

Declaration of conflicting interests

The authors declared no potential conflicts of interest with respect to the research, authorship, and/or publication of this article.

Provenance and peer review

Not commissioned; externally peer reviewed.

Supplemental material

Supplemental material for this article is available online.

References

1. Buysse DJ. Insomnia. *JAMA* 2013; 309: 706–16.
2. Kraus SS and Rabin LA. Sleep America: managing the crisis of adult chronic insomnia and associated conditions. *J Affect Disord* 2012; 138: 192–212.
3. Yang P and Chen Y. *China guidelines for the prevention and treatment of insomnia*. Beijing: People's Medical Publishing House, 2012:1–34.
4. Fischer J, Dogas Z, Bassetti CL, et al. Standard procedures for adults in accredited sleep medicine centres in Europe. *J Sleep Res* 2012; 21: 357–68.
5. Sun YJ, Yuan JM and Yang ZM. Effectiveness and safety of moxibustion for primary insomnia: a systematic review and meta-analysis. *BMC Complement Altern Med* 2016; 16: 217.
6. Zhang YF, Zhou KL, Lou YY, et al. Investigation of the binding interaction between estazolam and bovine serum albumin: multi-spectroscopic methods and molecular docking technique. *J Biomol Struct Dyn* 2016:1–10.
7. Lengge S, Wang YH, Gerile W, et al. The effect of Mongolian medical acupuncture on cytokines and neurotransmitters in the brain tissue of insomniac rats. *Eur J Integr Med* 2015; 7: 492–8.
8. Chen Y. *Experimental treatment of Mongolian medicine [M]*: 105. Hohehot: Press of Inner Mongolian University, 2008.
9. Kong M and Xing C S. Xiaoyaosan intervenes the changes of 5-HT1A receptor and 5-HT2A receptor of the hippocampus of model rats with sleep disorder of depression. *Chin J Experi Tradi Med Formula* 2010; 16: 157–60.
10. He F and Li Y. The treatment of insomnia using Mongolian warm acupuncture. *Chin J Ethomed Ethnophar* 2011:6–7.
11. Zhao L and Sun J. The treatment of insomnia using warm acupuncture and super-laser as well as Tianwanbuxin pill. *Chin J Nat Med* 2015; 24: 383–4.
12. Wang M, Yue Y and Li J. Observation of the efficacy of the treatment of sub-healthy insomnia using warm acupuncture at back-shu and ear acupoint. *Am J Chin Med* 2011; 43: 98–9.
13. Jian J. Clinical study of the treatment of insomnia using Mongolian warm acupuncture combined with Mongolian drug of Sugmel-3 decoction. *World Lat Med Infor* 2016; 135.
14. Xiao LY, Liu WA, Wu QM, et al. [Influence of herbal-cake-separated moxibustion on contents of 5-HT, DA and NE in hypothalamus in rats with functional dyspepsia of liver stagnation and spleen deficiency syndrome]. *Zhen Ci Yan Jiu* 2016; 41: 60–4.
15. Lob HE, Song J, Hurr C, et al. Deletion of p22phox-dependent oxidative stress in the hypothalamus protects against obesity by modulating β3-adrenergic mechanisms. *JCI Insight* 2017; 2: e87094.
16. Jang SH and Kwon HG. The direct pathway from the brainstem reticular formation to the cerebral cortex in the ascending reticular activating system: a diffusion tensor imaging study. *Neurosci Lett* 2015; 606: 200–3.
17. Arab Z, Shariati AR, Asayesh H, et al. A sham-controlled trial of acupressure on the quality of sleep and life in haemodialysis patients. *Acupunct Med* 2016; 34: 2–6.

18. Livingston WS, Rusch HL, Nersesian PV, et al. Improved sleep in military personnel is associated with changes in the expression of inflammatory genes and improvement in depression symptoms. *Front Psychiatry* 2015; 6: 1–15.

19. Heinzelmann M G. Epigenetic mechanisms shape the biological response to trauma and risk for PTSD: acritical review. *Nurs Res Pract* 2013; 10.

20. Fukuchi M, Fujii H, Takachi H, et al. Activation of tyrosine hydroxylase (TH) gene transcription induced by brain-derived neurotrophic factor (BDNF) and its selective inhibition through Ca(2+) signals evoked via the N-methyl-D-aspartate (NMDA) receptor. *Brain Res* 2010; 1366: 18–26.

21. Yang L, Jiang Y, Wen Z, et al. Over-expressed EGR1 may exaggerate ischemic injury after experimental stroke by decreasing BDNF expression. *Neuroscience* 2015; 290: 509–17.

22. Iacopetti P, Michelini M, Stuckmann I, et al. Expression of the anti-proliferative gene TIS21 at the onset of neurogenesis identifies single neuroepithelial cells that switch from proliferative to neuron-generating division. *Proc Natl Acad Sci U S A* 1999; 96: 4639–44.

23. Michael R, Dolsen BA and Lauren D. Insomnia as a transdiagnostic process in psychiatric disorders. *Curr Psychiatry Rep* 2014; 16: 471.

24. Luxton DD, Greenburg D, Ryan J, et al. Prevalence and impact of short sleep duration in redeployed OIF soldiers. *Sleep* 2011; 34: 1189–95.

25. Church D, Hawk C, Brooks AJ, et al. Psychological trauma symptom improvement in veterans using emotional freedom techniques: a randomized controlled trial. *J Nerv Ment Dis* 2013; 201: 153–60.

26. Lopresti AL and Drummond PD. Obesity and psychiatric disorders: commonalities in dysregulated biological pathways and their implications for treatment. *Prog Neuropsychopharmacol Biol Psychiatry* 2013; 45: 92–9.

27. Prather AA, Marsland AL, Hall M, et al. Normative variation in self-reported sleep quality and sleep debt is associated with stimulated pro-inflammatory cytokine production. *Biol Psychol* 2009; 82: 12–17.

28. Chennaoui M, Sauvet F, Drogou C, et al. Effect of one night of sleep loss on changes in tumor necrosis factor alpha (TNF-α) levels in healthy men. *Cytokine* 2011; 56: 318–24.

29. Axelsson J, Rehman JU, Akerstedt T, et al. Effects of sustained sleep restriction on mitogen-stimulated cytokines, chemokines and T helper 1/ T helper 2 balance in humans. *PLoS One* 2013; 8: e82291.

Int J Clin Exp Med 2019;12(5):6300-6312
www.ijcem.com /ISSN:1940-5901/IJCEM0087620

Original Article
Effects of Mongolian medical warm acupuncture on model rats with insomnia based on positron emission tomography-computed tomography (PET-CT)

Lidao Bao[1*], Hongwei Yuan[2*], Lengge Si[3], Sha Li[1], Agula Bo[3]

Departments of [1]Pharmacy, [2]Pathology, Affiliated Hospital of Inner Mongolia Medical University, Hohhot, Inner Mongolia, China; [3]Mongolian Medicine School, Inner Mongolia Medical University, Hohhot, Inner Mongolia, China. *Equal contributors and co-first authors.

Received October 30, 2018; Accepted February 8, 2019; Epub May 15, 2019; Published May 30, 2019

Abstract: Objective: Insomnia is one of the most common sleep disorders, with a very high morbidity. Mongolian medicine is characterized by a unique theory, presenting favorable therapeutic effects in the treatment of insomnia. In Mongolian medicine, warm acupuncture is ubiquitously applied for treatment of insomnia. It can invigorate bodily functions, regulate qi, blood, and somatostatin, strengthen immunity, and prevent and treat multiple diseases. The current study aimed to explore the effects of Mongolian medical warm acupuncture on cerebral glucose metabolism in insomnia rats using the PET-CT technique. Materials and methods: Rats were injected with para-chlorophenylalanine (PCPA) to establish the insomnia model. Rats were randomly divided into the normal group, model group, and warm acupuncture group, which received tail intravenous injections of 18F-FDG for scanning imaging of PET/CT. Expression of NDRG2 was detected with Western blotting. Differential expression of microRNAs in the brain tissues of the insomnia rats, before and after Mongolian medical warm acupuncture, was detected for qPCR verification. Plasmids were transfected to neurocytes of the rats for dual-luciferase reporter assay examination. Expression of NDRG2 was detected with the immunohistochemical method. Relevant cytokines and neurotransmitters were detected with ELISA. Results: Glucose metabolism in the Mongolian medical warm acupuncture group was strengthened, compared with that in the model group. Present results showed significant differences in the effects of Mongolian medical warm acupuncture, which plays a promoting role in cerebral function activity of model rats with insomnia via activating most regions inhibited in the brain. Chip data analysis found that expression of 156 miRNAs in the rats treated with Mongolian medical warm acupuncture was obviously altered. Of which, levels of miR-181a were increased by 3.2 times, compared with those in the model group. In silico analysis with TargetScan, PicTar, and miRanda showed that miR-181a and NDRG2 might have a target regulation relationship. Results of luciferase assay in 293T cells indicated no significant changes in the MUT-NDRG2-3'UTR group, while fluorescence intensity in the WT group was decreased significantly, following addition of miR-181a mimics. Western blotting results indicated that expression of NDRG2 in neuronal cells of the model rats with insomnia was significantly downregulated at 72 hours, after addition of miR-181a mimics, compared to that in the scramble group (P<0.01). Administration of warm acupuncture reduced volume shrinkage. Rod-like fusion occurred in NDRG2-positive cells of the rats, while expression of NDRG2, particularly in the neuron cytoplasm, was downregulated, compared to that in model group. Levels of IL-1, IL-2, IL-6, and TNF-α in the warm acupuncture group increased significantly, compared with those in the model group (P<0.05). Warm acupuncture significantly increased levels of GABA and reduced levels of Glu, compared with the insomnia model group. Conclusion: Mongolian medical warm acupuncture plays a promoting role in glucose metabolism in the brain of the model rats with insomnia. It upregulates levels of miR-18 and reduces NDRG2 levels, providing an academic basis for modern development of the traditional ethnic medicine.

Keywords: Mongolian medical warm acupuncture, PET-CT, insomnia, immediate central mechanism

Introduction

Insomnia indicates an unfavorable quality or amount of sleep, failing to meet normal physiological needs. It influences social function, as well. It is currently one of the most common sleep disorders, with a very high morbidity [1]. According to the World Health Organization, about 1/3 of the population suffers from sleep disorders. The percentage of people with vari-

附　录

Original Article

Ⓦ Thieme

Research on Treating Insomnia Accompanied With Depression by Mongolian Medical Warm Acupuncture

Untersuchung der Behandlung von Insomnie in Verbindung mit einer Depression mittels heißer Akupunktur nach Mongolischer Medizin

Authors
Lidao Bao[1]*, Sha Li[1]*, Qiu Jin[2], Lengge Si[2], Agula Bo[1]

Affiliations
1 Department of Pharmacy, Affiliated Hospital of Inner Mongolia Medical University, Hohhot, Inner Mongolia, P. R. China
2 Mongolian Medicine School, Inner Mongolia Medical University, Hohhot, Inner Mongolia, P. R. China

Key words
Mongolian medical, warm acupuncture, insomnia, depression

Schlüsselwörter
Heiße Akupunktur nach Mongolischer Medizin, Insomnie, Depression

Received 16.08.2017
Accepted 03.07.2018

Bibliography
DOI https://doi.org/10.1055/a-0658-1675
Phys Med Rehab Kuror 2018; 28: 358–364
© Georg Thieme Verlag KG Stuttgart · New York
ISSN 0940-6689

Correspondence
Lidao Bao & Agula Bo
Mongolian Medicine School
Inner Mongolia Medical University
Hohhot
Inner Mongolia
010110
P. R. China
agula_bo@163.com

ABSTRACT

Objective To observe the therapeutic effect of Mongolian medical warm acupuncture in treating the patients with insomnia accompanied with depression and discuss the mechanism of action of Mongolian medical warm acupuncture in treating insomnia.

* These authors contributed equally to this work and should be considered co-first authors.

Method 50 patients with insomnia accompanied with depression were clinically selected and randomly divided into the Mongolian medical warm acupuncture group and the drug group (trazodone) of 25 each. The patients in the Mongolian medical warm acupuncture group were subjected to acupoint stimulation (Xin acupoint, Dinghui acupoint, and Heyi) for 30 min once a day. 100mg of trazodone were administered to the patients in the drug group. The patients in both groups were treated for 4 weeks. The patients in both groups were compared in terms of Pittsburgh sleep quality index, sleep quality, daytime functions, self-rating depression scale etc.

Result There was a significant difference in total score of Pittsburgh sleep quality index (PSQI) between the patients in the Mongolian medical warm acupuncture group before treatment (16.83 ± 3.68) and those after treatment (8.18 ± 3.78)(P < 0.01). The scores of sleep quality and daytime functions of the patients in the Mongolian medical warm acupuncture group (6.76 ± 2.76) were superior to those in the drug group (5.89 ± 2.87)(P < 0.05). The self-rating depression scale (SDS) scores of the patients in the Mongolian medical warm acupuncture group after treatment (0.54 ± 0.89) decreased significantly when compared with those before treatment (P < 0.01). There was no significant difference in clinical therapeutic effect between both groups (P = 0.0812 > 0.05). The obvious curative rate in the Mongolian medical warm acupuncture group (75.58 %) was significantly superior to that in the drug group (49.77 %) (P = 0.0382 < 0.05). The Asberg side effect rating scale (SERS) score in the drug group after treatment (6.11 ± 2.06) was significantly higher than that in the Mongolian medical warm acupuncture group (4.15 ± 1.98) (P < 0.05).

Conclusion Mongolian medical warm acupuncture has therapeutical effect on insomnia accompanied with depression and Mongolian medical warm acupuncture has better therapeutical effect and fewer side effects than trazodone. Mongolian medical warm acupuncture has certain sedative-hypnotic and anti-depressive effects applies to insomnia accompanied with suppression.

ZUSAMMENFASSUNG

Ziel Feststellung der therapeutischen Wirkung von heißer Akupunktur nach Mongolischer Medizin in der Behandlung von

358

Bao L et al. Mongolian Medical Warm Acupuncture treat insomnia... Phys Med Rehab Kuror 2018; 28: 358–364

Hindawi
Evidence-Based Complementary and Alternative Medicine
Volume 2018, Article ID 6571320, 8 pages
https://doi.org/10.1155/2018/6571320

Hindawi

Research Article
Research on Roles of Mongolian Medical Warm Acupuncture in Inhibiting p38 MAPK Activation and Apoptosis of Nucleus Pulposus Cells

Sha Li,[1] Lidao Bao [ID],[1] Lengge Si,[2] Xiaohui Wang,[1] and Agula Bo [ID][2]

[1]Department of Pharmacy, Affiliated Hospital of Inner Mongolia Medical University, Hohhot, Inner Mongolia 010059, China
[2]Mongolian Medicine School, Inner Mongolia Medical University, Hohhot, Inner Mongolia 010110, China

Correspondence should be addressed to Lidao Bao; baolidao2017@163.com and Agula Bo; agula_bo@163.com

Received 31 March 2018; Revised 9 July 2018; Accepted 30 July 2018; Published 9 August 2018

Academic Editor: Cristina Nogueira

Background. Mongolian medical warm acupuncture has a desirable therapeutic effect on sciatica. Apoptosis of the nucleus pulposus cells is considered to play an important role in sciatica. Evidence has demonstrated that oxidative stress and its induced activation of the signaling pathways play important roles in sciatica. However, further research is expected to reveal whether Mongolian medical warm acupuncture can inhibit the apoptosis of nucleus pulposus cells and oxidative stress. *Objective.* To study the effect of the p38 MAPK pathway activated by the generated ROS on apoptosis and the expression of the genes related to the balance of the extracellular matrix metabolism during treatment of sciatica with Mongolian medical warm acupuncture. *Method.* The volume of the active oxygen generated in the nucleus pulposus cells was detected following intervention of Mongolian medical warm acupuncture. The p38 MAPK phosphorylation level was detected with Western blot. The genes are related to the metabolism of the nucleus pulposus extracellular matrix. *Result.* Mongolian medical warm acupuncture reduced the active oxygen within the nucleus pulposus cells and inhibited the activation of the p38 MAPK pathway (P=0.013). Meanwhile, it upregulated the gene expression of Type II collagen, aggrecan, Sox-9, and tissue matrix metalloproteinase reagent 1 (P-0.015; P=0.025; P=0.031; P=0.045) and downregulated the gene expression of matrix metalloproteinase 3 (P=0.015). *Conclusion.* Mongolian medical warm acupuncture may inhibit apoptosis of nucleus pulposus cells and activation of the extracellular matrix decomposition metabolism pathway and promote its anabolism. This process may rely on the oxidative stress matrix of the p38 MAPK pathway.

1. Introduction

Sciatica is a chronic process that influences some compositional, structural, and functional changes in intervertebral disc [1]. It is one of the major causes of lumbago. It can lead to loss of labor ability in many patients [2]. The intervertebral disc is the largest nonvascular tissue in the body. In addition to the end plate, the intervertebral disc mainly comprises two different categories of anatomical structures, i.e., internal nucleus pulposus and peripheral anulus fibrosus [3]. Apoptosis of the nucleus pulposus cells is considered to play an important role in sciatica [4]. Sciatica belongs to "white vein diseases". In Mongolian medicine, it is believed that prevalence of Badagan and qi and blood operating disorders are the common pathological results arising from various

pathogenic factors and the pathological basis of onset of pain. The three major factors lose their balance thus leading to ache, numbness, and muscular atrophy of lower limbs [5]. Treatment at the acupoints or joints aims to eliminate evils for supporting healthy energy, promote blood circulation for removing blood stasis, relax muscles and tendons and remove obstruction from meridians, relieve swelling and pain, and regulate the immune functions [6].

Previous research has indicated that excessive ROS (reactive oxygen species) can not only directly oxidize and damage DNA, protein, and lipid and but also activate a large number of stress-sensitive pathways [7] in the cells as signal molecules, such as p38 MAPK pathways, c-Jun N-terminal kinase (JNK) pathway [8], extracellular signal-regulated protein kinase (ERK) pathway, and nuclear factor-kappa B NF-B

Wissenschaft und Forschung

♆Thieme

Research on the Mechanism of Mongolian Medical Warm Acupuncture in Alleviating Insomnia by Increasing the BCL-2/BAX Ratio and Decreasing the Hormones Related to the Central HPA Axis of the Stress Response

Untersuchung der Wirkungsweise der heißen Akupunktur nach Mongolischer Medizin bei der Linderung von Schlafstörungen durch Erhöhung des BCL-2/BAX Verhältnisses und Senkung der mit der zentralen HPA-Achse assoziierten Hormonspiegel bei der Stressantwort

Authors
Lidao Bao[1], Hongwei Yuan[2], Lengge Si[3], Yuehong Wang[3], Yingsong Chen[3], Agula Bo[3]

Affiliations
1 Department of Pharmacy, Affiliated Hospital of Inner Mongolia Medical University, Hohhot, Inner Mongolia, P. R. China
2 Department of Pathology, Affiliated Hospital of Inner Mongolia Medical University, Hohhot, Inner Mongolia, P. R. China
3 Mongolian Medicine School, Inner Mongolia Medical University, Hohhot, Inner Mongolia, P. R. China

Key words
insomnia, Mongolian medical warm acupuncture, 5HT1A, 5HT2, D2, HPA axis

Schlüsselwörter
Schlaflosigkeit, heiße Akupunktur nach Mongolischer Medizin, 5HT1A, 5HT2, D2, HPA-Achse

received 04.07.2017
accepted 16.08.2017

Bibliography
DOI https://doi.org/10.1055/s-0043-118484
Phys Med Rehab Kuror 2017; 27: 290–297
© Georg Thieme Verlag KG Stuttgart · New York
ISSN 0940-6689

Correspondence
Prof. Lidao Bao and Prof. Agula Bo
Department of Pharmacy
Affiliated Hospital of Inner Mongolia Medical University
1 Tongdaobei Road, Hohhot, Inner Mongolia, P. R. China
010059 Hohhot
China
baolidao2017@163.com

ABSTRACT

Background Mongolian medical warm acupuncture is efficacious in treatment of insomnia but the mechanism still remains unclear. There is no research on the effect on the changes in expression of mRNA in the receptors of 5HT, DA, 5HT1α, 5HT2α, and DRD2 and the levels of hormones related to the central HPA axis in the stress response.

Objective To further explain the mechanism of Mongolian medical warm acupuncture in insomnia treatment and its role in protecting cerebral neurons, elaborate the effect of Mongolian medical warm acupuncture on the changes in expression of 5HT, DA, 5HT1α, and 5HT2α at different sites in the brains of the PCPA-induced insomnia model rats and the levels of hormones related to the central HPA axis in the stress response.

Method 72 Wistar rats were randomly divided into blank group, model group, Mongolian medical warm acupuncture group, and diazepam group of 18 each. The rats were intraperitoneally injected with PCPA (400 mg/kg) for 2 consecutive days to induce insomnia. The sleep latency and sleep duration before and after treatment were observed. The content of 5HT in the hypothalamus and hippocampus was measured with the ELISA method. The content of mRNA in the 5HT1A and 5HT2A receptors in the hypothalamus and hippocampus with the qPCR technique. The content of DA in the hypothalamus and corpus striatum was determined with the ELISA method. The content of ELISA in the hypothalamus and the content of ACTH in the serum of the insomnia rats were determined with the ELISA method. The changes in content of the BCL-2 and BAX proteins in the hippocampus were observed with the immunohisto-chemical method.

Result PCPA intraperitoneal injections were able to prolong the sleep latency of the rats and shorten the sleep duration (P < 0.05) when compared with the blank group. Mongolian medical warm acupuncture was able to alleviate the tendency of decreasing weight gain arising from insomnia (P < 0.05).

290

EXPERIMENTAL AND THERAPEUTIC MEDICINE 14: 289-297, 2017

Mechanism of Mongolian medical warm acupuncture in treating insomnia by regulating miR-101a in rats with insomnia

AGULA BO[1], LENGGE SI[1], YUEHONG WANG[1], LIDAO BAO[1,2] and HONGWEI YUAN[3]

[1]College of Traditional Mongolia Medicine, Inner Mongolia Medical University, Hohhot, Inner Mongolia 010110; Departments of [2]Pharmacy and [3]Pathology, Affiliated Hospital of Inner Mongolia Medical University, Hohhot, Inner Mongolia 010059, P.R. China

Received October 31, 2016; Accepted March 20, 2017

DOI: 10.3892/etm.2017.4452

Abstract. MicroRNAs (miRNAs or miRs) and the target genes before and after warm acupuncture at the genetic level were assessed, and the cytokines and neurotransmitters related to insomnia were studied. Male Sprague-Dawley rats were used to create PCPA insomnia rat models and randomly divided into the normal, model, warm acupuncture, and drug groups. The Dinghui Acupoint, Heyi Acupoint, and Xin Acupoint were inserted in the Mongolian medicine warm acupuncture group. The differential expression profile of microRNA in the brain tissue of the insomnia rats was determined before and after Mongolian medicine warm acupuncture for establishment of miR-101a mimics and inhibitor. qPCR was used to detect the expression level of miR-101a. Western blotting was used to detect the expression level of PAX8. The rats receiving Mongolian medicine warm acupuncture had 141 miRNAs with differential expression compared with the normal rats. The expression level of miR-101a in the cells of the hippocampus of the insomnia rats transfected with miR-101a mimics increased significantly at 72 h (P<0.05). The activity of the neuronal cells transfected with miR-101a inhibitor increased significantly at 72 h (P<0.05). The western blotting result indicated that the expression of the PAX8 protein in the neuronal cells of the insomnia model rats was inhibited and downregulated significantly at 72 h after addition of miR-101a mimics compared with that in the scramble added group (P<0.01). The levels of the interleukins IL-1, IL-2, and IL-6 and the tumor necrosis factor-α in the hypothalamus, hippocampus, and prefrontal cortex decreased significantly compared with those in the blank control group (P<0.05). The levels of noradrenaline, dopamine, and glutamic decreased significantly following warm acupuncture or western medicine treatment (P<0.05). In conclusion, this study demonstrates that the upregulation of miR-101a in the rats treated with warm acupuncture is directly associated with PAX8 regulation.

Introduction

Insomnia is a subjective experience characterized by a difficulty in falling asleep and/or staying asleep, which results in the failure of sleep quality or quantity to meet an individual's normal physiological needs and affects their social functions. It is the most common sleep disorder with very high rates of morbidity (1). According to an investigation by the World Health Organization, ~1/3 of the world's population suffers from sleep disorders (2). The percentage of people with various types of sleep disorders in China is significantly higher (35%) than the rest of the world (27%). Thus, effective prevention and treatment of insomnia is a main focus of research in the world (3).

In clinical treatment, hypnotics are primarily used in modern medicine. This drug treatment may be accompanied by many side effects. It is not an ideal therapeutic regimen due to its poor long-term efficacy and addiction, and tolerance, in the case of long-term administration (4). Mongolian medicine has a unique mechanism and good efficacy in treatment of insomnia. In Mongolian medicine, it is believed that the imbalance among Heyi, Xila, and Badagan, predominance of Heyi in the heart and white meridian, and Heyi blood intermingling arising from dysfunctions are the basic etiology and pathogenesis. Such negative emotions as tension, worry, fear, depression and anxiety; and social environment, diet, daily life and movement conditions are external factors. In the Mongolian medicine, the treatment of insomnia mainly focuses on relieving Heyi and regulating Heyi, Xila, and Badagan (5-7). The warm needling therapy is one of most common methods for the treatment of insomnia in Mongolian medicine as it functions in warming and smoothing meridians, regulating *qi* and blood, regulating

Correspondence to: Dr Agula Bo or Dr Lengge Si, College of Traditional Mongolia Medicine, Inner Mongolia Medical University, Jinshan Economic and Technological Development Zone, Hohhot, Inner Mongolia 010110, P.R. China
E-mail: bagulaimmu@163.com
E-mail: silengge2016@163.com

Key words: warm acupuncture, insomnia, miR-101a, Mongolian medicine

附 录

Hindawi Publishing Corporation
Evidence-Based Complementary and Alternative Medicine
Volume 2016, Article ID 6190285, 10 pages
http://dx.doi.org/10.1155/2016/6190285

Research Article

Clinical Trial Research on Mongolian Medical Warm Acupuncture in Treating Insomnia

Agula Bo,[1] Lengge Si,[1] Yuehong Wang,[1] Lan Xiu,[2] Rihan Wu,[3] Yutang Li,[4] Rigenjiya Mu,[1] Latai Ga,[1] Mei Miao,[3] Fu Shuang,[3] Yunhua Wu,[1] Qiu Jin,[1] Suocai Tong,[1] Gerile Wuyun,[1] Wurihan Guan,[1] Rigen Mo,[3] Sileng Hu,[1] Lixia Zhang,[1] Rui Peng,[1] and Lidao Bao[1,5]

[1] *College of Traditional Mongolian Medicine, Inner Mongolia Medical University, Hohhot 010110, China*
[2] *Department of Mongolian Medicine, Affiliated Hospital of Inner Mongolia University for the Nationalities, Tongliao 028000, China*
[3] *Department of Mongolia Medicine, Inner Mongolia International Mongolian Hospital, Hohhot 010010, China*
[4] *Department of Mongolia Medicine, Affiliated People's Hospital of Hospital of Inner Mongolia Medical University, Hohhot 010010, China*
[5] *Department of Pharmacy, Affiliated Hospital of Inner Mongolia Medical University, Hohhot 010059, China*

Correspondence should be addressed to Agula Bo; bagulaimmu@163.com and Lidao Bao; baolidao237@163.com

Received 16 March 2016; Accepted 15 August 2016

Academic Editor: Waris Qidwai

Objective. Insomnia is one of the most common sleep disorders. Hypnotics have poor long-term efficacy. Mongolian medical warm acupuncture has significant efficacy in treating insomnia. The paper evaluates the role of Mongolian medical warm acupuncture in treating insomnia by investigating the Mongolian medicine syndromes and conditions, Pittsburgh sleep quality index, and polysomnography indexes. *Method*. The patients were diagnosed in accordance with International Classification of Sleep Disorders (ICSD-2). The insomnia patients were divided into the acupuncture group (40 cases) and the estazolam group (40 cases). The patients underwent intervention of Mongolian medical warm acupuncture and estazolam. The indicators of the Mongolian medicine syndromes and conditions, Pittsburgh sleep quality index (PSQI), and polysomnography indexes (PSG) have been detected. *Result*. Based on the comparison of the Mongolian medicine syndrome scores between the warm acupuncture group and the drug treatment group, the result indicated $P < 0.01$. The clinical efficacy result showed that the effective rate (85%) in the warm acupuncture group was higher than that (70%) in the drug group. The total scores of PSQI of both groups were approximated. The sleep quality indexes of both groups decreased significantly ($P < 0.05$). The sleep quality index in the Mongolian medical warm acupuncture group decreased significantly ($P < 0.01$) and was better than that in the estazolam group. The sleep efficiency and daytime functions of the patients in the Mongolian medical warm acupuncture group improved significantly ($P < 0.01$). The sleep time was significantly extended ($P < 0.01$) in the Mongolian medical warm acupuncture group following PSG intervention. The sleep time during NREM in the Mongolian warm acupuncture group increased significantly ($P < 0.01$). The sleep time exhibited a decreasing trend during REM and it decreased significantly in the Mongolian warm acupuncture group ($P < 0.01$). The percentage of sleep time in the total sleep time during NREM3+4 in the Mongolian medical warm acupuncture group increased significantly. *Conclusion*. Mongolian medical warm acupuncture is efficient and safe in treating insomnia. It is able to better improve the patients' sleep time and daytime functions. It is better than that in the estazolam group following drug withdrawal in terms of improving the sleep time. It is more effective in helping the insomnia patients than hypnotics.

1. Introduction

Insomnia is a subjective experience of sleep with its quality or amount insufficient to meet the physiological needs as a result of difficulties in sleep onset and/or sleep maintenance. It can influence the social functions. It is one of the most common sleep disorders [1]. The clinical data have shown that long-term insomnia will cause increased morbidity rates of many disease such as heart diseases, hypertension, hyperlipidemia, senile dementia, depression, and anxiety. Therefore [2], the

Available online at www.sciencedirect.com

ScienceDirect

ELSEVIER　　　European Journal of Integrative Medicine 7 (2015) 492–498

European Journal of
INTEGRATIVE
MEDICINE

www.elsevier.com/eujim

Research paper

The effect of Mongolian medical acupuncture on cytokines and neurotransmitters in the brain tissue of insomniac rats

Lengge Si[a], Yuehong Wang[b], Gerile Wuyun[b], Lidao Bao[c,*], B. Agula[a,b,**]

[a] School of Preclinical Medicine, Beijing University of Chinese Medicine, Beijing 100029, PR China
[b] College of Mongolian Medicine, Inner Mongolia Medical University, Hohhot 010110, PR China
[c] Department of Pharmacy, Affiliated Hospital of Inner Mongolia Medical University, Hohhot 010059, PR China

Received 14 January 2015; received in revised form 27 May 2015; accepted 27 May 2015

Abstract

Introduction: Mongolian medical acupuncture (MMA) is thought to have a significant therapeutic effect on insomnia. The effect of MMA on levels of interleukins (ILs) and neurotransmitters in insomniac rats was investigated and the potential mechanism operating for insomnia is discussed.
Methods: SD rats in 6 groups (control group 1, control group 2, normal acupuncture group, insomnia group, insomnia + acupuncture group, and insomnia + Western medicine group) were intraperitoneally injected with p-chlorophenylalanine to provide an insomniac model. "Dinghui, Heyi and Xin acupoints" were stimulated with needles to observe the locomotor activities of insomniac rats (injected with pentobarbital sodium) and their sleep time. Levels of interleukin (IL)-1, IL-2, and IL-6, and tumor necrosis factor (TNF)-α in the brain prefrontal lobe cortex, hypothalamus, and hippocampus tissue were measured by enzyme linked immunosorbent assay. Noradrenaline (NE), dopamine (DA), 5-hydroxytryptamine (5-HT), glutamic acid (Glu) and γ-aminobutyric acid (GABA) levels were measured by HPLC-ECD, and acetyl choline (Ach) level was determined by HPLC-RE-ECD.
Results: Insomniac rats experienced quietness, reduced activities and recovery of sleep time, drinking and eating and mental state after MMA stimulation. MMA significantly prolonged the sleep time induced by pentobarbital sodium. Levels of IL-1, IL-2, IL-6 and TNF-α significantly increased compared with those of insomniac models ($P < 0.01$). Levels of NE, DA, and Glu decreased significantly ($P < 0.01$), whereas those of 5-HT, GABA, and Ach increased significantly ($P < 0.01$).
Conclusions: MMA significantly decreased the cerebral excitability of insomniac rats. It promoted sleep probably by regulating the contents of cytokines and neurotransmitters in brain tissues.
© 2015 Elsevier GmbH. All rights reserved.

Keywords: Mongolian medical acupuncture; Interleukin; Insomnia; γ-Aminobutyric acid

1. Introduction

A study by World Health Organization has indicated that approximately 27% of global people are bothered by sleep-related diseases. Results from international epidemiological investigations have shown that approximately 17% of the global population suffer from severe insomnia each year [1,2].

* Corresponding author.
** Corresponding author at: College of Mongolian Medicine, Inner Mongolia Medical University, Hohhot 010110, PR China. Tel.: +86 4716636945.
E-mail addresses: lidao_bao@163.com (L. Bao), bagulaimmu@163.com (B. Agula).

http://dx.doi.org/10.1016/j.eujim.2015.05.008
1876-3820/© 2015 Elsevier GmbH. All rights reserved.

Insomnia may cause daytime functional defects, significantly decrease the quality of life, and lead to severe negative effect on individuals and the society [3,4]. In Western medicine, barbiturates and benzodiazepines have commonly been used to treat insomnia [5]. Drug therapy, which is often accompanied by different degrees of side effects and drug dependence, is not an ideal therapeutic method.

Sleep–wake is a coordinated, integrated physiological process involving multiple systems and centers, following a complex mechanism. It is largely associated with special nervous structures such as sleep-activating cells in the preoptic region of the brainstem reticular system, histamine neurons in the tuberomammillary nucleus, neurotransmitters closely

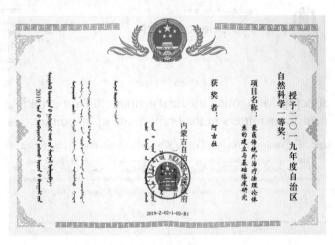

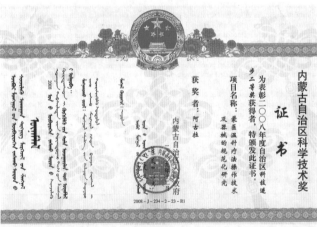

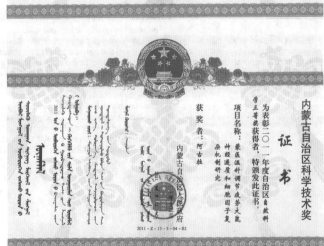

二、蒙医温针疗法研究相关重要成果证书

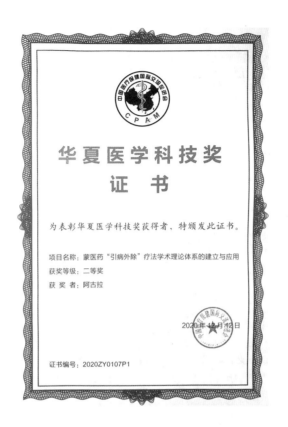

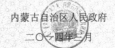

证书号第1943885号

实用新型专利证书

实用新型名称：电热温针器

发 明 人：阿古拉;乌兰;唐大鸣;陈英松;朝鲁门

专 利 号：ZL 2011 2 0058078.0

专利申请日：2011 年 03 月 08 日

专 利 权 人：内蒙古医学院

授权公告日：2011 年 09 月 21 日

　　本实用新型经过本局依照中华人民共和国专利法进行初步审查，决定授予专利权，颁发本证书并在专利登记簿上予以登记，专利权自授权公告之日起生效。

　　本专利的专利权期限为十年，自申请日起算。专利权人应当依照专利法及其实施细则规定缴纳年费。本专利的年费应当在每年 03 月 08 日前缴纳，未按照规定缴纳年费的，专利权自应当缴纳年费期满之日起终止。

　　专利证书记载专利权登记时的法律状况，专利权的转移、质押、无效、终止、恢复和专利权人的姓名或名称、国籍、地址变更等事项记载在专利登记簿上。

局长

2011 年 09 月 21 日

第 1 页（共 1 页）

证书号第5406317号

实用新型专利证书

实用新型名称：一种蒙医用电热温针装置

发 明 人：阿古拉;包立道;斯楞格;王月洪

专 利 号：ZL 2016 2 0154017.7

专利申请日：2016 年 03 月 01 日

专 利 权 人：阿古拉

授权公告日：2016 年 08 月 10 日

　　本实用新型经过本局依照中华人民共和国专利法进行初步审查，决定授予专利权，颁发本证书并在专利登记簿上予以登记，专利权自授权公告之日起生效。

　　本专利的专利权期限为十年，自申请日起算。专利权人应当依照专利法及其实施细则规定缴纳年费。本专利的年费应当在每年 03 月 01 日前缴纳，未按照规定缴纳年费的，专利权自应当缴纳年费期满之日起终止。

　　专利证书记载专利权登记时的法律状况，专利权的转移、质押、无效、终止、恢复和专利权人的姓名或名称、国籍、地址变更等事项记载在专利登记簿上。

局长
申长雨

第 1 页（共 1 页）

证书号第4625504号

实用新型专利证书

实用新型名称：蒙医多媒体人体穴位模型

发 明 人：陈英崧;阿古拉;朝鲁门;嘎拉台;乌云格日勒

专 利 号：ZL 2014 2 0811029.3

专利申请日：2014 年 12 月 18 日

专 利 权 人：内蒙古医科大学

授权公告日：2015 年 09 月 16 日

　　本实用新型经过本局依照中华人民共和国专利法进行初步审查，决定授予专利权，颁发本证书并在专利登记簿上予以登记，专利权自授权公告之日起生效。

　　本专利的专利权期限为十年，自申请日起算，专利权人应当依照专利法及其实施细则规定缴纳年费。本专利的年费应当在每年 12 月 18 日前缴纳，未按照规定缴纳年费的，专利权自应当缴纳年费期满之日起终止。

　　专利证书记载专利权登记时的法律状况。专利权的转移、质押、无效、终止、恢复和专利权人的姓名或名称、国籍、地址变更等事项记载在专利登记簿上。

局长
申长雨

第 1 页 (共 1 页)

证书号第3186707号

外观设计专利证书

外观设计名称：蒙医针灸铜人穴位模型（多媒体）

设 计 人：包金荣;阿古拉;乌云格日乐;嘎拉台

专 利 号：ZL 2014 3 0340408.4

专利申请日：2014 年 09 月 15 日

专 利 权 人：内蒙古医科大学

授权公告日：2015 年 04 月 22 日

　　本外观设计经过本局依照中华人民共和国专利法进行初步审查，决定授予专利权，颁发本证书并在专利登记簿上予以登记，专利权自授权公告之日起生效。

　　本专利的专利权期限为十年，自申请日起算，专利权人应当依照专利法及其实施细则规定缴纳年费。本专利的年费应当在每年 09 月 15 日前缴纳，未按照规定缴纳年费的，专利权自应当缴纳年费期满之日起终止。

　　专利证书记载专利权登记时的法律状况。专利权的转移、质押、无效、终止、恢复和专利权人的姓名或名称、国籍、地址变更等事项记载在专利登记簿上。

局长
申长雨

第 1 页 (共 1 页)